Pocket Prescriber
Psychiatry

T0321255

Pocket Prescriber Psychiatry

Second Edition

Edited by

Matt Butler MRes MRCPsych
Wellcome Trust Doctoral Clinical Research Fellow, Institute of
Psychiatry, Psychology and Neuroscience and Specialist Registrar in
Psychiatry, South London and Maudsley NHS Foundation Trust

Timothy RJ Nicholson MBBS BSc MSc PhD MRCP MRCPsych
Reader in Neuropsychiatry, Institute of Psychiatry Psychology and
Neuroscience, King's College London, and Honorary Consultant
Neuropsychiatrist, South London and Maudsley NHS Foundation Trust

Jonathan P Rogers MA MB BChir PhD MRCP MRCPsych FHEA
Clinical Lecturer, Division of Psychiatry, University College London

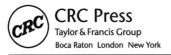

CRC Press is an imprint of the
Taylor & Francis Group, an **informa** business

Second edition published 2024
by CRC Press
2385 NW Executive Center Drive, Suite 320, Boca Raton, FL 33431

and by CRC Press
4 Park Square, Milton Park, Abingdon, Oxon, OX14 4RN

CRC Press is an imprint of Taylor & Francis Group, LLC

© 2024 selection and editorial matter, Jonathan P Rogers, Matt Butler and Timothy RJ Nicholson; individual chapters, the contributors

First edition published 2019

ISBN: 9781032397412 (pbk)
ISBN: 9781032677521 (ebk)

DOI: 10.1201/9781032677521

Typeset in Warnock Pro
by Evolution Design & Digital Ltd (Kent)

CONTENTS

CONTRIBUTORS

David S Baldwin, Prof MA DM FRCPsych
Professor of Psychiatry
Faculty of Medicine
University of Southampton

Stuart Benefield, MPharm MRPharmS
Pharmacist
South London and Maudsley NHS
    Foundation Trust

**David Coghill, Prof BSc (Med Sci) MB
    ChB MD**
Financial Markets Foundation Chair of
    Developmental Mental Health
Departments of Paediatrics and
    Psychiatry
Faculty of Medicine Dentistry and Health
    Sciences
University of Melbourne

**Fiona Cresswell, Dr MBChB BSc PhD
    MRCP DTM&H DipGUM DipHIV
    PGCert Epi**
Academic Clinical Lecturer
Global Health and Infection
Brighton and Sussex Medical School

**Paul Deslandes, Dr BPharm PhD MRSB
    CBiol**
Senior Lecturer
University of South Wales

**Olubanke Dzahini, MSc BPharm
    DipPharmPrac MRPharmS MCMHP**
Principal Pharmacist
South London and Maudsley NHS
    Foundation Trust
Institute of Pharmaceutical Science
King's College London

**Siobhan Gee, Dr MPharm PGDip
    MFRPSII PhD**
Interim Deputy Director of Pharmacy
South London and Maudsley NHS
    Foundation Trust
Honorary Senior Lecturer
Faculty of Life Sciences and Medicine
King's College London

**Jeremy Hall, Prof MA MB BChir MPhil
    PhD FRCPsych**
Director, Neuroscience and Mental
    Health Innovation Institute
Cardiff University

**Ryhana Haniff, BSc (Pharmacy) PGDip
    MRPharmS**
Clinical Pharmacist
Royal Free London NHS Foundation
    Trust

Zarah Haniff, MPharm MSc MRPharmS
PhD Fellow and Pharmacist
Institute of Psychiatry, Psychology and
    Neuroscience
King's College London

**Jules Haste, BSc DipClinPharm
    MRPharmS, MCMHP**
Principal Pharmacist
Sussex Partnership NHS Foundation
    Trust

Hubertus Himmerich, Dr SARCPsych
Clinical Senior Lecturer in Eating
    Disorders
King's College London

Frank Holloway, Dr FRCPsych
Emeritus Consultant Psychiatrist
South London and Maudsley Hospital
    NHS Foundation Trust

Annie Lane, MPharm
Principal Pharmacist
South London and Maudsley NHS
  Foundation Trust

**Anne Lingford-Hughes, Prof MA PhD
BM BCh FRCPsych**
Professor of Addiction Biology and Hon
  Consultant Psychiatrist
Imperial College London and CNWL
  NHS Foundation Trust

**R Hamish McAllister-Williams, Prof BSc
MB ChB PhD MD FRCPsych**
Professor of Affective Disorders
Institute of Neuroscience
Newcastle University

**Stirling Moorey, Dr BSc MBBS MA
FRCPsych**
Consultant Psychiatrist in CBT (retired)
South London and Maudsley NHS
  Foundation Trust

**Akshay Nair, Dr MA BMBCh MRCPsych
PhD**
Consultant Neuropsychiatrist
St. George's University Hospitals NHS
  Foundation Trust

Marianne Novak, Dr MBChB MRCP PhD
Consultant Neurologist
St. George's University Hospitals NHS
  Foundation Trust
Kingston Hospital NHS Foundation Trust
University College London Hospital NHS
  Foundation Trust

John T O'Brien, Prof FMedSci
Foundation Professor of Old Age
  Psychiatry
Department of Psychiatry
University of Cambridge

**David Okai, Dr MD(Res) MRCPsych
DipCBT**
Consultant Neuropsychiatrist
South London and Maudsley NHS
  Foundation Trust
Senior Lecturer
King's College London

Edward Palmer, Dr BSc (Hons) MBBS
Academic Clinical Fellow in Psychiatry
Institute for Mental Health
University of Birmingham

Neha Pathak, Dr MBBS PhD
Specialty Trainee in Community Sexual
  and Reproductive Health
Guy's & St Thomas' NHS Foundation
  Trust

Tom Pollak, Dr PhD MRCPsych NIHR
Clinical Lecturer
King's College London
Honorary Consultant Neuropsychiatrist
South London and Maudsley NHS
  Foundation Trust

Deborah Robson, Dr PhD
Senior Lecturer in Tobacco Harm
  Reduction
National Addiction Centre, Addictions
  Department and NIHR ARC South
  London
Institute of Psychiatry, Psychology and
  Neuroscience
King's College London

**James Rucker, Dr MBBS MRCPsych
MSc PhD**
Senior Clinical Lecturer
Institute of Psychiatry, Psychology and
  Neuroscience
King's College London

Liz Sampson, Prof MBChB MRCPsych MSc MD
Professor Consultant Liaison Psychiatrist
Division of Psychiatry
University College London
Department of Psychological Medicine
Royal London Hospital
East London NHS Foundation Trust

Tim Segal, Dr MA, MBBS, MRCPsych
Clinical Lead for Neuropsychiatry
South London and Maudsley NHS
    Foundation Trust

Hugh Selsick, Dr BSc (Hons) MBBCh
Consultant in Psychiatry and Sleep
    Medicine
Insomnia and Behavioural Sleep Medicine
    Clinic
Royal London Hospital for Integrated
    Medicine
University College London Hospitals

Peter Tyrer, Prof MD FRCPsych FMedSci
Emeritus Professor of Community
    Psychiatry
Imperial College London

**Rachel Upthegrove, Prof MBBS
    FRCPsych PhD**
Professor of Psychiatry and Youth Mental
    Health
Institute for Mental Health
University of Birmingham
Consultant Psychiatrist
Early Intervention in Psychosis Service
Birmingham Women's and Children's
    NHS Foundation Trust

**Allister Vale, Prof MD FRCP FRCPE
    FRCPG FFOM FAACT FBTS FBPhS
    FEAPCCT Hon FRCPG**
Clinical Pharmacologist and Toxicologist
City Hospital, Birmingham and
    University of Birmingham

Immo Weichert, Dr MRCP
Acute Physician
Acute Medicine Department
Ipswich Hospital
East Suffolk and North Essex NHS
    Foundation Trust

Angelika Wieck, Dr MD, FRCPsych
Honorary Perinatal Consultant
    Psychiatrist
Greater Manchester Mental Health NHS
    Foundation Trust
Honorary Senior Lecturer
University of Manchester

**Allan H Young, Prof MB ChB MPhil PhD
    FRCPsych FRCPC FRSB**
Director, Centre for Affective Disorders
Institute of Psychiatry, Psychology and
    Neuroscience
King's College London

FOREWORD

Forty years ago, when I qualified as a doctor, the psychotropic drugs available for use in clinical practice included lithium, 'conventional neuroleptics' (such as chlorpromazine and haloperidol), tricyclic antidepressants, monoamine oxidase inhibitors and benzodiazepines. Subsequent decades saw the appearance of selective serotonin reuptake inhibitors, developed based on prevailing views of the aetiology of depression, and anticipated to be better tolerated and safer than tricyclics when taken in overdose. In parallel, knowledge of the greater effectiveness of clozapine and its reduced liability for extrapyramidal adverse effects encouraged the development of 'second-generation' antipsychotics, and their subsequent widespread adoption into clinical care. However, some of the expectations relating to emerging medications were dashed with widespread awareness of treatment-emergent adverse effects such as sexual dysfunction with SSRIs or weight gain and impaired glucose tolerance with newer antipsychotics.

Clinicians and patients together came to realise that a more nuanced approach is needed when considering the balance of potential benefits and possible risks associated with psychotropic drug treatment, both across and within classes of medication. Rather than being swayed by the findings of high-profile single randomised controlled trials, current and emerging 'evidence' is beheld differently: study findings are synthesised and appraised in a more sophisticated manner through systematic reviews and network meta-analyses, resulting in a wealth of data. Unfortunately, this can sometimes be hard to comprehend. This is where clinical guidelines come in: evidence is distilled and marshalled to inform key treatment decisions, from whether to start medication to when and how it should be stopped. The British Association for Psychopharmacology (BAP) regularly produces and updates such clinical guidance, relating to most mental disorders, and these have been adopted enthusiastically in many countries. However, doctors and non-medical prescribers need a succinct summary of the principal recommendations within these guidelines relating to key treatment decisions; this is where the *Pocket Prescriber Psychiatry* comes in.

This revision retains many features of the previous edition, such as quick-to follow summary boxes and tables which facilitate comparisons between competing options. It draws on updated guidance (including recently published guidelines relating to catatonia, which are anticipated to influence both psychiatric and neurological practice) and places increased emphasis on important aspects of prescribing in the perinatal period. Increased attention is paid to the management of co-morbid physical health concerns in patients with severe mental illness, and more consideration is given to tapering of psychotropic medication when treatment courses are concluded. In addition, the chapter relating to management of psychiatric emergences has been reformatted to make it more immediately relevant to the needs of on-call psychiatrists and their patients. Matt Butler, Timothy Nicholson and Jonathan Rogers have worked tirelessly to produce this new and extended version of the *Pocket Prescriber* and I trust it will prove both indispensable to hard-pressed clinicians and beneficial in improving outcomes for their patients.

Professor David Baldwin
President (2022/2024)
British Association for Psychopharmacology

ACKNOWLEDGEMENTS

This edition is dedicated to Prof Donald Singer in memoriam.

Our thanks to all those who have supported, enthused and inspired us throughout the years. Many of you have also contributed to this book.

Thanks to Ellen for being great. Thanks to Daryl Clare, Michael Wilde and Kurt Willoughby for showing us how to achieve our goals.

Thanks to the British Association for Psychopharmacology for their collaboration on this and the previous edition of the book.

And thanks to every reader for making this a worthwhile endeavour! We hope you enjoy reading it as much as we enjoyed putting it together.

HOW TO USE THIS BOOK

STANDARD LAYOUT OF DRUGS

DRUG/TRADE NAME
Class/action: More information is given for generic forms, especially for the original and most commonly used drug(s) of each class.
Use: indication^x (doses correlated below).
CI: contraindications; **L** (liver failure), **R** (renal failure), **H** (heart failure), **P** (pregnancy), **B** (breastfeeding). *Allergy to active drug or any excipients (other substances in the preparation) not specifically mentioned in, but relevant to, all monographs.*
Caution: **L** (liver failure), **R** (renal failure), **H** (heart failure), **P** (pregnancy), **B** (breastfeeding), **E** (elderly patients). If a contraindication is given for a drug caution is also inherently implied.
SE: side effects; not an exhaustive list: chosen based on expert opinion if common and/or serious.
Warn: information to give to patients before starting drug.
Monitor: parameters that need to be monitored during treatment.
Interactions: included only if common or potentially serious; $\uparrow/\downarrow$**P450** (induces/inhibits cytochrome P450 metabolism), **W+** (increases effect of warfarin), **W−** (decreases effect of warfarin).
Dose: dose^x (for use^x). *NB: Doses are for adults only.*

Important points highlighted at end of drug entry.

Resources that appear fundamental do not always agree and it is sometimes impossible to determine from first principles why they say the things they do. In this book, the SPC and the BNF have been the primary sources of pharmacological knowledge. Where there are irreconcilable differences, we have usually given priority to the SPC.

Use/dose^{NICE}: National Institute for Health and Care Excellence (NICE) guidelines exist for the drug (basics often in the *British National Formulary* [BNF] – see https://www.nice.org.uk for full details).

Dose^{BNF/SPC}: Dose regimen complicated; please refer to BNF and/or SPC (Summary of Product Characteristics sheet; the manufacturer's information sheet enclosed with drug packaging – can also be viewed at or downloaded from https://www.medicines.org.uk/emc). **Asterisks (*)** and **daggers (')** denote links between information within local text.
Other sources:
^{BAP} Guidance from the British Association for Psycho-pharmacology
^{MPG} The Maudsley Prescribing Guidelines in Psychiatry, 14E
^{SIGN} Scottish Intercollegiate Guidelines Network
^{UKTIS} UK Teratology Information Service
^{UKDILAS} UK Drugs in Lactation Advisory Service
^{NEPTUNE} Novel Psychoactive Treatment: UK Network
^{TOXBASE} Clinical toxicology database of the National Poisons Information Service

Only relevant sections are included for each drug. **Trade names** (in **SOLID GREY** font) are given only if found regularly on drug charts or if a non-proprietary (generic, non-trade-name) drug does not yet exist.
Indications of antibiotics are changeable and vary widely: consult up-to-date local guidelines.

↑/↓ electrolytes refers to serum levels, unless stated otherwise.

KEY

☠ Potential dangers highlighted with skull and crossbones

▼ New drug or new indication under intense surveillance by the Committee on Safety of Medicines (CSM): *important to report all suspected drug reactions via Yellow Card Scheme* (accurate as going to press: from European Medicines Agency list)

☺ *Good for:* reasons to give a certain drug when choice exists

☹ *Bad for:* reasons to not give a certain drug when choice exists

⇒ Causes/goes to

∴ Therefore

Δ Change/disturbance

Ψ Psychiatric

↑ Increase/high

↓ Decrease/low

DOSES

od	once daily	nocte	at night
bd	twice daily	mane	in the morning
tds	three times daily	prn	as required
qds	four times daily	stat	at once

ROUTES

im	intramuscular	po	oral
inh	inhaled	pr	rectal
iv	intravenous	sc	subcutaneous
ivi	intravenous infusion	top	topical
neb	via nebuliser	sl	sublingual

Routes are presumed PO, unless stated otherwise.

LIST OF ABBREVIATIONS

5-ASA	5-aminosalicylic acid
5-HT	5-hydroxytryptamine (= serotonin)
A&E	accident and emergency
AAC	antibiotic-associated colitis, often *C. difficile*
Ab	antibody
abdo	abdomen/abdominal
ABG	arterial blood gases
ABPM	ambulatory blood pressure monitoring
ACC	American College of Cardiology
ACCP	American College of Chest Physicians
ACE-i	angiotensin-converting enzyme (ACE) inhibitor
ACh	acetylcholine
ACS	acute coronary syndrome
ADHD	attention deficit hyperactivity disorder
ADP	adenosine diphosphate
AF	atrial fibrillation
Ag	antigen
AHA	American Heart Association
AIE	autoimmune encephalitis
AKI	acute kidney injury
ALL	acute lymphoblastic leukaemia
ALP	alkaline phosphatase
ALS	adult life support (algorithms of the European Resuscitation Council)
ALT	alanine (-amino) transferase
AMI	acute myocardial infarction
AMTS	abbreviated mental test score (same as MTS)
ANA	anti-nuclear antigen
APTT	activated partial thromboplastin time
ARB	angiotensin receptor blocker
ART	antiretroviral therapy
ARDS	adult respiratory distress syndrome
AS	aortic stenosis
ASAP	as soon as possible

assoc	associated
AST	aspartate transaminase
AV	arteriovenous
AVM	arteriovenous malformation
AVN	atrioventricular node
BAP	British Association for Psychopharmacology
BBB	bundle branch block
BCSH	British Committee for Standards in Haematology
BCT	broad complex tachycardia
BD	twice daily
BF	blood flow
BG	serum blood glucose in mmol/L; *see also* CBG (capillary blood glucose)
BHS	British Hypertension Society
BIH	benign intracranial hypertension
BIPAP	bilevel/biphasic positive airway pressure
BM	bone marrow (*NB:* BM is often used, confusingly, to signify finger-prick glucose; CBG [capillary blood glucose] is used for this purpose in this book)
BMI	body mass index = weight (kg)/height (m)^2
BNF	British National Formulary
BP	blood pressure
BPAD	bipolar affective disorder
BPH	benign prostatic hypertrophy
BPSD	behavioural and psychological symptoms of dementia
BTS	British Thoracic Society
Bx	biopsy
C	constipation
Ca	cancer
Ca^{2+}	calcium
CAH	congenital adrenal hyperplasia
CBF	cerebral blood flow
CBG	capillary blood glucose in mmol/L (finger-prick testing)
CCB	calcium channel blocker
CCF	congestive cardiac failure

CCU	coronary care unit
cf	compared with
CHF	congestive heart failure
CI	contraindicated
CK	creatine kinase
CKD	chronic kidney disease
CLL	chronic lymphocytic leukaemia
CML	chronic myelogenous leukaemia
CMV	cytomegalovirus
CNS	central nervous system
CO	cardiac output
COCP	combined oral contraceptive pill
COPD	chronic obstructive pulmonary disease
COX	cyclo-oxygenase
CPR	cardiopulmonary resuscitation
CRF	chronic renal failure
CRP	C-reactive protein
CSF	cerebrospinal fluid
CSM	Committee on Safety of Medicines
CT	computerised tomography
CTO	Community Treatment Order
CVA	cerebrovascular accident
CVD	cardiovascular disease
CVP	central venous pressure
CXR	chest X-ray
D	diarrhoea
$D_{1/2/3 ...}$	dopamine receptor subtype$_{1/2/3 ...}$
D&V	diarrhoea and vomiting
DA	dopamine
DCT	distal convoluted tubule
dfx	defects
DI	diabetes insipidus
DIC	disseminated intravascular coagulation
DKA	diabetic ketoacidosis
DM	diabetes mellitus
DMARD	disease-modifying anti-rheumatic drug

DOAC	direct oral anticoagulant
dt	due to
DWI	diffusion-weighted (imaging); specialist magnetic resonance imaging (MRI) mostly used for stroke/transient ischaemic attack (TIA)
Dx	diagnosis
EØ	eosinophils
e'lyte	electrolyte
EBV	Epstein–Barr virus
ECG	electrocardiogram
ECT	electroconvulsive therapy
EF	ejection fraction
ENT	ear, nose and throat
EPSE	extrapyramidal side effects
ERC	European Resuscitation Council
ESC	European Society of Cardiology
esp	especially
ESR	erythrocyte sedimentation rate
exac	exacerbates
FBC	full blood count
FDG	fluorodeoxyglucose
Fe	iron
FFP	fresh frozen plasma
FGA	first-generation antipsychotic
FHx	family history
FiO$_2$	inspired O$_2$ concentration
FRIII	fixed rate intravenous insulin infusion
fx	effects
G6PD	glucose-6-phosphate dehydrogenase
GABA	γ-aminobutyric acid
GBS	Guillain–Barré syndrome
GCS	Glasgow Coma Scale
GFR	glomerular filtration rate
GI	gastrointestinal
GIK	glucose, insulin and K$^+$ infusion
GMC	General Medical Council (of United Kingdom)

GORD	gastro-oesophageal reflux disease
GTN	glyceryl trinitrate
GU	genitourinary
h	hour(s)
H(O)CM	hypertrophic (obstructive) cardiomyopathy
Hb	haemoglobin
HB	heart block
HBPM	home blood pressure monitoring
Hct	haematocrit
HDL	high-density lipoprotein
HF	heart failure; *see also* CHF (congestive heart failure)
HHS	hyperosmolar hyperglycaemic state
HIT	heparin-induced thrombocytopenia
HIV	human immunodeficiency virus
HLA	human leucocyte antigen
HMG-CoA	3-hydroxy-3-methyl-glutaryl coenzyme A
HONK	hyperosmolar non-ketotic state; *see also* HHS (hyperosmolar hyperglycaemic state)
HR	heart rate
hrly	hourly
HSV	herpes simplex virus
Ht	height
HTN	hypertension
HUS	haemolytic uraemic syndrome
Hx	history
IBD	inflammatory bowel disease
IBS	irritable bowel syndrome
IBW	ideal body weight
ICD	impulse control disorder
ICP	intracranial pressure
ICU	intensive care unit
IHD	ischaemic heart disease
IL-2	interleukin-2
IM	intramuscular
inc	including
INH	inhaled

INR	international normalised ratio (prothrombin ratio)
IOP	intraocular pressure
IPT	interpersonal therapy
ITP	immune/idiopathic thrombocytopenic purpura
ITU	intensive therapy unit
IUD	intrauterine device
IV	intravenous
IVDU	intravenous drug user
IVI	intravenous infusion
IVIG	intravenous immunoglobulins
Ix	investigation
JBDS	Joint British Diabetes Societies
JVP	jugular venous pressure
K⁺	potassium (serum levels unless stated otherwise)
LØ	lymphocytes
LA	long-acting
LBBB	left bundle branch block
LDL	low-density lipoprotein
LF	liver failure
LFTs	liver function tests
LG1	leucine-rich glioma-inactivated 1
LMWH	low-molecular-weight heparin
LP	lumbar puncture
LVF	left ventricular failure
MØ	macrophages
mane	in morning
MAOI	monoamine oxidase inhibitor
MAP	mean arterial pressure
MCA	middle cerebral artery/Mental Capacity Act
MCV	mean corpuscular volume
metab	metabolised
MG	myasthenia gravis
MHA	Mental Health Act
MHRA	Medicines and Healthcare Products Regulatory Agency (UK)
MI	myocardial infarction

MIBG	metaiodobenzylguanidine
MMF	mycophenolate mofetil
MMSE	Mini-Mental State Examination
MPG	*The Maudsley Prescribing Guidelines in Psychiatry*, 14th Edition
MR	modified release (drug preparation)†
MRI	magnetic resonance imaging
MRSA	methicillin-resistant *Staphylococcus aureus*
MS	multiple sclerosis
MSK	muskuloskeletal
MUST	malnutrition universal screening tool
Mx	management
N	nausea
N&V	nausea and vomiting
NØ	neutrophils
NA	noradrenaline (norepinephrine)
Na⁺	sodium (serum levels unless stated otherwise)
NBM	nil by mouth
NCT	narrow complex tachycardia
NDRI	noradrenaline and dopamine reuptake inhibitor
neb	via nebuliser
NEPTUNE	Novel Psychoactive Treatment: UK Network
NGT	nasogastric tube
NH	non-Hodgkin's (lymphoma)
NICE	National Institute for Health and Care Excellence
NIDDM	non-insulin-dependent diabetes mellitus
NIHSS	National (US) Institute of Health Stroke Scale
NIV	non-invasive ventilation
NMDA	N-methyl-D-aspartate
NMJ	neuromuscular junction
NMS	neuroleptic malignant syndrome
NO	nitric oxide
nocte	at night
NPIS	National Poisons Information Service
NPV	negative predictive value
NSAID	non-steroidal anti-inflammatory drug

NSTEMI	non-ST elevation myocardial infarction
NYHA	New York Heart Association
OCD	obsessive-compulsive disorder
OCP	oral contraceptive pill
OD	once daily
OGD	oesophagogastroduodenoscopy
OTC	over-the-counter
p'way(s)	pathway(s)
PAN	polyarteritis nodosa
PBC	primary biliary cirrhosis
PCI	percutaneous coronary intervention
PCOS	polycystic ovary syndrome
PCP	*Pneumocystis carinii* pneumonia
PCV	packed cell volume
PDA	patent ductus arteriosus
PE	pulmonary embolism
PEA	pulseless electrical activity
PEF	peak expiratory flow
PEG	percutaneous endoscopic gastrostomy
PET	positron emission tomography
PG(x)	prostaglandin (receptor subtype x)
phaeo	phaeochromocytoma
PHx	past history (of)
PID	pelvic inflammatory disease
PML	progressive multifocal leukoencephalopathy
PMR	polymyalgia rheumatica
PO	by mouth (oral)
PO_4	phosphate (serum levels, unless stated otherwise)
PPI	proton pump inhibitor
PR	rectal
prep(s)	preparation(s)
PRN	as required
PSA	prostate-specific antigen
Plt	platelet(s)
PT	prothrombin time
PTH	parathyroid hormone

PTSD	post-traumatic stress disorder
PU(D)	peptic ulcer (disease)
PUO	pyrexia of unknown origin
PVD	peripheral vascular disease
Px	prophylaxis
QDS	four times daily
QT(c)	QT interval (corrected for rate)
RA	rheumatoid arthritis
RAS	renal artery stenosis
RBF	renal blood flow
r/f	refer
RF	renal failure
RID	relative infant dose
RLS	restless legs syndrome
ROSIER	recognition of stroke in emergency room scale for diagnosis of stroke/transient ischaemic attack (TIA)
RR	respiratory rate
RRT	renal replacement therapy
RSV	respiratory syncytial virus
RTI	respiratory tract infection
RV	right ventricle
RVF	right ventricular failure
Rx	treatment
SAH	subarachnoid haemorrhage
SAN	sinoatrial node
SBE	subacute bacterial endocarditis
SC	subcutaneous
SCLE	subacute cutaneous lupus erythematosus
SE(s)	side effect(s)
sec	second(s)
SGA	second-generation antipsychotic
SIADH	syndrome of inappropriate antidiuretic hormone
SIGN	Scottish Intercollegiate Guidelines Network
SJS	Stevens–Johnson syndrome
SL	sublingual
SLE	systemic lupus erythematosus

SMI	serious mental illness
SOA	swelling of ankles
SOB (OE)	shortness of breath (on exertion)
SPC	summary of product characteristic sheet
SPECT	single photon emission computed tomography scan
spp	species
SR	slow/sustained release (drug preparation)
SSRI	selective serotonin reuptake inhibitor
SSS	sick sinus syndrome
stat	at once
STEMI	ST elevation myocardial infarction
supp	suppository
SVT	supraventricular tachycardia
Sx	symptoms
SZ	schizophrenia
$T_{1/2}$	half-life
T2DM	type 2 diabetes mellitus
T_3	triiodothyronine/liothyronine
T_4	thyroxine ($\uparrow$/$\downarrow$ T_4 = hyper-/hypothyroid)
TB	tuberculosis
TCA	tricyclic antidepressant
TDS	three times daily
TE	thromboembolism
TEDS	thromboembolism deterrent stockings
TEN	toxic epidermal necrolysis
TFTs	thyroid function tests
TG	triglyceride
THC	delta-9-tetrahydrocannabinol
TIA	transient ischaemic attack
TIBC	total iron-binding capacity
T_{max}	time of peak concentration of a drug
TNF	tumour necrosis factor
top	topical
TOXBASE	the primary clinical toxicology database of the National Poisons Information Service
TPMT	thiopurine methyltransferase

TPR	total peripheral resistance
TTA(s)	(drugs) to take away, i.e. prescriptions for inpatients on discharge/leave (aka TTO)
TTP	thrombotic thrombocytopenic purpura
U&Es	urea and electrolytes
UA(P)	unstable angina (pectoris)
UC	ulcerative colitis
UDS	urine drug screen
UKTIS	UK Teratology Information Service
UKDILAS	UK Drugs in Lactation Advisory Service
URTI	upper respiratory tract infection
USS	ultrasound scan
UTI	urinary tract infection
UV	ultraviolet
V	vomiting
VE(s)	ventricular ectopic(s)
VF	ventricular fibrillation
vit	vitamin
VLDL	very-low-density lipoprotein
VRIII	variable rate intravenous insulin infusion
VT	ventricular tachycardia
VTE	venous thromboembolism
VZV	varicella zoster virus (chickenpox/shingles)
w	with
w/in	within
w/o	without
WCC	white cell count
WE	Wernicke's encephalopathy
wk(s)	week(s)
wkly	weekly
WPW	Wolff–Parkinson–White syndrome
Wt	weight
xs	excess
ZE	Zollinger–Ellison syndrome

HOW TO PRESCRIBE SAFELY

Take time/care to ↓ risk to patients (and protect yourself).
Always check the following are correct for all prescriptions:
patient, indication and drug, **legible** format (generic name, clarity, handwriting, **identifiable signature**, your contact number), dosage, frequency, time(s) of day, date, duration of treatment, route of administration.

DO

- Make a clear, accurate record in the notes of all medicines prescribed, and indication, written at the time of prescription.
- Complete allergy box and agreed relevant labels and e-alerts.
- Include on all drug charts and TTAs the patient's surname and given name, date of birth, date of admission and consultant (if possible use a printed label for patient details).
- **PRINT** (i.e. use uppercase) all drugs as approved (generic) names, e.g. 'IBUPROFEN' *not* '**nurofen**'.
- State dose, route and frequency, giving strength of solutions/creams.
- Write microgram in full; avoid abbreviations such as mcg or μ.
- Abbreviate the word gram to 'g' (rather than 'gm' which is easily confused with mg).
- Write the word 'units' in full, preceded by a space; abbreviating to 'U' can be misread as zero (a 10-fold error).
- Document weight: guides dosing and GFR calculation.
- Write quantities <1 g in mg (e.g. 400 mg *not* 0.4 g).
- Write quantities <1 mg in micrograms (e.g. 200 micrograms *not* 0.2 mg).
- Write quantities <1 microgram in nanograms (e.g. 500 nanograms *not* 0.5 micrograms).
- Do not use trailing zeroes (10 mg *not* 10.0 mg).
- Precede decimal points with another figure (e.g. 0.8 mL *not* .8 mL), and only use decimals where unavoidable.
- Check and recheck calculations.

- Provide clear additional instructions, e.g. for monitoring, review of antibiotic route and duration, maximum daily/24 h dose for as required drugs.
- Specify solution to be used and duration of any iv infusions/injections.
- Avoid using abbreviated/non-standard drug names.
- Avoid writing 'T' (tablet sign) for non-tablet formulations, e.g. sprays.
- Amend a prescribed drug by drawing a line through it, date and initial this, then rewrite as new prescription.
- Review need for drugs, especially when rewriting a drug chart.
- Check and count number of drugs when rewriting a drug chart.
- Check when prescribing unfamiliar drug(s)/doses or drugs you were familiar with but have not prescribed recently.

IMPORTANT FURTHER ADVICE

1   Make sure choice of drug and dose are right for the patient, their condition and significant co-morbidity, with particular attention to age*, gender, weight, renal or liver dysfunction, risk of drug–drug and drug–disease interactions and risks in pregnancy (and those of childbearing age who may become pregnant) and during breastfeeding. Anticipate possible effects of over-the-counter and herbal medicines and lifestyle (e.g. smoking status, alcohol use and dietary salt intake).
    *Although arbitrary, age >65 years denotes 'elderly', effects of age can occur earlier/later and are continuous across age spectrum.

2   Common settings where drug problems occur are often predictable if you understand relevant risks, pathology, routes of drug metabolism (liver, P450, renal, etc.) and drug mechanisms of action. Take particular care with
    - Renal or liver disease.
    - Pregnancy/breastfeeding: use safest options (in the United Kingdom consider consulting the UK Teratology Information Service [tel: 0344 892 0909]).

- Prescribing or dispensing medicines that could be confused with others (e.g. sound or look similar). See MHRA for examples.
- NSAIDs/bisphosphonates and peptic ulcer disease.
- Asthma and β-blockers.
- Conditions worsened by antimuscarinic drugs (see p. 387: urinary retention/BPH, glaucoma, paralytic ileus.
- Rare conditions where drugs commonly pose risk, e.g. porphyria, myasthenia, G6PD deficiency, phaeo.

3   Always ensure informed consent; agreeing proposed prescriptions with the patient (or carer if patient has authorised their involvement in their care or lacks capacity); explaining proposed benefits, nature and duration of treatment; clarifying concerns; warning of possible, especially severe, adverse effects; highlighting recommended monitoring and review arrangements and stating what the patient should do in the event of a suspected adverse reaction. Only in extreme emergencies can it be justified to have not done this. For drugs with common potentially fatal/severe side effects, document that these risks have been explained to, and accepted by, the patient.

4   Seek legal advice on eligibility to prescribe and use unlicensed and off-label medicines, checking national guidance (in the UK, see MHRA and GMC guidance).

5   Prescribe with care. Prescribing should be for the benefit of the patient not the prescriber.

6   Keep up to date about medicines you are prescribing and the related conditions you are treating.

7   Follow CSM guidance on reporting suspected adverse reactions to black triangle drugs and other medicines (see https://yellowcard. mhra.gov.uk for links to Yellow Card reporting scheme and details of reported adverse drug reactions for specific medicines).

8   Ensure continuity of care by keeping the patient's GP (or other preferred medical adviser) informed about prescribing, monitoring and follow-up arrangements and responsibilities.

9   Check that appropriate previous medicines are continued and over-the-counter and herbal medicine use is recorded.

10 Patient Group Directions (prescribing in highly specific situations by healthcare professionals without a medical degree): the GMC advises these should be limited to situations where there is a 'distinct advantage for patient care … consistent with appropriate professional relationships and accountability'.

11 Be judicious. Some drugs are underused, whilst others are overused. Be confident, knowledgeable and curious when it comes to deciding when and when not to prescribe. Do not rely solely on received wisdom, but remember that experience can often be the best teacher.

12 Deprescribing should be part of routine patient care. It concerns withdrawing or reducing the dose of medicines, supervised by a healthcare professional. Its aim is to improve outcomes, e.g. by minimising polypharmacy. Deprescribing always involves shared decision-making with patients.

13 Keep up to date with GMC advice on prescribing (GMC guidelines: https://www.gmc-uk.org/ethical-guidance/ethical-guidance-for-doctors/good-practice-in-prescribing-and-managing-medicines-and-devices).

14 All sedative medications may impair driving and the ability to operate machinery. Warn patients of this risk.

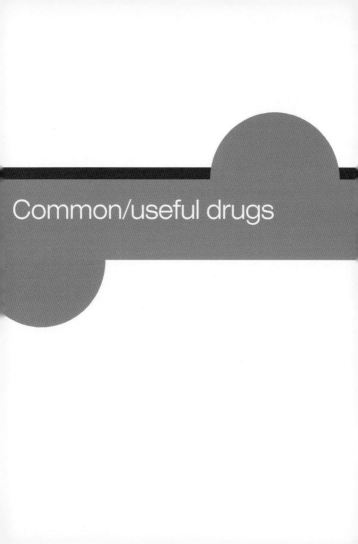

Common/useful drugs

ACAMPROSATE

Modifies GABA transmission $\Rightarrow$ ↓pleasurable fx of alcohol ∴ ↓s craving and relapse rate.

Use: maintaining alcohol abstinence supported by counselling.

CI: R/P/B.

Caution: L (if severe).

SE: GI upset, pruritus, rash, Δ libido.

Dose: 666 mg tds po if age 18–65 years (avoid outside this age range) and >60 kg (if <60 kg, give 666 mg mane then 333 mg noon and nocte). *Start ASAP after alcohol stopped. Usually give for 1 year.*

ACETYLCYSTEINE (*N*-ACETYLCYSTEINE, NAC)/PARVOLEX

Precursor of glutathione, which detoxifies metabolites of paracetamol.

Use: paracetamol od.

Caution: asthma* and atopy.

SE: allergy: rash, bronchospasm*, anaphylactoid reactions (esp if ivi too quick**).

Dose: initially 150 mg/kg in 5% glucose 200 mL as ivi over 60 min, then 50 mg/kg in 500 mL over 4 h, then 100 mg/kg in 1 L over 16 h. *NB:* use max Wt of 110 kg for dose calculation, even if patient weighs more. Ensure not given too quickly**. See p. 406 for Mx of paracetamol od and treatment line graph.

ACICLOVIR (previously ACYCLOVIR)

Antiviral. Inhibits DNA polymerase *only in infected cells:* needs activation by viral thymidine kinase (produced by herpes species).

Use: *IV:* severe HSV or varicella zoster virus (VZV) infections, e.g. meningitis, encephalitis and in immunocompromised patients (esp HIV – also used for Px); *po/top:* mucous membrane, genital, eye infections.

Caution: dehydration*, **R/E/P/B**.

SE: at ↑doses: AKI, encephalopathy (esp if dehydrated*). Also hypersensitivity, seizures, GI upset, blood disorders, skin reactions (including photosensitivity), headache, fever, dyspnoea, many non-specific neurological symptoms, ↓Pt, ↓WBC. Rarely Ψ reactions and hepatotoxicity.

Interactions: ↑s fx/toxicity of theophylline/aminophylline; ↑risk of lithium toxicity with high-dose aciclovir iv.

Dose: 5 mg/kg tds ivi over 1 h (10 mg/kg tds ivi if HSV encephalitis or VZV in immunocompromised patients); po/top.[SPC/BNF] Rx duration varies by indication and may be longer if immunocompromised: consult specialist guidelines.

☠ ivi leaks ⇒ severe local inflammation/ulceration. ☠

AGOMELATINE/VALDOXAN

Antidepressant: synthetic melatonin analogue; melatonin receptor (MT_1/MT_2) agonist re-synchronises circadian rhythms and ↑s NA/DA in frontal cortex via $5-HT_{2C}$ antagonism.

Use: depression, esp if risk of inconsistent use (↓risk of withdrawal syndrome) or prominent insomnia/poor appetite.

CI: dementia, transaminases >3× upper limit of normal, and see interactions that follow, **L**.

Caution: Hx mania (bipolar), **R/P/B/E**.

SE: GI upset (N, D and C, abdo pain), **headache**, Δ LFTs (↑transaminases in 5%; usually transient), drowsiness, sweating, anxiety, suicidal behaviour.

Monitor: LFTs before and 3, 6, 12 and 24 wks after starting. Repeat if dose↑.

Interactions: levels ↑↑ by strong CYP1A2 inhibitors (e.g. fluvoxamine, ciprofloxacin – avoid), ↑ by moderate inhibitors (e.g. propranolol, enoxacin, oestrogens) and ↓ by smoking.

Dose: 25 mg nocte (can ↑ to 50 mg nocte after 2 wks).

ALENDRONATE (ALENDRONIC ACID)

Bisphosphonate: ↓s osteoclastic bone resorption.

Use: osteoporosis Rx and Px (esp if on corticosteroids).

CI: delayed GI emptying (esp achalasia and oesophageal stricture/other abnormalities), ↓Ca^{2+}, unable to sit/stand upright ≥30 min, **R** (if severe)/**P/B**.

Caution: upper GI disorders (inc gastritis/PU), **R**.

SE: oesophageal reactions*, GI upset/distension, $\downarrow Ca^{2+}$, $\downarrow po_4$ (transient), PU, hypersensitivity (esp skin reactions), myalgia. Rarely osteonecrosis of jaw and femoral stress fractures (discontinue drug and consider no further bisphosphonates).

Warn: take upright with full glass of water on an empty stomach; stay upright ≥30 min after administration. Stop tablets and seek medical attention if symptoms of oesophageal irritation. Dental review if dental hygiene poor.

Dose: 10 mg mane[SPC/BNF] (10 mg od dosing can be given as once-wkly 70 mg tablet *if for post-menopausal osteoporosis*. Once-wkly doses unlicensed in men but may ↑ compliance).

ALFACALCIDOL
1-α-hydroxycholecalciferol: partially activated vit D.
Use: severe vit D deficiency 2° to CRF.
CI/SE: $\uparrow Ca^{2+}$ and metastatic calcification.
Caution: nephrolithiasis, granulomatosis Dx (e.g. sarcoidosis), E/P/B.
Monitor: Ca^{2+} and po_4: monitor levels wkly, watch for symptoms (esp N&V), rash, nephrocalcinosis.
Interactions: fx $\downarrow$d by barbiturates, anticonvulsants; $\uparrow$d by thiazides; avoid magnesium-containing antacids and other vit D analogues.
Dose: initially 1 microgram (= 1000 nanograms) od po; maintenance 250–1000 nanograms od po; adjust dose to avoid hypercalcaemia.
NB: $\downarrow$dose in elderly (initial dose 500 nanograms).

ALISKIREN
Direct renin inhibitor ($\downarrow$s angiotensinogen $\Rightarrow$ angiotensin I).
Use: essential HTN.
CI: angioedema, potent P-glycoprotein inhibitors (*ciclosporin, itraconazole, quinidine), ACE-i/ARB, P/B.
Caution: not recommended with ACE-i, ARBs, dehydration (risk of $\downarrow$BP), RAS, diuretics, $\downarrow Na^+$ diet, **$\uparrow K^+$, moderate potent

P-glycoprotein inhibitors (*ketoconazole, clari-/teli-/erythromycin, verapamil, amiodarone), DM***, R (if GFR <30 mL/min)/H/P/B/E.
SE: diarrhoea, dizziness, ↓BP, ↑K⁺, ↓GFR. Rarely rash, angioedema, ↓Hb.
Monitor: U&Es esp **↑K⁺ if taking ACE-i, ARBs, K⁺ sparing diuretics, K⁺ salts (inc dietary salt substitutes) or heparin. Check BG/HbA₁C regularly***.
Interactions: fruit juice; ↓s furosemide levels. Levels ↓ by irbesartan; levels ↑ by keto-/itraconazole. fx ↓ by NSAIDs. fx ↑ by P-glycoprotein inhibitors (see *CI/Caution).
Dose: initially 150 mg od, ↑ing to 300 mg od if required.

ALLOPURINOL

Xanthine oxidase inhibitor: ↓s uric acid synthesis.
Use: Px of gout, renal stones (urate or Ca²⁺ oxalate) and other ↑urate states (esp 2° to chemotherapy).
CI: acute gout: can worsen – do not start drug during attack (but do not stop drug if acute attack occurs during Rx).
Caution: R (↓dose), L (↓dose and monitor LFTs), P/B.
SE: GI upset, ☠ **severe skin reactions** ☠ (*stop if drug rash develops and allopurinol is implicated* – can reintroduce cautiously if mild reaction and no recurrence). Rarely neuropathy (and many non-specific neurological symptoms), blood disorders, RF, hepatotoxicity, gynaecomastia, vasculitis.
Warn: report rashes, maintain good hydration; ↑risk acute attacks just after initiating.
Interactions: ↑s fx/toxicity of azathioprine (and possibly other cytotoxics, esp ciclosporin), chlorpropamide and theophyllines. ↑levels of vidarabine and didanosine. Level ↓d by salicylates and probenecid. ↑rash with ampicillin and amoxicillin, **W+**.
Dose: initially 100 mg od po (↑ if required to max of 900 mg/day in divided doses of up to 300 mg) after food. Usual dose 300 mg/day.
NB: ↓dose if ↑s fx other drugs or LF or RF.
Initial Rx can ↑gout: give colchicine or NSAID (naproxen or ibuprofen – *not aspirin*) Px until ≥1 month after urate normalised.

ALPRAZOLAM/XANAX

Short-acting benzodiazepine: GABA$_A$ receptor positive allosteric modulator.

Use: short-term use in anxiety.

CI: respiratory depression, marked neuromuscular respiratory weakness inc unstable myasthenia gravis, sleep apnoea, acute pulmonary insufficiency, chronic psychosis, depression (do not give alprazolam alone), **L** (if severe).

Caution: respiratory disease, muscle weakness (inc MG), Hx of drug/alcohol abuse, personality disorder, organic brain diseases, prolonged use (and abrupt withdrawal thereafter), **L** (mild-to-moderate insufficiency)/**R**/**P**/**B**/**E**. Can produce paradoxical effects.

SE: **respiratory depression (rarely apnoea), drowsiness, dependence** (problematic, as short half-life). Also ataxia, amnesia, headache, vertigo, GI upset, jaundice, ↓BP, ↓HR, visual/libido/urinary disturbances, blood disorders, paradoxical disinhibition in Ψ disorder.

Warn: sedation ↑ by alcohol. Do not stop suddenly, as can ⇒ withdrawal.

Interactions: P450 inhibitors/inducers may ↑/↓ effects; levels ↑ by aprepitant, crizotinib, diltiazem, dronedarone, erythromycin, fluconazole, imatinib, isavuconazole, netupitant, nilotinib, posaconazole, verapamil.

Dose: 250–500 micrograms po tds, ↑ if necessary up to 3 mg po od (elderly: 250 micrograms bd/tds).

Not prescribable in NHS primary care.

AMANTADINE

Weak DA agonist; ↑s release and ↓s reuptake of DA; NMDA antagonist.

Use: Parkinson's disease, dyskinesias[1] and post-herpetic neuralgia. Also used for fatigue in MS (unlicensed[NICE])[2].

CI: gastric ulcer (inc Hx of), epilepsy, **R** (if creatinine clearance <15 mL/min), **P**/**B**.

Caution: confused or hallucinatory states, **L**/**H**/**E**.

SE: confusion, hallucinations, pedal oedema NMS-like syndrome.
Warn: Can ↓skilled task performance (esp driving). Stop drug slowly*. Monitor for emergent impulse control disorders.
Interactions: memantine ↑risk of CNS toxicity, anticholinergics.
Dose: 100–400 mg daily[SPC/BNF,1]; 200 mg daily[NICE,2]. *NB: ↓dose in* **RF, E ≥ 65 years.**
NB: stop slowly: risk of withdrawal syndrome.*

AMIODARONE

Class III antiarrhythmic: ↑s refractory period of conducting system; has ↓negative inotropic fx than other drugs and can give when others ineffective/CI.
Use: tachyarrhythmias: esp paroxysmal SVT, AF, atrial flutter, nodal tachycardias, VT and VF. Also in CPR/periarrest arrhythmias.
CI: ↓HR (sinus), sinoatrial HB, SAN disease or severe conduction disturbance w/o pacemaker, Hx of thyroid disease/iodine sensitivity, **P/B**.
Caution: porphyria, ↓K⁺ (↑risk of torsades), **L/R/H/E**.
SE: *Acute:* N&V (dose-dependent), ↓HR/BP. *Chronic:* rarely but seriously ↑ or ↓T₄, interstitial lung disease (e.g. fibrosis, *but reversible if caught early*), **hepatotoxicity, conduction disturbances** (esp ↓HR). *Common:* **malaise, fatigue,** photosensitive skin (rarely 'grey-slate'), corneal deposits ± 'night glare' (reversible), tremor, sleep disorders. *Less commonly:* optic neuritis (rare but can ↓vision), peripheral neuropathy, blood disorders, hypersensitivity.
Warn: avoid sunlight/use sunscreen (inc several months after stopping).
Monitor: TFTs and LFTs (baseline then 6 monthly). Also baseline K⁺ and CXR (watch for ↑SOB/alveolitis).
Interactions: Drugs that ↑QT. ↑s fx of phenytoin and digoxin. Other class III and many class Ia antiarrhythmics, antipsychotics, TCAs, lithium, erythromycin, co-trimoxazole, antimalarials, nelfinavir, ritonavir ⇒ ↑risk of ventricular arrhythmias. Verapamil, diltiazem and β-blockers ⇒ ↑risk of ↓HR and HB; CYP3A4 inhibition with statins ↑myopathy, **W+**.

Dose: po: load with 200 mg tds in first wk, 200 mg bd in second wk, then (usually od) maintenance dose according to response (long $T_{1/2}$: months before steady plasma concentration). *NB: initiate in hospital or specialist outpatient service*; **iv:** (extreme emergencies only) 300 mg in 10–20 mL 5% glucose over ≥3 min (do not repeat for at least 15 min); **ivi:** 5 mg/kg over 20–120 min (max 1.2 g/day).

☠ iv doses: give via central line (if no time for insertion, give via largest Venflon possible) with ECG monitoring. Avoid giving if severe respiratory failure or ↓BP (unless caused by arrhythmia), as can worsen. Avoid iv boluses if CCF/cardiomyopathy ☠.

AMISULPRIDE/SOLIAN

Atypical antipsychotic with selective D_2 receptor binding; low dose preferentially blocks presynaptic autoreceptors, but high dose blocks post-synaptic receptors.

Use: acute psychotic episode in schizophrenia[1], schizophrenia with predominantly negative symptoms[2].

CI: CNS depression, phaeo, prolactin-dependent tumours, prepubescent children, co-prescription with levodopa and ropinirole, **P/B**.

Caution: Parkinson's, drugs that ↑QTc, epilepsy, MG, glaucoma (angle-closure), ↑prostate, severe respiratory disease, jaundice, blood disorders, DM, dementia in the elderly.

Class SE: EPSE, ↑prolactin and assoc Sx, sedation, ↑Wt, ↑QTc, VTE, blood dyscrasias, ↓seizure threshold, NMS.

Monitor: ECG may be required, esp if (risk factors for) CVD or inpatient admission; prolactin concentration at start of therapy, 6 months and then yearly; physical health monitoring (cardiovascular disease risk) at least once/year.

Interactions: ↑risk of ↑QTc/torsade de pointes with β-blockers, calcium channel blockers, diuretics, stimulant laxatives, class 1A and III antiarrhythmics (e.g. quinidine, disopyramide, amiodarone, sotalol), ↑sedative fx of alcohol and ↓fx of levodopa, and ropinirole.

Dose: 400–800 mg po od in two divided doses (maximum 1.2 g od)[1], 50–300 mg po od[2].

AMITRIPTYLINE

TCA: blocks reuptake of NA (and 5-HT).

Use: depression[1] (esp if insomnia, ↓appetite, psychomotor slowing or agitation prominent. *NB:* ↑danger in od cf other antidepressants), neuropathic pain[2], migraine prophylaxis.

CI: recent MI (w/in 3 months), arrhythmias (esp HB), CCF, mania, porphyria **B, L** (if severe).

Caution: cardiac/thyroid disease, epilepsy*, glaucoma (angle-closure), ↑prostate, phaeo, porphyria, anaesthesia. Also Hx of mania, psychosis or urinary retention, **L/H/P/E**.

SE: antimuscarinic fx, cardiac fx (arrhythmias, HB, HR, postural ↓BP, dizziness, syncope: **dangerous in od**), ↑Wt, sedation (often ⇒ 'hangover'), seizures. Rarely mania, fever, blood disorders, hypersensitivity, Δ LFTs, ↓Na+ (esp in elderly), agitation, confusion, serotonin syndrome, neuroleptic malignant syndrome.

Interactions: ☠ MAOIs ⇒ HTN and CNS excitation. **Never give with, or <2 wks after, MAOI** ☠. Levels ↑d by SSRIs (risk of serotonin syndrome), phenothiazines and cimetidine. ↑risk of arrhythmias with amiodarone, pimozide (is CI), thioridazine and some class I antiarrhythmics. ↑risk of paralytic ileus with antimuscarinics. ↑s sedative fx of alcohol.

Dose: initially 25 mg bd (daily dose of 10–25 mg in elderly), ↑if required to max 75 mg bd[1]; initially 10 mg nocte ↑ing if required to 75 mg nocte[2].

> ☠ Overdose is associated with high rate of fatality. TCA overdose ⇒ dilated pupils, arrhythmias, ↓BP, hypothermia, hyperreflexia, extensor plantar responses, seizures, respiratory depression and coma ☠.

AMLODIPINE

Ca2+ channel blocker (dihydropyridine): as nifedipine, but ⇒ no ↓contractility or ↑HF.

Use: HTN, angina (esp 'Prinzmetal's' = coronary vasospasm).
CI: ACS, cardiogenic shock, significant aortic stenosis, **P/B**.
Caution: BPH (poly-/nocturia), acute porphyria, CHF, **L/E**.
SE: as nifedipine but ↑ankle swelling and possibly ↓vasodilator fx (headache, flushing and dizziness).
Interactions: care with inducers and inhibitors of CYP450 3A4; ↓simvastatin dose max 20 mg od; avoid grapefruit juice.
Dose: initially 5 mg od PO (↑ if required to 10 mg). *NB:* consider ↓dose in **LF**.

AMOXICILLIN
Broad-spectrum penicillin; good GI absorption (can give po and iv).
Use: consult local guidance on antibiotic choice.
CI/Caution/SE/Interactions: see Ampicillin.
Dose: e.g. 500–1000 mg tds PO/IV (mild/moderate infections usually 250–500 mg TDS PO). *NB:* ↓dose in **RF**.

AMPICILLIN
Broad-spectrum penicillin for iv use: has ↓GI absorption cf amoxicillin, which is preferred po.
Use: consult local guidance on antibiotic choice.
CI: penicillin hypersensitivity (*NB:* cross-reactivity with cephalosporins).
Caution: EBV/CMV infections, ALL, CLL (all ↑risk of rash), **R**.
SE: rash (erythematous, maculopapular: often does not reflect true allergy) more common in RF or crystal nephropathy, **N&V&D** (rarely AAC), hypersensitivity, CNS/blood disorders.
Interactions: levels ↑ by probenecid. ↑risk of rash with allopurinol. Can ↓fx of OCP (warn patient); ↑levels of methotrexate, **W+**.
Dose: most indications 250 mg^{-1} g qds po, 500 mg qds im/iv$^{SPC/BNF}$ (meningitis 2 g 4-hrly ivi[1]). *NB:* ↓dose in **RF**.

APIXABAN
Oral anticoagulant; direct inhibitor of activated factor X (factor Xa).

Use: Px of VTE following knee[1] or hip[2] replacement surgery, Rx of deep-vein thrombosis (DVT)[3], Rx of PE[3], Px of recurrent DVT[4] or PE[4], Px of stroke and systemic embolism in non-valvular AF and at ≥1 risk factor[5] (e.g. previous stroke or TIA, symptomatic HF, DM, HTN, or ≥75 years of age).

CI: active, clinically significant bleeding, risk factors for major bleeding[BNF], **L** (if severe)/**R** (if severe)/ **P/B**.

Caution: 🕱 anaesthesia with post-operative indwelling epidural catheter (risk of paralysis), see BNF 🕱; prosthetic heart valve (efficacy not established); **L**.

SE: anaemia, haemorrhage; nausea, skin reactions; administration site reactions; CNS haemorrhage, ↓BP; post-procedural haematoma, ↓Pt; wound complications.

Warn: carry alert card at all times.

Interactions: strong CYP450 inhibitors to be avoided.

Dose: start 12–24 hours after surgery 1.2–2.5 mg bd po[1,2] for 10–14 days[1] or 32–38 days[2]. Initially 10 mg bd for 7 days po, then maintenance 5 mg bd po[3]. 2.5 mg bd po, after completion of 6 months anticoagulant Rx[4]. 5 mg twice daily, reduce dose to 2.5 mg twice daily in patients with ≥2 of the following: ≥80 years of age, Wt <61 kg, or serum creatinine ≥133 micromol/L[5]. See SPC for how to change from, or to, other anticoagulants.

AQUEOUS CREAM Emulsifying ointment (phenoxyethanol in purified water). Topical cream used as emollient in dry skin conditions and as a soap substitute.

ARIPIPRAZOLE/ABILIFY

Atypical (third-generation) antipsychotic; *partial* D$_2$ (and 5-HT$_{1A}$) agonist ⇒ ↓dopaminergic neuronal activity. Also potent 5-HT$_{2A}$ antagonist.

Use: schizophrenia, mania (Px and acute Rx).

CI: hypersensitivity.

Caution: cerebrovascular disease, Hx or ↑risk of seizures, family Hx of ↑QT, **L/P/E**.

SE: EPSE (esp akathisia/restlessness, although generally ⇒ ↓EPSE than other antipsychotics), dizziness, sedation (or insomnia), blurred vision, fatigue, headache, GI upset, anxiety and ↑salivation. Rarely ↑HR, depression, orthostatic ↓BP. Very rarely skin/blood disorders, ↑QTc, DM, NMS, tardive dyskinesia, seizures and CVA.

Interactions: metab by P450 ∴ many: most importantly levels ↑ by itraconazole, HIV protease inhibitors, fluoxetine, paroxetine and levels ↓ by carbamazepine, rifampicin, rifabutin, phenytoin, primidone, efavirenz, nevirapine and St John's wort.

Dose: 10–15 mg po od (max 30 mg/od); 5.25–15 (usually 9.75) mg im as single dose repeated after ≥2 h if required (max three injections/day or combined im/po dose of 30 mg/day). *NB:* ↓dose in elderly; double dose with potent CYP3A4 inducers and halve dose with potent CYP3A4 or CYP2D6 inhibitors.

ASENAPINE

Atypical antipsychotic, less likely to cause ↑ weight than others in class. Given sublingually.

Use: Acute mania in bipolar disorder; licenced for schizophrenia in US.

Caution: as for other antipsychotics, plus dementia with Lewy bodies, **L/R/P/B/E.**

Class SE: EPSE, ↑prolactin and assoc Sx, sedation, ↑Wt, ↑QTc, VTE, blood dyscrasias, ↓seizure threshold, NMS.

Specific SE: Anxiety, nausea, taste altered; Uncommon: BBB, dysarthria, dysphagia, sexual dysfunction, syncope, Accommodation disorder, rhabdomyolysis.

Monitoring: BG* (± HbA1C) after 1 month then 4–6 monthly. LFTs, U&Es, FBC, prolactin (CK only if NMS suspected). Wt and lipids every 3 months for 1 year, then at least annually.

Interactions: metab by P450 (1A2) ∴ many, but most importantly, levels ↓d by carbamazepine and smoking. ↑risk of ↓NØ with valproate. Levels may be ↑d by ciprofloxacin, fluvoxamine. ↑risk of arrhythmias with drugs that ↑QTc. ↑risk of ↓BP with general anaesthetics and antihypertensives. ↓s fx of anticonvulsants. May ↑ paroxetine levels.

Dose: 5mg bd SL, increased to 10mg bd as necessary

ASPIRIN

NSAID. Inhibits COX-1 and COX-2 ⇒ ↓PG synthesis (∴ anti-inflammatory and antipyrexial) and ↓thromboxane A$_2$ (∴ anti-Plt aggregation).

Use: mild-to-moderate pain/pyrexia[1], IHD and thromboembolic CVA Px[2] and acute Rx[3]; see BNF for additional indications.

CI: <16 years old, unless specifically indicated (can ⇒ Reye's syndrome), PU (active or at analgesic dose PHx of), hypersensitivity to any NSAID, haemophilia, **R** (GFR <10 mL/min)/**L** (if severe)/**B**.

Caution: asthma, gout, any allergic disease*, dehydration, uncontrolled HTN, gout, G6PD deficiency, **L/R** (avoid if either severe)/**P/E**.

SE: GI irritation, bleeding (esp GI: ↑↑risk if also anticoagulated)**. Rarely hypersensitivity* (anaphylaxis, bronchospasm, skin reactions), AKI, hepatotoxicity, ototoxic in od.

Interactions: ↑GI bleeding with anticoagulants**, other NSAIDs (avoid), SSRIs and SNRIs. **W+**. Can ⇒ ↑levels of methotrexate, ↑fx of anticonvulsants and ↓fx of spironolactone.

Dose: 300–900 mg 4–6 hrly (max 4 g/day)[1], 75 mg od[2], 300 mg stat[3].

> Stop 7 days before surgery if significant bleeding is expected. If cardiac surgery or patient has ACS, consider continuing.

ATENOLOL

β-blocker: (mildly) cardioselective* (β$_1$ > β$_2$), ↑H$_2$O solubility ∴ ↓central fx** and ↑renal excretion***.

Use: HTN[1], angina[2], MI (within 12 h as early intervention)[3], arrhythmias[4].

CI/Caution/SE/Interactions: see Propranolol ⇒ ↓bronchospasm* (but avoid in all asthma/only use in COPD if no other choice) and ↓sleep disturbance/nightmares**.

Dose: 25–50 mg od po[1]; 100 mg od po[2]; 5 mg iv over 5 min, 50 mg po 15 min later, 50 mg po after 12 h, then 100 mg od po[3]; 50–100 mg od po[4] (for iv doses, see SPC/BNF). *NB:* **consider ↓dose in RF***.**

ATOMOXETINE

Noradrenaline reuptake inhibitor: exact mechanism unknown.
Use: ADHD.
CI: Rx with MAOI, phaeo, severe cerebro-/cardiovascular disease, **H**.
Caution: ↑QTc, aggressive behaviour, cerebro-/cardiovascular disease, emotional lability, epilepsy, hostility, HTN, mania, psychosis, susceptibility to angle-closure glaucoma.
SE: Headache, GI upset, ↓appetite, ↓growth rate, cardiac fx (↑HR, ↑BP, postural ↓BP, syncope), somnolence, Δmood, dizziness, rash. *Uncommonly* suicidal behaviour, ↑QTc.
Monitor: Depression, anxiety, tics, pulse, BP, Wt, Ht and appetite at start, after each dose Δ and every 6 months.
Interactions: levels ↑ by bupropion, cinacalcet, fluoxetine, panobinostat, paroxetine, terbinafine; ↑risk of SE with dexamfetamine, lisdexamfetamine, MAOIs.
Dose: adult (<70 kg): initially 500 microgram/kg po od for 7 days, maintenance 1.2 mg/kg od (maximum 1.8 mg/kg od/120 mg od); adult (>70 kg): initially 40 mg po od for 7 days, maintenance 80–100 mg od (maximum 120 mg od), may be given as single dose mane or in two divided doses with last dose no later than early evening.

ATORVASTATIN

HMG-CoA reductase inhibitor.
Use/CI/Caution/SE: see Simvastatin.
Interactions: ↑risk of myopathy includes with 🐟 fibrates 🐟, daptomycin, ciclosporin, nicotinic acid, itra-/posaconazole. Levels ↑ by clari-/telithromycin.
Dose: initially 10 mg nocte (↑ if necessary, at intervals 1 ≥4 wks, to max 80 mg). In CVD and post ACS aim for 80 mg daily[NICE].

L/R/H = Liver, Renal and Heart failure. **E** = elderly. **P** = pregnancy. **B** = breastfeeding.

AZITHROMYCIN

Macrolide antibiotic: see Erythromycin.
Use: consult local guidance on antibiotic choice.
CI: as erythromycin, plus **L** (if severe).
Caution/SE/Interactions: as erythromycin (*NB:* ↑**P450** ∴ many interactions) but ⇒ ↓GI SEs.
Dose: *500 mg od po for 3 days only* (continue for 5/7 for invasive strep, 7/7 for typhoid); 500 mg od po for 17 days for Lyme disease; for GU infections 1 g od po *as single dose.*

BACLOFEN

Skeletal muscle relaxant: ↓s spinal reflexes, general CNS inhibition at ↑doses.
Use: spasticity, if chronic/severe (esp 2° to MS or cord pathology).
CI: PU, porphyria, hereditary galactose intolerance.
Caution: Ψ disorders, epilepsy, Hx of PU, Parkinson's, porphyria, DM, hypertonic bladder sphincter, respiratory/cerebrovascular disease, **L/R/P/E**.
SE: sedation, ↓**muscle tone, nausea, urinary dysfunction**, GI upset, ↓BP. Others rare: ↑spasticity (*stop drug!*), multiple neurological/Ψ symptoms, cardiac/hepatic/respiratory dysfunction.
Warn: may ↓skilled tasks (esp driving), ↑s fx of alcohol.
Interactions: fx ↑ by TCAs. May ↑fx of antihypertensives.
Dose: 5 mg tds po (after food) ↑ing, if required, to max of 100 mg/day. *NB:* ↓**dose in RF.** In severe cases, can give by intrathecal pump (see SPC/BNF).

Stop gradually over ≥1–2 wks to avoid withdrawal symptoms: confusion, ↑spasticity, Ψ reactions, fits, ↑HR.

BECLOMETASONE/BECOTIDE

Inh corticosteroid: ↓s airway oedema and mucous secretions.
Use: chronic asthma not controlled by short-acting β₂ agonists alone, i.e. symptoms ≥3× week.
Caution: TB (inc quiescent).

SE: oral candidiasis (2° to immunosuppression: ↓d by rinsing mouth with H_2O after use), **hoarse voice**. Rarely glaucoma, hypersensitivity. ↑doses may ⇒ adrenal suppression, Cushing's, ↓bone density, lower RTI, ↓growth (controversial). Visual disturbance: systemic absorption more likely to occur with higher dose.

Dose: 200–2000 micrograms daily inh (normally start at 200 micrograms bd). Use high-dose inhaler if daily requirements are >800 micrograms.[SPC/BNF] Specify named product for CFC metered disc inhalers, as dose ranges from 50 to 400 micrograms/delivery. CFC-free pressurized metered dose inhalers are not interchangeable.

Rarely ⇒ paradoxical bronchospasm: can be prevented by switching from aerosol to dry powder forms or by using inh β_2 agonists.

BENDROFLUMETHIAZIDE

Thiazide diuretic: ↓s Na^+ (and Cl) reabsorption from DCT ⇒ Na^+ and H_2O loss and stimulates K^+ excretion.

Use: oedema[1] (2° to HF or low-protein states), HTN[2] (in short term by ↓ing fluid volume and CO; in long term by ↓ing TPR).

CI: ↓K^+ (refractory to Rx), ↓Na^+, ↓Ca^{2+}, Addison's disease, ↑urate (if symptoms), **L/R** (if either severe, otherwise caution).

Caution: porphyria, and can worsen gout, DM or SLE, **P/B/E**.

SE: dehydration (esp in elderly), ↓BP (esp postural), ↓K^+, GI upset, impotence, ↓Na^+, alkalosis (with ↓Cl), ↓Mg^{2+}, ↑Ca^{2+}, ↑urate/gout, ↑glucose, lipid metabolism (esp ↑cholesterol), rash, photosensitivity, blood disorders (inc ↓Pt, ↓NØ), pancreatitis, intrahepatic cholestasis, hypersensitivity reactions (inc severe respiratory and skin reactions), arrhythmias.

Interactions: ↑s lithium levels. fx ↓ by **NSAIDs** and oestrogens. If ↓K^+ can ↑toxic fx of many drugs (esp digoxin, NSAIDs, corticosteriods, drugs that may prolong QTc and many antiarrhythmics). ↑risk of ↓Na^+ with carbamazepine; ↑risk of ↓K^+ with amphotericin. ↑risk of allopurinol hypersensitivity.

Dose: initially 5–10 mg mane po[1], then ↓dose *frequency* (i.e. omit days) if possible; 2.5 mg od po[2,3] (little benefit from ↑doses).

BENPERIDOL

Butyrophenone typical antipsychotic: dopamine antagonist, selective for D_2 receptor; some weaker binding to 5-HT receptors.

Use: antisocial sexual behaviour.

CI: Parkinson's disease, EPSEs, depression, ↓GCS, phaeo.

Caution: dementia, drugs that ↑QTc, epilepsy, MG, glaucoma (angle-closure), ↑prostate, severe respiratory disease, jaundice, blood disorders, DM, stroke risk factors, **P**.

Class SE: EPSE, ↑prolactin and assoc Sx, sedation, ↑Wt, QT prolongation, VTE, blood dyscrasias, ↓seizure threshold, NMS.

Warn: Photosensitivity at high doses. Extrapyramidal effects and withdrawal syndrome in neonate when used during third trimester. ↑fx of alcohol.

Monitor: prolactin at start, 6 months, then yearly. Regular FBC and LFTs during long-term treatment.

Interactions: ↑risk of ↓BP with atenolol, alcohol, amantadine, amitriptyline, amlodipine, aripiprazole, bendroflumethiazide, bromocriptine, candesartan, chlorpromazine, clozapine, haloperidol; CNS depressant effects with agomelatine, alcohol, alprazolam, amisulpride, aripiprazole, buprenorphine, cannabis extract, chlorphenamine, chlorpromazine, clozapine, codeine; ↓effects of amantadine, apomorphine, bromocriptine, levodopa (severe), ropinirole.

Dose: 0.25–1.5 mg po od in divided doses; elderly: initially 0.125–0.75 mg po od in divided doses.

BENZYLPENICILLIN SODIUM (= PENICILLIN G)

Penicillin with poor po absorption ∴ only given im/iv: used mostly against streptococcal (esp *S. pneumoniae*) and neisserial (esp *N. gonorrhoeae*, *N. meningitidis*) infections.

Use: (usually in conjunction with other agents) severe skin infections (esp cellulitis, wound infections, gas gangrene), meningitis, endocarditis, ENT infections, pneumococcal pneumonia.

CI: penicillin hypersensitivity (*NB:* cross-reactivity with cephalosporins common).

Caution: Hx of allergy, false +ve glycosuria, **R***.

SE: hypersensitivity (inc fever, arthralgia, rashes, urticaria, angioedema, anaphylaxis, serum sickness–like reactions, haemolytic ↓Hb, interstitial nephritis), **diarrhoea** (rarely AAC). Rarely blood disorders (↓Pt, ↓NØ, coagulation disorders), CNS toxicity (inc convulsions, esp at ↑doses or if RF*). ↑doses can ⇒ ↓K⁺ (and ↑Na⁺).

Interactions: levels ↑d by probenecid. ↑risk of rash with allopurinol. Can ↓fx of OCP. ↓Excretion of methotrexate.

Dose: 600 mg–1.2 g qds iv (or im/ivi). If very severe, give 2.4 g every 4 h (only as iv/ivi). *NB: ↓dose in RF.*

BETAMETHASONE CREAM (0.1%)/BETNOVATE

'Potent' strength topical corticosteroid (rarely used as weaker 0.05% or 0.025% preparations).

Use: inflammatory skin conditions, in particular, eczema.

CI: untreated infection, rosacea, acne.

SE: skin atrophy, worsening of infections, acne.

Dose: apply thinly one to two times per day. Use 'ointment' in dry skin conditions.

BIMATOPROST EYE DROPS

Topical PG analogue for glaucoma; see Latanoprost.

Use/CI/Caution/SE: see Latanoprost.

Dose: 1 drop od.

BISOPROLOL

β-blocker, cardioselective (β₁ > β₂).

Use: HTN[1], angina[2], HF[3].

CI/Caution/SE/Interactions: as propranolol, but also CI in HF needing inotropes or if SAN block; caution if psoriasis.

Dose: Initially 5mg od po[1,2] (maintenance 5–20 mg od); initially 1.25 mg od po[3] (↑ing slowly to max 10 mg od).[SPC/BNF] *NB: ↓dose in LF or RF.*

BOWEL PREPARATIONS/(E.G. PICOLAX)

Bowel-cleansing solutions for preparation for GI surgery/Ix.
CI: GI obstruction/ulceration/perforation, ileus, gastric retention,
toxic megacolon/colitis, acute IBD, rhabdo, hypermagnesemia,
dehydrated patients, **H**.
Caution: UC, DM, heart disease, reflux oesophagitis, ↑risk of
regurgitation/aspiration (e.g. ↓swallow/gag reflex/GCS), **R/P**.
SE: nausea, abdo pains, vomiting, electrolyte disturbance.
Dose: see SPC/BNF.

BRIMONIDINE EYE DROPS

Topical α_2 agonist: ↓s aqueous humour production ∴ ↓s IOP.
Use: open-angle glaucoma, ocular HTN (esp if β-blocker or PG
analogue CI or fails to ↓IOP).
Caution: postural ↓BP/HR, Raynaud's, cardiovascular disease
(esp IHD), cerebral insufficiency, depression*, **P/B** (avoid)/**R/L**.
SE: sedation, headache, dry mouth, HTN, blurred vision, **local
reactions** (esp discomfort, pruritus, hyperaemia, follicular
conjunctivitis). Rarely palpitations, depression*, hypersensitivity.
Interactions: ☠ MAOIs, TCAs, mianserin (or other
antidepressants affecting NA transmission) are CI. ☠
Dose: 1 drop bd of 0.2% solution. Also available as od
combination drop with timolol 0.5% (Combigan).

BRINZOLAMIDE

Topical carbonic anhydrase inhibitor for glaucoma. Similar to
dorzolamide (↓s aqueous humour production).
CI: hyperchloraemic acidosis, **R** (GFR <30 mL/min)/**L**.
Caution: **P/B**.
Dose: 1 drop bd/tds. Also available as od combination drop with
timolol 0.5% (Azarga).

BROMOCRIPTINE

DA agonist; ↓s pituitary release of prolactin and growth
hormone.

Use: endocrine disorders[1] (e.g. prolactinoma, galactorrhoea, acromegaly) and NMS (unlicensed). Rarely used for parkinsonism if L-dopa insufficient/not tolerated.

CI: SMI cardiac valvulopathy, hypersensitivity to ergot alkaloids, uncontrolled HTN. Also HTN/IHD post-partum or in puerperium.

Caution: cardiovascular disease, PU, porphyria, Raynaud's disease, serious Ψ disorders (esp psychosis, impulse control), **P/B**.

SE: GI upset, postural ↓BP (esp initially and if ↑alcohol intake), **behavioural Δs** (confusion, agitation, psychosis), ↑**sleep** (sudden onset/daytime). Rarely but seriously **fibrosis**: pulmonary, cardiac, retroperitoneal (can ⇒ AKI).

Warn: of ↑sleep. Report persistent cough or chest/abdo pain.

Monitor: BP, ESR, U&Es, CXR; pituitary size and visual fields (pregnancy and[1]); Rx > 6 m: gynaecological cytology.

Interactions: levels ↑ by ery-/clarithromycin and octreotide. Opposing action to antipsychotics. May inhibit CYP3A4: caution with PIs for HIV.

Dose: 1–30 mg/day. *NB:* **consider ↓dose in LF.**

BUDESONIDE

Inh corticosteroid for asthma[1]; similar to beclometasone but stronger (approximately double the strength per microgram). Also available po or as enemas for IBD[2] (see BNF).

Caution: **L.**

Dose: 200–800 micrograms bd inh (aerosol or powder) or 1–2 mg bd neb[1].

BUMETANIDE

Loop diuretic: inhibits Na^+/K^+ pump in ascending loop of Henle.

Use/CI/Caution/SE/Monitor/Interactions: as furosemide; also headaches, gynaecomastia and at ↑doses can ⇒ myalgia.

Dose: 1 mg mane po (500 micrograms may suffice in elderly), ↑ing if required (5 mg/24 h in severe cases of oedema only; ↑ by adding a lunchtime dose, then ↑ing each dose).

NB: give iv in severe oedema; bowel oedema ⇒ ↓po absorption.

BUPRENORPHINE

Partial agonist at μ-opioid receptor and antagonist at κ-opioid receptors ⇒ ↓neuronal excitability.

Use: moderate-to-severe pain[1], adjunct in treatment of opioid dependence[2]. *NB:* Subutex and Espranor are brands of oral buprenorphine; Suboxone is a combination of buprenorphine and naloxone designed to prevent injection. Buvidal is a long-acting injection. Sixmo is a subcutaneous implant.

CI: acute respiratory depression, acute severe obstructive airways disease, ↑risk of paralytic ileus, delayed gastric emptying, biliary colic, acute alcoholism, ↑ICP (respiratory depression ⇒ CO_2 retention and cerebral vasodilation ⇒ ↑ICP), phaeo, **H** (if 2° to chronic lung disease).

Caution: ↓consciousness, ↓respiratory reserve, obstructive airways disease, ↓BP/shock, acute abdo, biliary tract disorders (*NB:* biliary colic is CI), pancreatitis, bowel obstruction, IBD, ↑prostate/urethral stricture, arrhythmias, ↓T_4, adrenocorticoid insufficiency, MG, **L** (can ⇒ coma)/**R/P/B/E**. For *patch*, fever or external heat (⇒ Δs in absorption), other opioids within 24 h. For *opioid dependence*, hep B/C infection, abnormal LFTs.

SE: fatigue, sleep disorders, anxiety, ↓appetite, depression, diarrhoea, dyspnoea, GI discomfort, muscle weakness, oedema, tremor.

Warn: do not take other opioids within 24 h of patch removal (long duration of action).

Monitor: baseline and regular LFTs in[2].

Interactions: ↑risk of withdrawal if given with other opioids; ↑levels with atazanavir, clarithromycin, cobicistat, darunavir, fosamprenavir, idelalisib, itraconazole, ketoconazole, lopinavir, ritonavir, saquinavir, tipranavir, voriconazole; ↑risk of CNS excitation/depression with isocarboxazid, phenelzine, tranylcypromine; ↓fx with nalmefene.

Dose: Varies by preparation: consult BNF or specialist literature.

☠Do not confuse the formulations of transdermal patches which are available as 72-hour, 96-hour and 7-day patches☠.

BUPROPION/ZYBAN

NA and to lesser extent DA reuptake inhibitor (NDRI) developed as antidepressant, but also ↑s success of giving up smoking.

Use: (adjunct to) smoking cessation[1], depression (unlicensed use)[2].

CI: CNS tumour, acute alcohol/benzodiazepine withdrawal, Hx of seizures*, eating disorders, bipolar disorder, **L** (if severe cirrhosis)/**P/B**.

Caution: if ↑risk of seizures*: alcohol abuse, Hx of head trauma and DM, **R/H/E**.

SE: seizures*, **insomnia** (and other CNS reactions, e.g. anxiety, agitation, depression, fever, headaches, tremor, dizziness), decreased appetite. Also ↑HR, AV block, ↑ or ↓BP**, chest pain, hypersensitivity (inc severe skin reactions), GI upset, ↑Wt, mild antimuscarinic fx (esp **dry mouth**).

Monitor: BP**.

Interactions: ↓P450 ∴ many interactions, but importantly CNS drugs, esp if ↓seizure threshold*, e.g. antidepressants (☠ MAOIs; avoid together, including <2 wks after MAOI ☠), antimalarials, antipsychotics (esp risperidone), quinolones, sedating antihistamines, systemic corticosteroids, theophyllines, tramadol; ↓tamoxifen activation. Ritonavir ⇒ ↓plasma level of bupropion. ↓dose of CYP2B6 mod antiarrhythmics. Inhibits CYP2D6 so drugs metabolised by this pathway should be initiated at lower doses, e.g. type 1C antiarrhythmics, metoprolol, certain antidepressants. Metabolised by CYP2B6, so inihbitors such as orphenadrine, clopidogrel may ↑levels and inducers such as carbamazepine, phenytoin, ritonavir may reduce levels.

Dose: 150 mg od for 6 days then 150 mg bd for max 9 wks (↓dose if elderly or ↑seizure risk). Start 1–2 wks before target date of stopping smoking[1]; 150 mg od, ↑ to 300 mg if no improvement after 4 wks[2]. *NB:* max 150 mg/day in LF or RF.

BUSPIRONE HYDROCHLORIDE

5-HT$_{1A}$ receptor partial agonist ⇒ ↓firing rate of 5-HT-containing neurons in dorsal raphe.

Use: anxiety (short-term use); does not assist benzodiazepine withdrawal.

CI: epilepsy, acute alcohol intoxication, hypnotics, analgesics or antipsychotic drugs, **P**.

Caution: angle closure glaucoma, myasthenia gravis, drug dependence, **L/R**.

SE: dizziness, headache, anxiety, GI upset, agitation, sweating.

Interactions: metab by P450 ∴ ↓dose to 2.5 mg bd when used with potent CYP3A4 inhibitors; ↑levels with atazanavir, clarithromycin, cobicistat, darunavir, fosamprenavir, idelalisib, itraconazole, ketoconazole, linezolid, lopinavir, ritonavir, saquinavir, tipranavir, voriconazole; ↓levels with carbamazepine, enzalutamide, fosphenytoin, mitotane, phenobarbital, phenytoin, primidone, rifampicin; ↑risk of ↑BP with phenelzine, isocarboxazid, tranylcypromine.

Dose: 5 mg po bd/tds, ↑ at intervals 2–3 days, usual dose 15–30 mg od in divided doses, max 45 mg od.

CALCIFEROL

Vit D_2: needs renal (1) and hepatic (25) hydroxylation for activation.

Use: prophylaxis[1] and treatment[2] of vit D deficiency.

CI: ↑Ca^{2+}, metastatic calcification. **P** (only high doses).

Caution: **R** (if high 'pharmacological'* doses used), **B**.

SE: ↑Ca^{2+}. If over-Rx: GI upset, weakness, headache, polydipsia/polyuria, anorexia, RF, arrhythmias.

Monitor: Ca^{2+} (esp if N&V develops or ↑doses in RF*).

Interactions: fx ↓ by anticonvulsants and ↑ by thiazides.

Dose: 400 units od[1]; different loading regimens can be used to achieve a cumulative total of approximately 300 000 units divided into daily or weekly doses over 6–10 wks, then 800–2000 units daily[2]. Numerous preparations available, many with calcium carbonate component – too numerous to mention.

---

* *NB:* 400 units = 10 mg. Specify strength of tablet required to avoid confusion.[SPC/BNF]

CALCIUM CARBONATE

Use: osteoporosis, $\downarrow Ca^{2+}$, $\uparrow po_4$ (esp 2° to RF; binds po_4 in gut $\Rightarrow$ $\downarrow$absorption).

CI: conditions assoc with $\uparrow Ca^{2+}$ (in serum or urine).

Caution: sarcoid, Hx of kidney stones, phenylketonuria, **R**.

SE: GI upset, $\uparrow Ca^{2+}$ (serum or urine), $\downarrow$HR, arrhythmias.

Interactions: fx $\uparrow$ by thiazides, fx $\downarrow$ by corticosteroids, $\downarrow$s absorption of tetracyclines (give ≥2 h before or 6 h after) and bisphosphonates.

Dose: as required up to 40 mmol/day in osteoporosis if $\downarrow$dietary intake, e.g. Calcichew (standard 12.5 mmol or 'forte' 25 mmol tablets), Cacit (12.5 mmol tablets), Calcium 500 (12.5 mmol tablets) or Adcal (15 mmol tablets). Multiple other preparations available.

CANDESARTAN

Angiotensin II antagonist.

Use: HTN[1] or HF[2] (when ACE-i not tolerated).

CI: cholestasis, **L** (if severe)/**P/B**.

Caution/SE/Interactions: see Losartan.

Dose: initially 8 mg od[1] (4 mg if LF, 4 mg if RF/intravascular volume depletion) $\uparrow$ing at 4 wk intervals if necessary to max of 32 mg od; initially 4 mg od[2] $\uparrow$ing at intervals ≥2 wks to 'target dose' of 32 mg od (or max tolerated). *NB:* **$\downarrow$dose in LF.**

CARBAMAZEPINE/TEGRETOL

Antiepileptic, mood stabiliser, analgesic; $\downarrow$s synaptic transmission.

Use: epilepsy[1] (generalised tonic-clonic and partial seizures, but may exacerbate absence/myoclonic seizures), Px bipolar disorder[2] (if unresponsive to lithium), neuralgia[3] (esp post-herpetic, trigeminal and DM related).

CI: unpaced AV conduction dfx, Hx of BM suppression, acute porphyria.

Caution: cardiac disease, Hx of skin disorders (HLA-B*1502 in Han Chinese or Thai origin have $\uparrow$risk of SE – esp SJS), Hx of haematological drug reactions, glaucoma, **L/R/P** ($\Rightarrow$ neural tube dfx* ∴ $\Rightarrow$ folate Px and screen for dfx)/**B**.

Dose-related SE: N&V, headache, drowsiness, dizziness, vertigo, ataxia, visual Δ (esp double vision): control by ↓ing dose, Δ dose times/spacing or use of MR preparations**.

Other SE: skin reactions (transient erythema common), blood disorders (esp ↓WCC*** – often transient, ↓Pt, aplastic anaemia), ↑γ-GT (usually not clinically relevant), oedema, ↓Na⁺ (inc SIADH), HF, arrhythmias. Many rarer SEsᴿᴾᶜ/ᴮᴺᶠ, including suicidal thoughts/behaviour.

Warn: watch for signs of liver/skin/haematological disease.

Monitor: U&Es, LFTs, FBC, TFTs if T₄ Rx, ± serum levels (optimum therapeutic range = 4–12 mg/L). Vit D level.

Interactions: ↑**P450** – interacts with many drugs, check at time of prescribing. May cause failure of OCP; ↓levels of thyroid hormones if on hypothyroid Rx; fx are ↑d by **ery-/clarithromycin**, isoniazid, verapamil and diltiazem; and fx are ↓d by phenytoin, phenobarbitone. 🚫 **CI with MAOIs,** 🚫 **W–**.

Dose: dosing frequency depends on preparation, usual initial doses range between 100 and 200 mg od/bd (↑ slowly to max of 1.6 g/day[2,3] or 2 g/day[1]).

CARIPRAZINE
Atypical antipsychotic; selective partial agonist D₃ > D₂.

Use: schizophrenia.

Caution: akathisia, tardive dyskinesia, Parkinson's, NMS, suicidal ideation and behaviour, ↑QTc (although ↓than most antipsychotics), epilepsy, MG, glaucoma (angle-closure), ↑prostate, severe respiratory disease, jaundice, blood disorders, DM, BPSD.

SE: as with all antipsychotics plus anxiety, akathisia/EPSEs, bradyphrenia, drooling, eye/vision disorders, gait abnormalities, HTN, MSK stiffness, nausea, abnormal reflexes, sleep disorders, speech impairment, bruxism. Uncommon: anaemia, cardiac conduction disorder, delirium, depression ± suicidality, dysaesthesia, eosinophilia, eye irritation, GORD, hiccups, pruritus, sexual dysfunction, thirst, urinary disorders, vertigo. Rarely or very rarely: cataract, dysphagia, hypothyroidism, memory loss, rhabdomyolysis. Frequency unknown: hepatotoxicity.

Interactions: metab by P450 ∴ many.
Dose: 1.5 mg od, increased in steps of 1.5 mg; max 6 mg per day.

CEFACLOR

Oral second-generation cephalosporin.
Use: consult local guidance on antibiotic choice.
CI: cephalosporin hypersensitivity.
Caution: if at ↑risk of **AAC** (e.g. recent other antibiotic use,
↑age, severe underlying disease, ↑hospital/nursing home stay, GI
surgery, conditions/drugs that ↓gastric acidity [esp PPIs]), penicillin
hypersensitivity (up to 10% also allergic to cephalosporins), R/P/B
(but appropriate to use*).
SE: GI upset (esp N&D, but also **AAC**), **allergy** (anaphylaxis, fever,
arthralgia, skin reactions [inc severe]), **AKI, interstitial nephritis**
(reversible), hepatic dysfunction, blood disorders, CNS disturbance
(inc headache).
Interactions: levels ↑ by probenecid, mild **W+**.
Dose: dependent on indication and preparation; consult local
guidance. For example, 375 mg bd for gram ± bacterial infections;
250 mg tds po (500 mg tds in severe infections; max 4 g/day). *NB:
↓dose in RF.

Cephalosporins can ⇒ false-positive Coombs and urine glucose tests.

CEFALEXIN

Oral first-generation cephalosporin.
Use/CI/Caution/SE/Interactions: see Cefaclor and AAC
warning.
Dose: 250 mg qds or 500 mg bd/tds po (↑ in severe infections to
max 1.5 g qds). For Px of UTI, give 125 mg po nocte. *NB:* ↓dose
in RF.

CEFRADINE

Oral or parenteral first-generation cephalosporin.
Use: as cefaclor.
CI/Caution/SE/Interactions: see Cefaclor and AAC warning.

Dose: po: 250–500 mg qds *or* 500 mg–1 g bd (max 1 g qds).
NB: ↓dose in RF.

CEFTRIAXONE

Parenteral third-generation cephalosporin.
Use: consult local guidance on antibiotic choice.
CI/Caution/SE/Interactions: as cefaclor and **AAC warning**,
plus **L** (if coexistent RF), **R** (if severe), caution if dehydrated, young
or immobile (can precipitate in urine or gallbladder). Rarely ⇒
pancreatitis and ↑PT.
Dose: various dosing regimes depending on indication, e.g. 1 g
od im/iv/ivi (max 4 g/day); 1–2 g im/iv/ivi at induction; 2 g iv od or
21 days. *NB:* ↓dose in RF.

Max im dose = 1 g per site; if total >1 g, give at divided sites.

CEFUROXIME

Parenteral and oral second-generation cephalosporin: good for some
Gram –ve infections *(H. influenzae, N. gonorrhoeae)* and better than
third-generation cephalosporins for Gram +ve infections (esp *S. aureus*).
Use: consult local guidance on antibiotic choice.
CI/Caution/SE/Interactions: see Cefaclor and **AAC warning**.
Dose: 250–500 mg bd po[1]; 250 mg bd po[2]; 250 mg bd po[3]; 750 mg
tds/qds iv/im[4] (1.5 g tds/qds iv in very severe infections and 3 g tds
if meningitis); 1.5 g iv at induction (+750 mg iv/im tds for 24 h if
high-risk procedure)[5]. *NB:* ↓dose in RF.

CELECOXIB

NSAID which selectively inhibits COX-2 ∴ ↓GI SEs (COX-1
mediated).
Use: osteoarthritis/RA[NICE], ankylosing spondylitis.
CI: IHD, cerebrovascular disease, peripheral arterial
disease, *active* bleeding/PU, PVD, hypersensitivity to aspirin or
any other NSAID (inc asthma, angioedema, urticaria, rhinitis),
sulphonamide hypersensitivity, IBD, **L** (if severe)/**R** (GFR <30)/**H**
(moderate-severe)/**P/B**.

Caution: Hx of PU/GI bleeding, left ventricular dysfunction, HTN (monitor BP), ↑cardiovascular risk (e.g. DM, ↑lipids, smokers), oedema **H** (mild), asthma. **R***/**L** (if either mild-to-moderate)/**E**.

SE/Interactions: as ibuprofen, but ⇒ ↓PU/GI bleeding (but only if not in combination with aspirin) and ⇒ ↑risk of MI/CVA. Very rarely ⇒ seizures. Also, fluconazole ⇒ ↑serum levels and rifampicin ⇒ ↓serum levels. Mild **W+**.

Dose: 100–200 mg bd po. ↓dose in RF*. Consider gastroprotective Rx.COX-2 inhibitors and ↑risk of cardiovascular complications:

> **COX-2 inhibitors and ↑risk of cardiovascular complications:**
> CSM advises assessment of cardiovascular risk and use in preference to other NSAIDs only if at ↑↑risk of GI ulcer, perforation or bleeding. Use lowest effective dose and duration.

CETIRIZINE

Non-sedating antihistamine: selective peripheral H$_1$ antagonist.
Use: symptomatic relief from allergy (esp hay fever, urticaria).
CI: acute porphyria, **P/B**.
Caution: epilepsy, ↑prostate/urinary retention, glaucoma, pyloroduodenal obstruction, **R/L**.
SE: mild antimuscarinic fx (see p. 387), very mild rare sedation, headache.
Dose: 10 mg od po. ↓dose in RF.

CHLORAMPHENICOL EYE DROPS

Topical antibiotic, with no significant systemic fx, for superficial bacterial eye infections (e.g. conjunctivitis), or as prophylaxis, e.g. post-operatively or for corneal abrasions. Can rarely ⇒ aplastic anaemia; grey baby syndrome.
CI: personal/family Hx of aplastic anaemia.
SE: angioedema, BM disorders, ocular pain, fever, paraesthesia, skin reactions.

Dose: 1 drop of 0.5% solution every 2 h for the first 48 h and every 4 h thereafter. Can give as 1% ointment qds (or nocte only if using drops in daytime as well).

CHLORDIAZEPOXIDE/LIBRIUM

Long-acting benzodiazepine: GABA$_A$ receptor positive allosteric modulator.

Use: anxiety, short-term use (esp in alcohol withdrawal).

CI/Caution/SE/Interactions: see Diazepam.

Dose: 10 mg tds po for anxiety, ↑ing if required to max of 100 mg/day.

NB: ↓**dose in RF, LF and elderly**. ↑dose if benzodiazepine-resistant or in initial Rx of alcohol withdrawal (see reducing regimen on p. 252).

CHLORPHEN(IR)AMINE/PIRITON

Antihistamine: H$_1$ antagonist (peripheral *and central* ∴ sedating).

Use: allergies[1] (esp drug reactions, hay fever, urticaria), anaphylaxis[2].

CI: hypersensitivity to any antihistamine.

Caution: pyloroduodenal obstruction, urinary retention/↑prostate, thyrotoxicosis, asthma, bronchitis/bronchiectasis, severe HTN/CVD, glaucoma, epilepsy, **R/L/P/B**.

SE: drowsiness (rarely paradoxical stimulation), **antimuscarinic fx** (esp dry mouth; see p. 387), GI upset, arrhythmias, ↓BP, skin and hypersensitivity reactions (inc bronchospasm, photosensitivity). If given iv can cause transient CNS stimulation.

Warn: driving may be impaired.

Interactions: can ↑phenytoin levels. ↑fx by alcohol. ↑risk serotonin syndrome. ☠ **MAOIs** can ⇒ ↑↑antimuscarinic fx (SPC says chlorphenamine CI if MAOI given within 2 wks but evidence unclear). ☠

Dose: 4 mg 4–6 hrly po[1] (max 24 mg/24 h) ↓E; 10 mg iv over 1 min[2] (can ↑ to 20 mg, max 40 mg/24 h).

CHLORPROMAZINE/LARGACTIL

Phenothiazine ('typical') antipsychotic: dopamine antagonist (D_1 and $D_3 > D_2$ and D_4). Also blocks serotonin ($5\text{-}HT_{2A}$), histamine (H_1), adrenergic ($\alpha_1 > \alpha_2$) and muscarinic receptors, causing many SEs.

Use: schizophrenia, acute sedation (inc mania, severe anxiety, violent behaviour); intractable hiccups.

CI: CNS depression (inc coma), elderly patients with dementia, Hx of blood dyscrasias, phaeochromocytoma, MG, citalopram/escitalopram, angle-closure glaucoma, hypothyroidism, **H**.

Caution: Parkinson's, drugs that ↑QTc, epilepsy, MG, phaeo, glaucoma (angle-closure), ↑prostate, severe respiratory disease, jaundice, blood disorders, predisposition to postural ↓BP, ↑ or ↓temperature. Avoid direct sunlight (⇒ photosensitivity), **L**.

SE: sedation, extrapyramidal fx, antimuscarinic **fx**, seizures, ↑**Wt**, ↓BP (esp postural), ECG Δs (↑QTc), arrhythmias, endocrine fx (menstrual Δs, galactorrhoea, gynaecomastia, sexual dysfunction), Δ LFTs/jaundice, blood disorders (inc agranulocytosis, ↓WCC), ↓ or ↑temperature (esp in elderly), rash/↑pigmentation, neuroleptic malignant syndrome. Do not crush tablets (contact hypersensitivity; also possible from iv solution).

Monitor: FBC, BP.

Interactions: may ↑sedation caused by alcohol and sedative medications. May ↑hypotension caused by other medications, fx ↑d by TCAs (esp antimuscarinic fx), lithium (esp extrapyramidal fx), ritonavir, cimetidine and β-blockers (esp arrhythmias with sotalol; propranolol fx also ↑d by chlorpromazine). Avoid artemether/lumefantrine and drugs that ↑QTc or risk of ventricular arrhythmias (e.g. disopyramide, moxifloxacin).

Dose: 25–300 mg tds po[SPC/BNF]; 25–50 mg tds/qds im (painful, and may ⇒ ↓BP/↑HR). *NB:* ↓dose in elderly (approximately **1/3–1/2** adult dose but 10 mg od po may suffice) or if severe **RF**.

CHLOROQUINE

Antimalarial: inhibits protein synthesis and DNA/RNA polymerases.

Use: malaria Px[1] (only as Rx[2] if 'benign' spp (i.e. *P. ovale/vivax/malariae*); *P. falciparum* often resistant. Rarely for RA, SLE.[BNF]

Caution: QTc prolongation, cardiomyopathy, G6PD deficiency, severe GI disorders, can worsen psoriasis and MG, neurological disorders (esp epilepsy*), **L** (avoid other hepatotoxic drugs), **R/P**.
SE: GI upset, headache (mild, transient), **visual** Δ (rarely retinopathy**), **seizures***, hypersensitivity/skin reactions (inc pigment Δs), hair loss. Rarely **BM suppression**, cardiomyopathy. Arrhythmias common in od.
Monitor: FBC, vision** (ophthalmology review if long-term Rx).
Interactions: absorption ↓ by antacids. ↑risk of arrhythmias with amiodarone and moxifloxacin (use is contraindicated). ↑risk of convulsions with mefloquine. ↑s levels of digoxin and ciclosporin. ↓s levels of praziquantel.
Dose: Px[1]: 310 mg once-wkly as base (*specify on prescription: do not confuse with* **salt** *doses*); start 1 wk before arrival, continue 4 wks after leaving. Used mostly in conjunction with other drugs, depending on local resistance patterns.[SPC/BNF] **Rx**[2]: see SPC/BNF. *NB:* ↓**dose in RF**.

CIMETIDINE

As ranitidine, but ↑↑interactions (↓**P450** and **W+**) and ↑gynaecomastia ∴ prescribed rarely.
Caution: P/B.
Dose: 400 mg bd (can ↑ to 4 hrly[SPC/BNF]). *NB:* ↓**dose if LF or RF**.

CIPROFLOXACIN

(Fluoro)quinolone antibiotic: inhibits DNA gyrase; 'cidal' with broad spectrum, but particularly good for Gram −ve infections.
Use: consult local guidance on antibiotic choice.
Caution: seizures (inc Hx of, or predisposition to), MG (can worsen), ↑QTc (inc drugs that predispose to), G6PD deficiency, children/adolescents (theoretical risk of arthropathy), avoid ↑urine pH, DM or dehydration*, **R**.
SE: GI upset (esp N&D, sometimes AAC), pancreatitis, **neuro-Ψ fx** (esp confusion, seizures; also headache, dizziness, hallucinations, sleep and mood Δs), **tendinitis ± rupture** (esp if elderly or taking steroids), chest pain, oedema, **hypersensitivity** (rash, pruritus,

fever), QTc prolongation. Rarely hepatotoxicity, RF/interstitial nephritis, crystalluria*, blood disorders, ↑glucose, skin reactions (inc photosensitivity**, SJS, TEN). Slightly raised risk of aortic aneurysm, aortic dissection, cardiac valve regurgitation. Very rare cases of prolonged and potentially irreversible multi-organ reactions.

Warn: avoid UV light**, avoid ingesting Ca^{2+}-, Fe- and Zn-containing products (e.g. antacids***). May impair skilled tasks/driving.

Interactions: moderate CYP1A2 inhibitor: may affect clozapine and tizanidine (CI); increases levels of methotrexate. ↑s levels of theophyllines; NSAIDs ⇒ ↑risk of seizures; ↑s nephrotoxicity of ciclosporin; $FeSO_4$, Ca^{2+}-containing products, NB^{2+} and antacids*** ⇒ ↓po ciprofloxacin absorption (give 2 h before or 6 h after ciprofloxacin), drugs that ↑QTc, **W+**.

Dose: 250–750 mg bd po, 100–400 mg bd ivi (each dose over 1 h) according to indication[SPC/BNF] (250 mg bd po for 3 days for cystitis). *NB:* ↓dose if severe RF.

☠ Stop if tendinitis, severe neuro-Ψ fx or hypersensitivity. ☠

CITALOPRAM/CIPRAMIL

SSRI antidepressant.

Use: depression[1] (and panic disorder). Useful if polypharmacy, as ↓interactions and ↓cardio-/hepatotoxicity cf other SSRIs.

CI/Caution/SE/Warn: as fluoxetine, but risk of withdrawal syndrome if stopped abruptly. Can also ↑QTc (dose dependent); CI if ↑QTc (or congenital ↑QTc syndrome or taking other drugs that can ↑QT$_c$) and caution if ↑risk torsades de pointes (e.g. congestive HF, recent MI, bradyarrhythmias, predisposition to ↓K^+ or ↓Mg^{2+} dt concomitant illness or medicines; epilepsy, **P/B**.

Interaction: risk of serotonin syndrome with other serotonergic agents, selegiline and linezolid. ☠ **Never give with, or <2 wks after, MAOIs.** ☠

Dose: 20 mg od[1] ↑ing if necessary to max 40 mg (max 20 mg if elderly or **LF**).

CLARITHROMYCIN

Macrolide antibiotic: binds 50S ribosome.
Use: as erythromycin, part of triple therapy for *H. pylori*.
CI/Caution/SE/Interactions: as erythromycin, but ⇒ ↓GI SEs.
Dose: 250–500 mg bd po or 500 mg bd iv. *NB:* ↓**dose if RF.**

CLOBETASOL PROPIONATE 0.05% CREAM OR OINTMENT/DERMOVATE

Very-potent-strength topical corticosteroid.
Use: short-term Rx of severe inflammatory skin conditions (esp
discoid lupus, lichen simplex and palmar plantar psoriasis).
CI: untreated infection including *H. zoster*, rosacea, acne.
SE: skin atrophy, worsening of infections, acne (↑SEs cf less potent
topical steroids).
Dose: apply thinly od/bd up to 4 wks, usually specialist supervision.

CLOBETASONE BUTYRATE 0.05% CREAM OR OINTMENT/EUMOVATE

Moderately potent-strength topical corticosteroid.
Use: inflammatory skin conditions, esp eczema, dermatitis.
CI: untreated infection, rosacea, acne.
SE: skin atrophy, worsening of infections, acne.
Dose: apply thinly od/bd.

CLOMIPRAMINE

TCA; blocks reuptake of 5-HT and NA, ↑extracellular
concentrations in synaptic cleft, ↑serotonergic and noradrenergic
neurotransmission.
Use: depression[1], phobic and obsessional states[2], adjunctive
treatment of cataplexy with narcolepsy[3].
CI: mania, porphyria, arrhythmia, post-MI, severe liver disease,
MAOI, narrow-angle glaucoma, retention of urine.
Caution: chronic constipation, DM, epilepsy, Hx of bipolar
disorder/psychosis, hyperthyroidism, ↑intraocular pressure,
significant risk of suicide, phaeo, prostatic hypertrophy, angle-
closure glaucoma, urinary retention, cardiovascular disease **H**.

SE: antimuscarinic fx, cardiac fx (arrhythmias, HB, HR, postural ↓BP, dizziness, syncope: **dangerous in od**), ↑Wt, sedation (often ⇒ 'hangover'), seizures, GI upset, breast enlargement, paraesthesia, sexual dysfunction. Rarely blood disorders, hypersensitivity, Δ LFTs, ↓Na⁺ (esp in elderly), agitation, hallucination, Δ mood, confusion, NMS, abnormal muscle tone.

Warn: withdrawal effects may occur within 5 days of stopping treatment, worse after regular administration for 8 wks+. ↓dose gradually over 4 wks+. ↑effects of alcohol.

Interactions: metab by P450; ☠↑risk of serotonin syndrome with MAOI, e.g. isocarboxazid, moclobemide, phenelzine, selegiline, tranylcypromine (avoid with/for 14 days after stopping MAOI); Δ cardiac conduction with antiarrhythmic agents; hypokalaemia and ↑risk of QT prolongation and torsades de pointes with diuretics.

Dose: initially 10 mg po od at bedtime, ↑gradually/alternatively to 30–150 mg od in divided doses, max 250 mg od[1]; initially 25 mg po od, ↑gradually to 100–150 mg od over 2 wks, max 250 mg od[2]; start at 10 mg po od, ↑gradually to 10–75 mg od[3].

> ☠Overdose of TCA causes dry mouth, coma, hypotension, hypothermia, hyperreflexia, extensor plantar responses, convulsions, respiratory failure, cardiac conduction defects and arrhythmias. Dilated pupils and urinary retention also occur. ☠

CLONAZEPAM

Medium-acting benzodiazepine: GABA_A-receptor positive allosteric modulator.

Use: panic disorders (+/– agoraphobia) resistant to antidepressants/other anxiety disorders (unlicensed use)[1], epilepsy[2].

CI: coma, current alcohol/drug abuse, respiratory depression, sleep apnoea syndrome, MG, **L**.

Caution: porphyrias, airway obstruction, brain damage, cerebellar ataxia, depression, spinal ataxia, suicidal ideation.

SE: alopecia, ↓concentration, ↓coordination, ↑risk of fall, ↑risk of

fracture, ↓muscle tone, nystagmus, seizures, sexual dysfunction, skin reactions, speech impairment.
Warn: avoid in pregnancy (risk of neonatal withdrawal symptoms) and breastfeeding (present in milk).
Interactions: metab by P450; ↓levels of carbamazepine; ↓metabolism with ketoconazole; ↑levels of primidone, phenobarbital; Δ concentration of phenytoin.
Dose: 1–2 mg po od[1], initially 1 mg po od for 4 nights, ↑over 2–4 wks, usual dose 4–8 mg od at night, given in three to four divided doses if necessary[2].

☠ Overdose causes drowsiness, ataxia, dysarthria, nystagmus, respiratory depression and coma; can precipitate coma in hepatic impairment.
Do not confuse with clobazam when prescribing. ☠

CLONIDINE HYDROCHLORIDE

α_2-adrenergic receptor agonist ⇒ ↓noradrenaline release.
Use: Tourette syndrome and sedation (unlicensed)[1], HTN[2], Px of migraine/menopausal Sx[3], ADHD (unlicensed).
CI: severe slow dysrhythmia due to second/third degree HB/SSS **P/B**.
Caution: depression Hx, constipation, mild-to-moderate slow dysrhythmia, neuropathy, peripheral vascular disease (inc Raynaud's), cerebrovascular disease, **H**.
SE: sedation, postural ↓BP, dizziness, dry mouth, depression, headache, GI upset (N, V, C), sexual dysfunction.
Monitor: ECG advised.
Interactions: ↓antihypertensive fx with amitriptyline, clomipramine, dosulepin, doxepin, imipramine, lofepramine, nortriptyline. Mirtazapine may abolish effects in a dose-dependent manner.
Dose: initially 50–100 micrograms tds, increase dose every 2nd/3rd day, usual max dose 1.2 mg od.[2] Initially 50 micrograms bd for 2 weeks, increased if necessary to 75 micrograms bd. For unlicensed indications consult literature.

☠ In hypertension, must be withdrawn gradually to avoid severe rebound hypertension. ☠

CLOPIDOGREL

Antiplatelet agent: ADP receptor antagonist. ↑antiplatelet fx cf aspirin (but also ↑SEs).

Use: Px of atherothrombotic events if STEMI or NSTEMI (for 12 months in combination with aspirin, aspirin continued indefinitely), MI (within 'a few' to 35 days), ischaemic CVA (within 7 days to 6 months) or peripheral arterial disease. For use in ACS (see p. 422).

CI: active bleeding, L (if severe – otherwise caution), **P/B**.

Caution: ↑bleeding risk; trauma, surgery, drugs that ↑bleeding risk (*avoid with* **warfarin**), ↓fx by omeprazole, esomeprazole, fluvoxamine, fluoxetine, moclobemide, **R**.

SE: haemorrhage (esp GI or intracranial), **GI upset**, PU, pancreatitis, headache, fatigue, dizziness, paraesthesia, rash/pruritus, hepatobiliary/respiratory/blood disorders (↓NØ, ↑EØ, very rarely, TTP).

Monitor: for signs of occult bleeding (esp after invasive procedures); FBC if suspected bleeding.

Dose: 75 mg od. If not already on clopidogrel, usually load with 300 mg for ACS, then 75 mg od starting next day. If pre-PCI, load with 300–600 mg usually on morning of procedure. Varying durations depending on indication. Refer to BNF.

Stop 7 days before operations if antiplatelet fx not wanted (e.g. major surgery); discuss with surgeons doing operation.

CLOTRIMAZOLE/CANESTEN

Imidazole antifungal (topical).

Use: external candida infections (esp vaginal thrush).

Caution: can damage condoms and diaphragms.

Dose: bd/tds applications of 1% cream, continuing for 14 days after lesion healed. Also available as solution/spray for hairy areas, as pessary, and in 2% strength. See more.[BNF/SPC]

CLOZAPINE/CLOZARIL, ZAPONEX, DENZAPINE

Atypical antipsychotic: blocks dopamine ($D_4 > D_1 > D_2$ and D_3) and 5-HT_{2A} receptors. Potent antagonist at α-adrenergic, histaminergic and muscarinic receptors.

Use: schizophrenia[1], if resistant or intolerant (e.g. severe extrapyramidal fx) to two other antipsychotics, psychosis in Parkinson's[2].

CI: severe cardiac disorders (inc Hx of circulatory collapse, myocarditis, cardiomyopathy), coma/severe CNS depression, alcoholic/toxic psychosis, drug intoxication, Hx of agranulocytosis or $\downarrow$NØ, bone marrow disorders, paralytic ileus, uncontrolled epilepsy, **R/H** (if severe, otherwise caution), **L** (inc active liver disease), **B**.

Caution: Hx of epilepsy, cardiovascular disease, ↑prostate, glaucoma (angle-closure), P/E.

SE: ↑salivation (Rx with hyoscine hydrobromide), ↓BP and ↑HR (esp during initial titration), 💀 constipation 💀 (can ⇒ ileus/obstruction: have low threshold for giving laxatives), ↑Wt, sedation, ↓NØ* (3% of patients) and 💀 agranulocytosis 💀 (0.4%). Less commonly seizures, urinary incontinence, erectile dysfunction, **myocarditis/cardiomyopathy** (*stop immediately!*), hyperglycaemia, infections, **pneumonia** (*reduce dose/hold clozapine*), N&V, GORD, ↑BP, delirium, RF, ↓Pt. Rarely arrhythmias, hepatic dysfunction (*stop immediately!*), ↑TG, neuroleptic malignant syndrome, priapism.

Warn: to report symptoms of infection, e.g. fever, sore throat; to report changes in bowel habits, smoking habits; lifestyle advice to reduce risk of diabetes and CV disorders.

Monitor: FBC*, BP (esp during start of Rx), cardiac function (get baseline ECG/watch for persistent ↑HR). Drug levels can be taken 12 hours post-dose, although interpretation not straightforward (clinical value is disputed).

Interactions: care with all drugs that constipate, sedate, cause hypotension, ↑QT interval or ↓leucopoiesis (e.g. cytotoxics, sulphonamides/co-trimoxazole, chloramphenicol, penicillamine, carbamazepine, phenothiazines, esp depots). **metab by P450**: Caffeine, risperidone, fluoxetine, fluvoxamine, ciprofloxacin, ritonavir, OCP, cimetidine and erythromycin ↑clozapine levels. Smoking, carbamazepine, rifampicin and phenytoin ↓clozapine levels.

Dose: initially 12.5 mg nocte, ↑ing to 200–450 mg/day[SPC/BNF] (in 12.5–25 mg increments) usually given bd (max 900 mg/day); slower dose titration if >60 years.[1] 12.5 mg nocte, inc in steps of 12.5 mg up to twice wkly according to response, max 50 mg daily; in exceptional circumstances, inc by 12.5 mg wkly to max 100 mg od in one to two divided doses[2]. Monitor pre- and post-dose BP, HR, RR and temperature during initial titration. If abnormalities detected exclude serious causes.[†] If benign, titration may need to be slowed.

> If >2 days' doses missed, re-titration necessary. Get specialist advice.
> [†]Neutropenic sepsis, myocarditis, NMS, pneumonia.

> Monitoring of WBC, NØ and PLT is done by the manufacturers: in the United Kingdom, **Clozaril** Patient Monitoring Service (tel: 0845 7698269), **Denzapine** Monitoring Service (tel: 0333 2004141) or **Zaponex** Treatment Access System (tel: 0207 3655842). Register and then authorise/monitor baseline and subsequent FBCs*. *These are very useful resources for all clozapine questions.* Report any missed doses.

CO-AMOXICLAV/AUGMENTIN

Combination of amoxicillin + clavulanic acid (β-lactamase inhibitor). Reserve for when β-lactamase-producing strains known/ strongly suspected or other Rx has failed.

Use: consult local antibiotic prescribing guidelines.

CI/Caution/SE/Interactions: as ampicillin, plus higher risk of antibiotic-associated C. *difficile* infection; caution if anticoagulated, **L** (↑risk of cholestasis), **P**.

Dose: amoxicillin 250 mg/clavulanic acid 125 mg tds po (500 mg/125 mg tds po if severe); 1.2 g (expressed as co-amoxiclav) tds/qds iv/ivi.

CO-BENELDOPA/MADOPAR

Benserazide (peripheral DOPA-decarboxylase inhibitor) + L-dopa (precursor of dopamine).

Use: parkinsonism.

CI: glaucoma (closed-angle), taking MAO-A inhibitors, melanoma,[†] cardiovascular disease, severe psychosis, <25 years of age, **P/B/R/L**.

Caution: pulmonary/Ψ disease, glaucoma (open-angle), osteomalacia, Hx of PU or seizures, ventricular arrhythmias.

SE: dyskinesias, abdo upset, postural ↓BP, arrhythmias, drowsiness, aggression, Ψ disorders (confusion, depression, suicide, hallucinations, psychosis, hypomania, impulse control disorders), seizures, dizziness, headache, flushing, sweating, peripheral neuropathy, taste Δs, rash pruritus, can reactivate melanoma,[†] Δ LFTs, GI bleeding, blood disorders, dark body fluids (inc sweat).

Warn: can ⇒ daytime sleepiness (inc sudden-onset sleep).

Interactions: fx ↓d by neuroleptics, SEs ↑d by bupropion, **risk of ↑BP crisis with MAOIs** (but can give with MAO-B inhibitors and reversible MAO-AI moclobemide), ↓s iron absorption, risk of arrhythmias with halothane.

Dose: (expressed as levodopa only) initially 50 mg tds/qds immediate release, ↑ing total dose and number of doses in steps of 100 mg daily, according to response, to usual maintenance of 400–800 mg/day (↓ in elderly).[BNF/SPC] Available in dispersible form. If switching from MR levodopa to dispersible co-beneldopa, reduce dose by 30%.

CO-CARELDOPA/SINEMET

Carbidopa (peripheral DOPA-decarboxylase inhibitor) + L-dopa (precursor of dopamine).

Use: parkinsonism.

CI: glaucoma (closed-angle), taking MAO-A inhibitors, melanoma,[†] severe psychosis, **P/B**.

Caution: pulmonary/cardiovascular/Ψ disease, endocrine disorder, glaucoma (open-angle), osteomalacia, Hx of PU or seizures, ventricular arrhythmias, **L/R**.

SE: dyskinesias, abdo upset, postural ↓BP, arrhythmias, drowsiness, aggression, Ψ disorders (confusion, depression, suicide, hallucinations, psychosis, hypomania, impulse control disorders), seizures, dizziness, headache, flushing, sweating, peripheral neuropathy, taste Δs, rash/pruritus, can reactivate melanoma,† Δ LFTs, GI bleeding, blood disorders, dark body fluids (inc sweat).

Warn: can ⇒ daytime sleepiness (inc sudden-onset sleep).

Interactions: fx ↓d by neuroleptics, SEs ↑d by bupropion, **risk of ↑BP crisis with MAOIs** (but can give with MAO-B inhibitors and selective MAO-AI moclobemide), ↓s iron absorption, risk of arrhythmias with halothane.

Dose: (caribodopa/levodopa) initially 25/100 mg tds, ↑ing total dose and number of doses according to response up to 200/2000 mg daily in divided doses (usual maintenance of 400–800 mg/day); ↓ in elderly.^BNF/SPC Gel for enteral tube, increased in steps of 12.5/50 mg once daily.

CO-CODAMOL (30/500): = codeine 30 mg + paracetamol 500 mg per tablet.

Use/Caution/SE/Interactions: see Paracetamol and Codeine.

Warning: prescribe by dose, as also available as 8/500 and 15/500.

CI: P.

Dose: 2 tablets qds prn. *NB:* ↓dose if LF, RF or elderly.

CODEINE (PHOSPHATE)

Weak opiate analgesic. Mainly metabolised to morphine.

Use: mild/moderate pain, diarrhoea, antitussive.

CI: acute respiratory depression, risk of ileus, ↑ICP/head injury/coma, **P**.

Caution: all other conditions where morphine is either contraindicated or cautioned.

SE: as morphine, but milder. **Constipation** is the major problem: dose and length of Rx-dependent; anticipate this and give laxative Px as appropriate, esp in elderly. Also sedation, esp if LF.

Interactions: as morphine, ☠ MAOIs: do not give within 2 wks of. ☠

Dose: 30–60 mg up to 4-hrly po/im (max 240 mg/24 h). Genetic ultrarapid metabolisers risk serious toxicity, and poor metabolisers obtain little analgesia. Watch closely when initiating and adjust dose/change drug accordingly. *NB:* ↓**dose if LF, RF or elderly.**

CO-DYDRAMOL

Dihydrocodeine 10/20/30 mg + paracetamol 500 mg per tablet (10/500, 20/500, 30/500).
Dose: one to two tablets 4–6 hrly, max qds po; max dose paracetamol 1 g qds, codeine 60 mg qds. Usually prescribed 2 tablets qds (prn). *NB:* ↓**dose if LF, RF** or elderly.

CO-TRIMOXAZOLE/SEPTRIN

Antibiotic combination preparation: 5-to-1 mixture of sulphamethoxazole (a sulphonamide) + trimethoprim ⇒ synergistic action.
Use: PCP; other uses limited dt SEs (also rarely used for toxoplasmosis and nocardiosis).
CI: porphyria, **L/R/P/B** (if either severe, otherwise caution).
Caution: blood disorders, asthma, G6PD deficiency, risk factors for ↓folate and hyperkalaemia, **E**.
SE: skin reactions (inc SJS, TEN), blood disorders (↓NØ, ↓Pt, ↓glucose, BM suppression, agranulocytosis) relatively common, esp in elderly. Also N&V&D (inc AAC), ↑K^+, nephrotoxicity, hepatotoxicity, hypersensitivity, anorexia, abdo pain, glossitis, stomatitis, pancreatitis, arthralgia, myalgia, SLE, pulmonary infiltrates, seizures, ataxia, myocarditis.
Interactions: ↑s phenytoin levels. ↑s risk of arrhythmias with amiodarone, crystalluria with methenamine, antifolate fx with pyrimethamine, agranulocytosis with clozapine and toxicity with ciclosporin, azathioprine, mercaptopurine and methotrexate. **W+**.
Dose: PCP Rx: 120 mg/kg/day po/ivi in two to four divided doses (PCP Px 480–960 mg od po). PCP Px.[BNF/SPC] *NB:* ↓**dose if RF.**

☠ Stop immediately if rash or blood disorder occurs. ☠

CYCLIZINE

Antihistamine antiemetic.

Use: N&V Rx/Px (esp 2° to iv/im opioids, but not first choice in angina/MI/LVF*), vertigo, motion sickness, labyrinthine disorders.

CI/Caution/SE/Warn: as chlorphenamine, but also avoid in severe HF* (may undo haemodynamic benefits of opioids). Antimuscarinic fx (see p. 387), are most prominent SEs.

Dose: 50 mg po/im/iv tds.

CYPROHEPTADINE HYDROCHLORIDE

Potent histamine H_1-receptor and $5-HT_2$-receptor antagonist; competes with serotonin and histamine for receptor binding.

Use: allergy[1], adjunct in treatment of moderate serotonin syndrome (unlicensed)[2].

CI: porphyria, **L**.

Caution: ↑prostate/urinary retention, obstruction at pyloric junction, ↑risk of angle-closure glaucoma, seizures, **P**.

SE: drowsiness, insomnia, dizziness, **antimuscarinic fx** (see p. 387), ataxia, GI upset, ↑Wt, paraesthesia, hyperhidrosis, Ψ fx (agitation, hallucination), cytopoenias, hypersensitivity reactions (inc bronchospasm, photosensitivity), arrhythmias, epistaxis, hepatic disorders, ↓BP, labyrinthitis, irregular menstruation, oedema, seizure, tinnitus, tremor.

Warn: ↑sedation with alcohol.

Interactions: ↓fx of citalopram, dapoxetine, escitalopram, fluoxetine, fluvoxamine, metyrapone, paroxetine, sertraline, and other antidepressants (opposes action); ↓absorption of levodopa.

Dose: 4 mg po tds, usual dose 4–20 mg od, max 32 mg od[1]; 12 mg po as a single dose, repeated once if necessary, for longer-acting serotonergic agents (e.g. fluoxetine) regular lower doses (e.g. 4 mg tds) should be used[2].

DABIGATRAN (ETEXILATE)

Oral anticoagulant; direct thrombin inhibitor. Rapid onset and does not require therapeutic monitoring (unlike warfarin).

Use: Px of VTE (after THR/TKR)[1]; Rx of DVT or PE and Px of recurrent DVT or recurrent PE[2]; non-valvular AF embolism Px[3].BNF

CI: active bleeding, impaired haemostasis, **L** (if severe), **P/B**.

Caution: bleeding disorders, active GI ulceration, recent surgery, bacterial endocarditis, anaesthesia with post-operative indwelling epidural catheter (risk of paralysis; give initial dose ≥2 h after catheter removal and monitor for neurological signs), Wt <50 kg, **R** (avoid if creatinine clearance <30 mL/min), **H/E**.

SE: haemorrhage, hepatobiliary disorders.

Monitor: for ↓Hb or signs of bleeding (stop drug if severe). Assess RF before initiating Rx and annually for patients and elderly with renal failure.

Interactions: P-gp inducers and inhibitors[SPC/BNF] **NSAIDs** ↑risk of bleeding. Levels ↑ by amiodarone*.

Dose: 110 mg (75 mg if >75 years old) 1–4 h after surgery, then 220 mg od (150 mg if >75 years old) for 10 days, to be taken from first day after knee replacement or 28–35 days from first day after hip replacement[1]; 150 mg po bd after at least 5 days parenteral anticoagulant[2] (>74 years old see BNF for dose); 150 mg po bd[3]. *NB: ↓dose in RF, elderly or if taking amiodarone or verapamil.*

DALTEPARIN SODIUM/FRAGMIN

Low-molecular-weight heparin.

Use: thromboprophylaxis and treatment of thrombosis. Note: not licensed for treatment of venous thromboembolism in pregnancy.

CI: bacterial endocarditis, major trauma, epidural/spinal anaesthesia (Rx dose), haemophilia, PU, recent cerebral haemorrhage, recent eye or CNS surgery, thrombocytopenia (inc HIT), mechanical prosthetic heart valve.

Caution: falls risk, bleeding risk, severe HTN, **E**.

SE: haemorrhage, HIT, skin reactions. Rarely: alopecia, hyperkalaemia (if other RF present), osteoporosis (long term), spinal haematoma.

Monitor: Plt count before and after starting, K^+ in those w/ RF.

Interactions: caution if combining with other meds which carry bleeding risk (inc SSRIs and some common analgesics). Caution with medications which $\uparrow K^+$.

Dose: varies widely by indication and patient weight: consult BNF/local guidelines.

DANTROLENE SODIUM

Postsynaptic muscle relaxant; $\downarrow$excitation-contraction coupling in skeletal muscle by binding to ryanodine receptor, $\downarrow$intracellular calcium concentration.

Use: chronic severe spasticity of voluntary muscle (malignant hyperthermia by rapid iv injection).

CI: acute muscle spasm.

Caution: $\uparrow$risk of hepatotoxicity if female, age >30 or daily dose >400 mg. **H/P/B**.

SE: $\downarrow$appetite, Ψ fx (depression, anxiety), $\downarrow$sleep, seizure, visual disturbance, pericarditis, pleural effusion with $\uparrow$eosinophils, resp depression, GI upset (N, V, abdo pain), hepatotoxicity, rash, fever.

Warn: may cause severe liver damage, discontinue if no response within 6–8 wks.

Monitor: LFTs at initiation and regularly during Rx.

Interactions: $\uparrow$neuromuscular blockade with vecuronium bromide; $\uparrow$sedation with CNS depressants; $\uparrow$muscle weakness with benzodiazepines; hepatoxicity with combined oral contraceptive pill (COCP) and hormone replacement therapy in females.

Dose: initially 25 mg po od, $\uparrow$dose at wkly intervals; usual dose 75 mg tds od, max 100 mg qds od.

DAPAGLIFLOZIN/FORXIGA

Antidiabetic (reversible SGLT2 inhibitor): ↓renal reabsorption of glucose and ↑urinary excretion of glucose.

Use: type 2 DM in combination with metformin if CVD (start metformin first), CKD.

CI: ketoacidosis, **P/B**.

Caution: risk factors for DKA (including ↓β-cell reserve, restricted food intake or severe dehydration, sudden ↓ in insulin, ↑insulin requirements due to acute illness, surgery or alcohol abuse); CVD (risk of ↓BP); **E** (risk of ↓BP); electrolyte disturbances; ↓BP; ↑Hct. Correct hypovolaemia before starting Rx. **L/R**.

SE: GI upset, back pain, dizziness, dyslipidaemia, hypoglycaemia (in combination with insulin or sulphonylurea), ↑risk of infection, rash, urinary disorders, thirst hypovolaemia, RF, balanitis, genital pruritus, ↓Wt. Rare: DKA, gangrene.

Dose: 10 mg od. Dose of concomitant sulfonylurea or insulin may need to be ↓d. ↓dose and caution in severe LF – ↑exposure risk. Not recommended if >75 yrs old.

> ☠ DKA on SGLT2 inhibitors may be atypical with only moderately ↑blood glucose. Warn patients of risk factors and signs and symptoms of DKA. Advise to seek immediate medical attention if they develop. Test for ↑ketones if signs or symptoms of DKA, even if plasma glucose near normal. Stop SGLT2 inhibitor if DKA is suspected or diagnosed. Do not restart SGLT2 inhibitor in patients with DKA during use, unless another cause for DKA is identified and resolved. Interrupt SGLT2 inhibitor treatment in patients in hospital for major surgery or acute, serious illness. Rx may be restarted once condition stabilised. ☠

▼ DEXAMFETAMINE SULPHATE (= DEXAMFETAMINE)

CNS stimulant; stimulates release of DA > NA and 5-HT from pre-synaptic nerve terminals.

Use: refractory ADHD (unlicensed use in adults)[1] if response to lisdexamfetamine but cannot tolerate prolonged fx[NICE], narcolepsy[2].

CI: agitation, cardiac/vascular disorders, Hx of alcohol/drug misuse, ↑thyroid, moderate-to-severe HTN, **H/P/B**.

Caution: some Ψ disorders (psychosis, BPAD, anorexia), seizures, mild HTN, tics, ↑risk of angle-closure glaucoma.

SE: ↓appetite, ↓Wt, ↓sleep, agitation, **cardiac fx** (↑HR, ↑BP, arrhythmia), GI upset, dry mouth, arthralgia, dizziness, headache.

Monitor: aggression early in Rx (↓dose or stop); pulse, BP, Wt, Ht at start of Rx, after dose Δ and at intervals ≤6 months.

Interactions: ☠️↑risk of hypertensive crisis with isocarboxazid, phenelzine, tranylcypromine, moclobemide, rasagiline, safinamide, selegiline (avoid with/for 14 days after stopping MAOI)☠️; ↓fx of apraclonidine, guanethidine; ↑level with fluoxetine, paroxetine, ritonavir, tipranavir; ↑risk of SE with atomoxetine, nabilone.

Dose: initially 5 mg po bd, ↑dose at wkly intervals, maintenance dose given in two to four divided doses, max 60 mg od[1]; initially 10 mg po od in divided doses, ↑ in steps of 10 mg every wk, maintenance dose given in two to four divided doses, max 60 mg od[2].

☠️Overdose causes wakefulness, excessive activity, paranoia, hallucinations, hypertension followed by exhaustion, convulsions, hyperthermia and coma.☠️

DEXMEDETOMIDINE

Central α₂-adrenoreceptor agonist.

Use: licensed for sedation in ITU, used off-label for agitation. Need anaesthetist with appropriate airway support (although limited effect on respiratory drive).

CI: acute CVD, 2nd or 3rd deg AV block, significant hypotension.

Caution: abrupt withdrawal, bradycardia, IHD/CVD, malignant hyperthermia, severe neuro disorders, spinal cord injury, **E**.

SE: agitation, arrhythmias, dry mouth, BM ↓/↑, BP ↓/↑, hyperthermia, MI, nausea/vomiting, respiratory depression. Rare: abdominal distension, dyspnoea/apnoea, AV block, hallucinations, hypoalbuminaemia, metabolic acidosis.

Dose: iv 0.2–1.4 micrograms/kg/h.

DIAMORPHINE (HEROIN HYDROCHLORIDE)

Strong opiate (1.5× strength of morphine if both given iv).
Use: severe pain (acute and chronic)[1], AMI[2], acute LVF[3].
CI/Caution/SE/Interactions: as morphine, but less nausea/↓BP
and does not interact with baclofen, gabapentin and ritonavir.
☠ **Respiratory depression** (esp elderly). ☠
Dose: Refer to pain control guidelines. 5–10 mg sc/im (or 1/4–1/2
this dose iv) up to 4 hrly[1]; 5 mg iv (at 1 mg/min) followed by further
2.5–5 mg if necessary[2]; 2.5–5 mg iv (at 1 mg/min)[3]. Can give via
sc pump in chronic pain/palliative care. *NB:* ↓**dose if elderly, LF or
RF**.[BNF/SPC]

DIAZEPAM

Long-acting benzodiazepine: GABA$_A$-receptor positive allosteric
modulator.
Use: seizures (esp status epilepticus[1], febrile convulsions), *short-
term* Rx of acute alcohol withdrawal[2], anxiety[3], insomnia[4] (if also
anxiety; if not, then shorter-acting forms preferred, as ⇒ ↓hangover
sedation). Also used for muscle spasm[5] and catatonia (unlicensed).
CI: respiratory depression, marked neuromuscular respiratory
weakness inc unstable myasthenia gravis, sleep apnoea, acute
pulmonary insufficiency, chronic psychosis, depression (do not give
diazepam alone), **L** (if severe).
Caution: respiratory disease, muscle weakness (inc MG), Hx of
drug/alcohol abuse, personality disorder, porphyria, **L/R/P/B/E**.
SE: respiratory depression (rarely apnoea), **drowsiness, dependence**.
Also ataxia, amnesia, headache, vertigo, GI upset, jaundice,
↓BP, ↓HR, visual/libido/urinary disturbances, blood disorders,
paradoxical disinhibition in Ψ disorder.
Warn: sedation ↑ by alcohol. Do not stop suddenly, as can ⇒
withdrawal.
Interactions: metab by P450 ∴ many: ery-/clari-/telithromycin,
quinu-/dalfopristin and flu-/itra-/keto-/posaconazole can ↑levels.
Sedative fx ↑ by antipsychotics, antidepressants, antiseizure medications
and antiretrovirals. Can ↑fx of zidovudine and sodium oxybate. ↑risk
of ↓HR/BP and respiratory depression with im olanzapine.

Dose: 10 mg iv, then 10 mg after 10 min if required, at rate of 1 mL (5 mg)/min for status epilepticus[1]; 10 mg im, then 10 mg after at least 4 h if required for acute alcohol withdrawal[2]; 2 mg tds po (↑ up to 30 mg/day)[3,5]; 5–15 mg nocte po[4]. *NB*: ↓dose if elderly, LF or RF. If chronic exposure to benzodiazepines, ↑doses may be needed; do not stop suddenly, as can ⇒ withdrawal – taper cautiously, speed depending on duration of use and indication. If giving iv, use Diazemuls, an emulsion, to avoid venous irritation.

> 🙐 **Respiratory depression:** rare in monotherapy, even at high doses. However, significantly increased risk if in combination with alcohol, opiates or other drugs which reduce respiratory drive. Monitor O_2 sats and have O_2 (± intubation equipment) at hand, caution with flumazenil – see p. 403. 🙐

DICLOFENAC/VOLTAROL

Medium-strength NSAID; non-selective COX inhibitor.

Use: pain/inflammation, esp musculoskeletal; RA, osteoarthritis, acute gout, migraine, post-op and dental pain.

CI/Caution/SE/Interactions: as ibuprofen, but ↑risk of PU/GI bleeds and thrombotic events (↓risk of PU/GI bleeds if given with misoprostol as Arthrotec). Avoid in IHD, CVD, CCF, peripheral artery disease, acute porphyria. Ciclosporin ⇒ ↑serum levels. No known interaction with baclofen. Mild **W+**.

Dose: 25–50 mg tds po or 75 mg bd po (or im, but for max of 2 days); 75–150 mg/day pr (**divided doses**). Rarely used iv.[BNF/SPC] MR and top preparations available.[BNF/SPC] *NB*: **avoid/↓dose in RF and consider gastroprotective Rx.**

DIGOXIN

Cardiac glycoside: ↓s HR by slowing AVN conduction and ↑ing vagal tone. Also weak inotrope.

Use: AF (and other SVTs), HF.

CI: HB (intermittent complete), second-degree AV block, VF, VT, HOCM (can use with care if also AF and HF), SVTs 2° to WPW.

Caution: recent MI, $\downarrow$K^{+*}/$\downarrow$T$_4$ (both $\Rightarrow$ $\uparrow$digoxin sensitivity*), SSS, rhythms resembling AF (e.g. atrial tachycardia with variable AV block), **R/E** ($\downarrow$dose), **P**.

SE: generally mild unless rapid ivi, xs Rx or od: **GI upset** (esp nausea), **arrhythmias/HB**, neuro-Ψ disturbances (inc visual Δs, esp blurred vision and yellow/green halos), fatigue, weakness, confusion, hallucinations, mood Δs. Also gynaecomastia (if chronic Rx), rarely $\downarrow$Pt, rash, $\uparrow$EØ. Serious toxicity treated with **DIGIBIND** or **DIGIFAB**.

Monitor: U&Es, digoxin levels. For po, 6 h post-dose after steady-state achieved; trough reading required (therapeutic range = 1–2 micrograms/L). For iv, INF 6 h post-dose.

Interactions: fx/toxicity $\uparrow$d by Ca^{2+} antagonists (esp verapamil), amiodarone, propafenone, quinidine, antimalarials, itraconazole, amphotericin, ciclosporin, St John's wort and diuretics (mostly via $\downarrow$K^{+*}), but also ACE-i/ARBs and spironolactone (despite potential $\uparrow$K$^+$). Cholestyramine and antacids can $\downarrow$digoxin absorption.

Dose: *non-acute AF/SVTs:* load with 125–250 micrograms bd po (maintenance dose 62.5–250 micrograms od). For HF: 62.5–125 micrograms od. *NB:* $\downarrow$**dose if RF, elderly or digoxin given <2 wks ago.**

Digoxin loading for acute AF/SVTs: *either* 750 micrograms–1 mg as ivi over 2 h *or* 500 micrograms po repeated 12 h later. Then follow non-acute schedule.

DIHYDROCODEINE see Codeine: similar-strength opioid.
Dose: 30 mg 4–6 hrly po (or up to 50 mg 4–6 hrly im/sc) with or after food. Maximum 240 mg in 24 h. $\downarrow$**dose if RF.**

DILATING EYE DROPS (for funduscopy). Generally safe but rarely $\Rightarrow$ angle-closure glaucoma (suspect if develops red painful eye with $\downarrow$vision and nausea; *ophthalmic emergency*). Dilation blurs vision. Driving unsafe for at least 4 h when both eyes dilated. Apply one drop and allow 15 min for effect.

1 **Tropicamide** 1%: Most common; CI in children <1 year old (use 0.5%)

2 **Phenylephrine 2.5% or 10%:** Frequently used in combination with tropicamide. 2.5% most common. 10% ↑s systemic SEs. CI if cardiac disease, HTN, ↑HR, aneurysms, ↑T_4

Consider cycloplegic forms (e.g. cyclopentolate 1%) for refraction in children or if analgesia required, e.g. corneal abrasions and uveitis (↓s ciliary spasm).

DILTIAZEM

Rate-limiting benzothiazepine Ca^{2+} channel blocker: ↓s HR and contractility* (but < verapamil) and ↓s BP. Also dilates peripheral/coronary arteries.
Use: Rx/Px of angina[1] (esp if β-blockers CI) and HTN[2].
CI: LVF* with pulmonary congestion, ↓↓HR, second-/third-degree AV block (without pacemaker), SSS, acute porphyria **P/B**.
Caution: first-degree AV block, ↓HR, ↑pr interval, **L/R/H**.
SE: headache, flushing, GI upset (esp N&C), oedema (esp ankle), ↓HR, ↓BP, gum hyperplasia. Rarely SAN/AVN block, arrhythmias, rash, hepatotoxicity, gynaecomastia.
Interactions: β-blockers and verapamil (can ⇒ asystole, AV block, ↓↓HR, HF). ↑s fx of digoxin, ciclosporin, theophyllines, carbamazepine and phenytoin. ☠ ↑risk of VF with iv dantrolene. ☠
Dose: 60 mg tds (↑ing to max of 360 mg/day)[1]; 180–480 mg/day in one or two doses[2] (suitable for HTN only as MR preparation: no non-proprietary forms exist and brands vary in clinical fx ∴ specify which is required[SPC/BNF]). If changing brands, monitor for SEs. *NB:* **consider ↓ing doses if LF or RF.**

DIPROBASE Paraffin-based emollient cream/ointment for dry skin conditions (e.g. eczema, psoriasis).

DISULFIRAM/ANTABUSE

Alcohol dehydrogenase inhibitor: ⇒ ↑systemic acetaldehyde ⇒ unpleasant SE when alcohol ingested (inc small amounts ∴ care with alcohol-containing medications, foods, toiletries).

Use: maintenance of abstinence in alcohol dependence (not recommended in active alcoholism).
CI: Hx of IHD or CVA, HTN, psychosis, ↑suicide risk, severe personality disorder, **H/P/B**.
Caution: DM, epilepsy, respiratory disease, **L/R**.
SE: only if alcohol ingested – N&V, flushing, headache, ↑HR, ↓BP (± collapse if xs alcohol intake).
Interactions: ↑s fx of phenytoin, ↑toxicity with paraldehyde, **W+**.
Dose: initially 200 mg od, ↑dose if needed: max 500 mg po od. Review patient on Rx every 2 wks for first 2 months, then monthly for next 4 months and then 6 monthly thereafter.

NB: must have consumed no alcohol within at least 24 h of first dose. Prescribe under specialist supervision.

DOCUSATE SODIUM
Stimulant laxative: ⇒ ↑GI motility (also a softening agent).
Use/Caution/SE: see Senna (CI if GI obstruction).
Dose: 100 mg up to TDS PO (max 500 mg/day). Also available as enemas.$^{SPC/BNF}$

▼ DOMPERIDONE
Antiemetic: D$_2$ antagonist – inhibits central nausea chemoreceptor trigger zone. Poor blood-brain barrier penetration ∴ ↓central SEs (extrapyramidal fx, sedation) cf other dopamine antagonists.
Use: N&V, esp 2° to chemotherapy, Parkinson's disease or migraine.
CI: prolactinoma, cardiac disease (inc conditions where cardiac conduction is, or could be, impaired), GI obstruction, drugs that ↓CYP3A4 or ↑QTc, **H/L**.
Caution: GI obstruction, **R/P/B/E**.
SE: ↑QTc, rash, allergy, ↑prolactin (can ⇒ gynaecomastia, galactorrhoea and hyperprolactinoma). Rarely ↓libido, dystonia and extrapyramidal fx.
Dose: 10 mg tds po, not available im/iv. *NB:* ↓**dose if RF.**

DONEPEZIL/ARICEPT

Acetylcholinesterase inhibitor (reversible).

Use: mild-to-moderately severe dementia in Alzheimer's disease.

CI: P/B.

Caution: supraventricular conduction dfx (esp SSS), ↑risk of PU (e.g. Hx of PU or NSAID), COPD/asthma, **L**.

Class SE: cholinergic fx, GI upset (esp initially), **insomnia** (if occurs, change dose to mane), **headache**, fatigue, dizziness, syncope, rash, Ψ disturbances. Rarely ↓ or ↑BP, seizures, PU/GI bleeds, SAN/AVN block, hepatotoxicity, extrapyramidal symptoms can worsen.

Interactions: metab by P450 ∴ inhibitors and inducers could ↑ or ↓levels, respectively.

Dose: 5 mg nocte (↑ to 10 mg after 1 month if necessary); specialist use only – need review for clinical response and tolerance.

DOSULEPIN HYDROCHLORIDE

TCA: blocks reuptake of NA (and 5-HT) through binding to noradrenaline transporter (NAT) and serotonin transport (SERT).

Use: depression (less suitable for prescribing).

CI: as for amitriptyline **L/H**.

Caution: as for amitriptyline **P/E**.

Class SE: antimuscarinic fx (constipation, dry mouth, blurred vision), **cardiac fx** (arrhythmias, HB↑, HR, postural ↓BP, dizziness, syncope: **dangerous in od**), ↑Wt, sedation (often ⇒ 'hangover'), seizures, Δ LFTs, ↓Na⁺ (esp in elderly), agitation, confusion, neuroleptic malignant syndrome.

Warn: discontinuation symptoms if stopped abruptly.

Monitor: elderly patients for cardiac and Ψ SE and electrolytes.

Interactions: ☠ Never give with, or ≤2 wks after, MAOIs; do not give MAOIs within 2 wks of stopping dosulepin; ☠ may interact with lithium to ↑SEs and/or cause serotonin syndrome (rare, in practice ADs and lithium commonly co-prescribed); ↑levels with bupropion, cinacalcet, dronedarone, fluoxetine, paroxetine, terbinafine; ↑fx of adrenaline, noradrenaline, phenylephrine; ↓fx of ephedrine.

Dose: initially 75 mg po od at bedtime (or in divided doses), ↑ gradually to 150 mg od.

> ☠ Overdose is associated with high rate of fatality, more so than for other TCAs. TCA overdose ⇒ dilated pupils, arrhythmias, ↓BP, hypothermia, hyperreflexia, extensor plantar responses, seizures, respiratory depression and coma. ☠

DOXAZOSIN/CARDURA

α_1-Blocker ⇒ systemic vasodilation and relaxation of internal urethral sphincter ∴ ⇒ ↓TPR[1] and ↑bladder outflow[2].

Use: HTN[1], BPH[2].

CI: postural ↓BP, anuria, **B**.

Caution: postural ↓BP, micturition syncope, pulmonary oedema due to aortic or mitral stenosis **L/H/P/E**.

SE: postural ↓BP (esp after first dose*), dizziness, headache, urinary incontinence (esp women), GI upset (esp N&V), drowsiness/fatigue, syncope, mood Δs, dry mouth, oedema, somnolence, blurred vision, rhinitis. Rarely erectile dysfunction, ↑HR, arrhythmias, hypersensitivity/rash.

Interactions: ↑s hypotensive fx of diuretics, β-blockers, Ca^{2+} antagonists, silden-/tadal-/vardenafil, general anaesthetics, moxisylyte and antidepressants.

Dose: initially 1 mg od (give first dose before bed*), then slowly ↑ according to response (max 16 mg/day[1] or 8 mg/day[2]). 4 mg or 8 mg od if MR preparation, as **Cardura XL**.

DOXEPIN HYDROCHLORIDE/SINEPIN

TCA: blocks reuptake of NA and 5-HT.

Use: depression (less suitable for prescribing).

CI: as for amitriptyline **L/H**.

Caution: as for amitriptyline **P/E**.

Class SE: antimuscarinic fx (constipation, dry mouth, blurred vision), **cardiac fx** (arrhythmias, HB, ↑HR, postural ↓BP, dizziness, syncope: **dangerous in od**), ↑Wt, sedation (often ⇒ 'hangover'), seizures, Δ LFTs, ↓Na$^+$ (esp in elderly), agitation, confusion, neuroleptic malignant syndrome.

Warn: discontinuation symptoms if stopped abruptly.

Monitor: elderly patients for cardiac and Ψ SE and electrolytes.

Interactions: ☠ Never give with, or ≤2 wks after, MAOIs; do not give MAOIs within 2 wks of stopping doxepin; ☠ ↑risk of NMS with lithium; ↑levels with bupropion, cinacalcet, dronedarone, fluoxetine, paroxetine, terbinafine; ↑fx of adrenaline, noradrenaline, phenylephrine; ↓fx of ephedrine.

Dose: initially 75 mg po od at bedtime (or in divided doses), maintenance 25–300 mg od, doses >100 mg given in three divided doses.

> ☠ Overdose is associated with high rate of fatality. TCA overdose ⇒ dilated pupils, arrhythmias, ↓BP, hypothermia, hyperreflexia, extensor plantar responses, seizures, respiratory depression and coma. ☠

DOXYCYCLINE

Tetracycline antibiotic: inhibits ribosomal (30S) subunit.

Use: consult local antibiotic prescribing guidelines.

CI/Caution/SE/Interactions: as tetracycline, but can give with caution if RF; also CI in SLE and achlorhydria. Can ⇒ anorexia, flushing, tinnitus, oesophageal ulceration and ↑ciclosporin levels.

Warn: avoid UV light and products containing Zn/Fe/Ca^{2+} (e.g. antacids); specifically, avoid taking around the same time (chelation), fine to take >1 h before or >2 h after. Swallow whole with plenty of fluid, while sitting or standing.

Dose: 100–200 mg od/bd.[SPC/BNF] *NB:* ↓**dose in RF.**

DROPERIDOL

Butyrophenone: DA antagonist (chemoreceptor trigger zone).

Use: post-operative N&V[1]; acute behavioural disturbance (unlicensed)[2].

CI: ↓HR, ↓GCS, electrolyte Δs (↓K$^+$, ↓Mg^{2+}), phaeo, ↑QTc.

Caution: Parkinson's, drugs that ↑QTc, epilepsy, MG, glaucoma (angle-closure), ↑prostate, jaundice, blood disorders, electrolyte Δs, alcohol misuse, respiratory disease.

SE: see Haloperidol, may prolong QTc (disputed in recent studies, but remains a CI).

Warn: avoid direct sunlight (photosensitisation) with ↑doses, ↑fx of alcohol.

Monitor: prolactin at initiation, 6 months, then annually. Continuous SpO$_2$ if ventricular arrhythmia risk; ECG if cardiovascular risk factors identified.

Interactions: metab by P450; ↑levels with CYP1A2/3A4 inhibitors, e.g. ciprofloxacin, diltiazem, erythromycin, fluconazole, indinavir, verapamil, cimetidine; ↑risks of torsades de pointes/QT prolongation with antiarrhythmics (quinidine, disopyramide, procainamide, amiodarone, sotalol), antibiotics (erythromycin, clarithromycin, sparfloxacin), antihistamines (astemizole, terfenadine), antipsychotics (chlorpromazine, haloperidol, pimozide, thioridazine), antimalarial agents (chloroquine, halofantrine), cisapride, domperidone, methadone, pentamidine; ↑EPSE with metoclopramide, neuroleptics; avoid alcohol.

Dose: 0.625–1.25 mg iv, dose to be given 30 min before end of surgery, then 0.625–1.25 mg every 6 h as required[1], 2.5–5 mg im initial dose then up to 10 mg im as required ideally in steps of 1.25 mg[2].

DULOXETINE/CYMBALTA

5-HT and noradrenaline reuptake inhibitor.

Use: depression[1], generalised anxiety disorder[2], diabetic neuropathy[3] (review need ≤3 monthly and stop if inadequate response after 2 months), stress urinary incontinence[4] (assess benefit/tolerability after 2–4 wks).

CI: R (if eGFR <30 mL/min/1.73 m^2), **L**.

Caution: cardiac disease, Hx mania, epilepsy, ↑IOP, ↑risk of glaucoma (angle-closure), bleeding disorder/on drugs ↑ing bleeding risk, **H/P/B/E**.

SE: GI upset (N&V&C), abdo pain, Wt Δ, ↓appetite, palpitations, hot flushes, insomnia, sexual dysfunction, suicidal behaviour.

Warn: patient not to stop suddenly.

Interactions: metabolism ↓ by ciprofloxacin, fluvoxamine. ↑5-HT fx with St John's wort and antidepressants (esp moclobemide and MAOIs; avoid concomitant use and do not start for 1 wk after stopping duloxetine). Avoid with artemether/lumefantrine. ↑risk CNS toxicity with sibutramine.

Dose: 60 mg od[1]; initially 30 mg od (↑ to max 120 mg/day if required)[2]; 60 mg od (↑ to bd if required)[3]; 40 mg bd[4]. *NB:* stop gradually over 1–2 wks to ↓risk of withdrawal fx.

EDOXABAN

DOAC: direct and reversible inhibitor of factor Xa.

Use: stroke prophylaxis in AF, prophylaxis/treatment of DVT ± PE.

CI: current bleeding, previous significant bleed or bleeding risk; antiphospholipid syndrome, CNS vascular malformations, PUD, hepatic disease, varices, malignancy at risk of bleeding, prosthetic heart valve, recent CNS injury or surgery, cerebral haemorrhage, uncontrolled HTN.

Caution: moderate/severe mitral stenosis, surgery.

SE: abdo pain, anaemia, dizziness, haemorrhage, headache, nausea, skin reactions. Uncommon: CNS haemorrhage, thrombocytopenia.

Interactions: ciclosporin, dronedarone, erythromycin or ketoconazole: use max 30 mg od. Caution if combining with other meds which carry bleeding risk (inc SSRIs and some common analgesics).

Dose: 30 mg od (<61 kg or creatinine clearance 15–50 ml/min), 60 mg od (≥61 kg).

EMPAGLIFLOZIN/JARDIANCE

Oral antidiabetic (reversible SGLT2 inhibitor): ↓renal reabsorption of glucose and ↑urinary excretion of glucose.

Use: type 2 DM in combination with metformin if CVD (start metformin first), CKD, adjunctive in symptomatic chronic HF with reduced ejection fraction.

CI: ketoacidosis, **R** (if severe), **L** (if severe), **P/B**.

Caution: monitor renal function before Rx, then risk factors for DKA (including ↓β-cell reserve; conditions leading to restricted food intake or volume depletion/severe dehydration including GI illness; sudden ↓ in insulin; ↑insulin requirements due to acute illness, surgery or alcohol abuse), CVD (risk of ↓BP), **E** > 75 years of age (risk of ↓BP); electrolyte disturbances; ↓BP, concomitant antihypertensive Rx (increased risk of ↓volume), HF and other concomitant use of diuretics, ↑Hct; complicated UTI – consider temporarily interrupting Rx. Correct hypovolaemia before starting Rx and at least annually on Rx.

SE: balanitis; hypoglycaemia (in combination with insulin or sulphonylurea); ↑risk of infection, pruritus, thirst, urinary disorders, hypovolaemia. Rarely DKA.

Dose: 10 mg od po, increased to 25 mg od if necessary and if tolerated. Doses of concomitant insulin or drugs that stimulate insulin secretion may need to be ↓. ↓dose in mild RF. Avoid in severe RF or LF.

> ☠ DKA on SGLT2 inhibitors may be atypical with only moderately ↑blood glucose. Warn patients of risk factors and signs and symptoms of DKA. Advise to seek immediate medical attention if they develop. Test for ↑ketones if signs or symptoms of DKA, even if plasma glucose near normal. Stop SGLT2 inhibitor if DKA is suspected or diagnosed. Do not restart SGLT2 inhibitor in patients with DKA during use, unless another cause for DKA is identified and resolved. Interrupt SGLT2 inhibitor treatment in patients in hospital for major surgery or acute, serious illness. Rx may be restarted once condition stabilised. ☠

ENALAPRIL/INNOVACE

ACE-i.

Use: HTN[1], LVF[2].

CI/Caution/SE/Interactions: as captopril, plus **L**.

Dose: initially 5 mg od[1] (2.5 mg od[2]) ↑ing according to response, usual maintenance 20 mg od, max 40 mg/day. *NB:* ↓dose if elderly, taking diuretics or RF.

ENOXAPARIN SODIUM/CLEXANE

Low-molecular-weight heparin.

Use: thromboprophylaxis and treatment of thrombosis.

CI: bacterial endocarditis, major trauma, epidural/spinal anaesthesia (Rx dose), haemophilia, PU, recent cerebral haemorrhage, recent eye or CNS surgery, thrombocytopenia (inc HIT), mechanical prosthetic heart valve.

Caution: falls risk, bleeding risk, severe HTN, ↓/↑ weight, **E**.

SE: haemorrhage, HIT, thrombosis, skin reactions, headache. Uncommon: hepatic disorders, injection site necrosis, intracranial haemorrhage. Rarely: alopecia, hyperkalaemia (if other RF present), osteoporosis (long term), spinal haematoma. Very rare: cutaneous vasculitis, eosinophilia.

Monitor: Plt count before and after starting, K^+ in those w/ RF.

Interactions: caution if combining with other meds which carry bleeding risk (inc SSRIs and some common analgesics). Caution with medications which ↑K^+.

Dose: Varies by indication and patient, usually 40 mg od sc for prophylaxis of DVT/PE.

ENSURE Protein and calorie supplement drinks.

EPADERM Paraffin-based emollient ointment for very dry skin (and as soap substitute).

EPROSARTAN

Angiotensin II antagonist; see Losartan.

Use: HTN.

CI: **L** (if severe), **P/B**.

Caution/SE/Interactions: see Losartan.

Dose: 600 mg od. ↓ if elderly, RF or LF.

ERYTHROMYCIN

Macrolide antibiotic: binds 50S ribosome.

Use: consult local antibiotic prescribing guidelines. Often used if allergy to penicillin. GI stasis (unlicensed).
CI: macrolide hypersensitivity or if taking simvastatin, pimozide, ergotamine or dihydroergotamine (see SPC for other drug CI).
Caution: ↑QTc (inc drugs that predispose), porphyria, MG, **L/R/P/B**.
SE: GI upset (very commonly diarrhoea; rarely AAC), **dry itchy skin**, hypersensitivity (inc SJS, TEN), arrhythmias (esp VT), chest pain, reversible hearing loss (dose-related, esp if RF), cholestatic jaundice.
Interactions: ↓P450 ∴ many; most importantly ↑s levels of ciclosporin, digoxin, theophyllines and carbamazepine, other drugs that ↑QTc, **W+**.
Dose: e.g. 250–1000 mg po qds; iv preparations available. To be taken before food.

NB: venous irritant ∴ give po if possible.

ERYTHROPOIETIN
Recombinant erythropoietin.
Use: ↓Hb 2° to CRF or chemotherapy (zidovudine or platinum containing). Also unlicensed use for myeloma, lymphoma and certain myelodysplasias. Three types: α (**Eprex**), β (**NeoRecormon**) and longer-acting darbepoetin (**Aranesp**).
SE: ↑BP (monitor – interrupt Rx if BP uncontrolled), ↑K⁺, headache, arthralgia, oedema, VTE. ☠ Rarely ⇒ severe rash; red cell aplasia (esp subcutaneous **Eprex** if RF, which is now CI). ☠
CI/Caution/Dose: specialist use only^{SPC/BNF}; given subcutaneously (self-administered) or iv (as inpatient). ↓Fe/folate (monitor), ↑Al, infections and inflammatory disease can ↓response. *NB: transfusion is first-line Rx for ↓Hb 2° to cancer chemotherapy.*

ESCITALOPRAM/CIPRALEX
SSRI (active enantiomer of citalopram).
Use: depression, OCD, anxiety disorders.
CI/Caution/SE/Warn/Interactions: as citalopram.

Dose: initially 10 mg OD, ↑ing if necessary to 20 mg od. *NB:* **start at 5 mg and max dose 10 mg in elderly; halve doses in LF and for most anxiety disorders.**

ESKETAMINE
S-enantiomer of ketamine.
Use: major depressive disorder.
CI/Caution/SE/Interactions: see ketamine.
Dose: by intranasal administration. 56 mg on day 1, then 56–84 mg twice weekly for weeks 1–4, then 56–84 mg once weekly for weeks 5–8, then 56–84 mg every 1–2 weeks from week 9 onwards. Elderly: same regimen but start at 28 mg.

ESOMEPRAZOLE/NEXIUM
PPI; as omeprazole, plus CI **R** (if severe).
Dose: 20 mg od po (40 mg od for first 4 wks, if for gastro-oesophageal reflux); 20–40 mg/day iv^SPC/BNF. *NB:* max 20 mg/day if severe LF.

EXENATIDE/BYETTA
SC antidiabetic (glucagon-like peptide-1 receptor agonist): ⇒ ↑insulin secretion and ↓glucagon secretion and ↓gastric emptying.
Use: type 2 DM – reserved for combination therapy when other treatment options have failed. Combined with metformin or a sulphonylurea, or both, or with pioglitazone, or with both metformin and pioglitazone, in patients who have not achieved adequate glycaemic control with these drugs alone or in combination. Initiation by specialist only.
CI: ketoacidosis; severe gastrointestinal disease, **B/P**.
Caution/Interactions: may cause ↓Wt >1.5 kg/wk, pancreatitis, **R/E**. With immediate-release exenatide some po drugs should be taken >1 h before, or 4 h after exenatide injection.^BNF
SE: GI upset, ↓appetite, asthenia, dizziness, headache, skin reactions. Less common: alopecia, burping, drowsiness, hyperhidrosis, RF, altered taste, angioedema. Rarely severe pancreatitis (discontinue permanently if occurs).

Dose: sc (IR or MR). See BNF for dosing. Dose of concomitant sulphonylurea may need to be ↓.

FELODIPINE/PLENDIL

Ca^{2+} channel blocker (dihydropyridine): as amlodipine but ⇒ ↓HF/−ve inotropic fx.

Use: HTN[1], angina Px[2].
CI: IHD (if unstable angina or within 1 month of MI), significant aortic stenosis, **H** (if uncontrolled)/**P**.
Caution: stop drug if angina/HF worsen, **L/B**.
SE: as nifedipine but ↑ankle swelling and possibly ↓vasodilator fx (headache, flushing and dizziness).
Interactions: metab by **P450** ∴ levels ↑ by cimetidine, erythromycin, ketoconazole and grapefruit juice. Hypotensive fx ↑ by α-blockers. Levels ↓ by primidone. ↑s fx of tacrolimus.
Dose: initially 5 mg od, ↑ if required to 10 mg (max 20 mg[1]).
NB: ↓dose if LF or elderly.

FENTANYL

Strong opioid; used in severe chronic/palliative pain (top/sl/buccal/nasal spray) and in anaesthesia (iv).
CI: acute respiratory depression, risk of ileus, ↑ICP/head injury/coma.
Caution: all other conditions where morphine is CI or cautioned, but better tolerated in RF. Also DM, cerebral tumour.
SE: as morphine but generally ↓N&V/constipation.
Warn: patients/carers of signs/symptoms of opiate toxicity; ☠ serious opioid toxicity from accidental exposure to patches. ☠
Interactions: as morphine but levels ↑ (not ↓) by ritonavir, levels ↑ by itra-/fluconazole and no known interaction with gabapentin. May ↑levels of midazolam.
Dose: patches (do not cut): last 72 h and come in six strengths: 12, 25, 37.5, 50, 75 and 100 mg, which denote release of microgram/h (approx equivalent to daily oral morphine of 30, 60, 90, 120, 180 and 240 mg, respectively). **Lozenges (buccal)** for 'breakthrough' pain as Actiq: initially 200 micrograms over 15 min, repeating after 15 min if needed and adjusting dose to give

max 4 lozenges daily (available as 200, 400, 600, 800, 1200 or 1600 micrograms).
Tablets: for 'breakthrough' pain as **Effentora** (buccal) or **Abstral** (sl) 100, 200, 400, 600 and 800 micrograms.^{SPC/BNF} *Only use if taking regular opioids (fatalities reported otherwise). If >4 doses/day needed, adjust background analgesia.* **Nasal spray:** for 'breakthrough' pain as **Instanyl** or **PecFent**.^{SPC/BNF} *NB:* ↓**dose if LF or elderly. No initial ↓dose needed in RF, but may accumulate over time. Unless given iv has prolonged onset/offset; use only when opioid requirements stable and cover first 12 h after initial Rx with prn short-acting opioid. Only for use if have previously tolerated opioids. If serious adverse reactions, remove patch immediately and monitor for up to 24 h. Fever/external heat can ⇒ ↑absorption (∴ ↑fx) from patches.

FERROUS FUMARATE

As ferrous sulphate, but ↓GI upset; available in UK as **Fersaday** (322 mg tablet od as Px or bd as Rx) (1 tablet of 210 mg od/bd Px; tds Rx) or **Galfer** (305 mg capsule od as Px/bd as Rx).

FERROUS GLUCONATE

As ferrous sulphate, but ↓GI upset. Px: 600 mg od; Rx: 1.2–1.8 g/day in two to three divided doses before food.

FERROUS SULPHATE

Oral Fe preparation.
Use: Fe-deficient ↓Hb Rx/Px.
Caution: P.
SE: dark stools (can confuse with melaena, which smells worse), GI upset (esp nausea; consider switching to ferrous gluconate/fumarate or take with food, but latter can ⇒ ↓absorption), Δ bowel habit (dose-dependent, usually constipation–important to note as risk of interactions, particularly with clozapine).
Interactions: thyroxine, tetracyclines.
Dose: Rx: 200 mg/tds^{BNF}. Px: 200 mg od/bd.

FINASTERIDE

Antiandrogen: 5-α-reductase inhibitor; prevents conversion of testosterone to more potent dihydrotestosterone.

Use: BPH[1] (↓s prostate size and symptoms), male-pattern baldness[2].

Caution: Ca prostate (can ⇒ ↓PSA and ∴ mask), obstructive uropathy, **P** (teratogenic; inadvertent absorption can occur via handling tablets or from contact with semen, in which it is excreted ∴ *those of childbearing potential must avoid handling crushed or broken tablets, and sexual partners of those on the drug must use condoms if, or likely to become, pregnant*).

SE: sexual dysfunction, testicular pain, gynaecomastia, hypersensitivity (inc swelling of lips/face), male breast cancer. Rare reports of depression and suicidal thoughts.[MHRA]

Dose: 5 mg od[1], 1 mg od[2].

FLUCLOXACILLIN

Penicillin (penicillinase-resistant).

Use: consult local antibiotic prescribing guidelines.

CI/Caution/SE/Interactions: as benzylpenicillin, plus CI if Hx of flucloxacillin-assoc jaundice/hepatic dysfunction and caution if LF, as rarely ⇒ hepatitis or **cholestatic jaundice** (may develop up to 2 months after Rx stopped).

Dose: 250–500 mg QDS PO/IM (or up to 2 g QDS IV). *NB:* ↓**dose in severe RF.**

FLUCONAZOLE

Triazole antifungal: good po absorption and CSF penetration.

Use: fungal meningitis (esp cryptococcal), candidiasis (mucosal, vaginal, systemic), other fungal infections (esp tinea, pityriasis).

CI: acute porphyria.

Caution: susceptibility to ↑QTc, **L/R/P/B**.

SE: GI upset, hypersensitivity (can ⇒ angioedema, TEN, SJS, anaphylaxis: if develops rash, stop drug or monitor closely), hepatotoxicity, headache. Rarely blood/metabolic (↑lipids, ↓K⁺) disorders, dizziness, seizures, alopecia.

Monitor: LFTs; stop drug if features of liver disease develop.
Interactions: ↓P450 ∴ many; most importantly, ↑s fx of theophyllines, ciclosporin, phenytoin and tacrolimus. Hepatotoxic drugs. Also ↓clopidogrel fx. **W+.**
Dose: 50–400 mg/day po or iv according to indication.[SPC/BNF] *NB:* ↓**dose in RF.**

FLUDROCORTISONE

Mineralocorticoid (also has very minimal glucocorticoid actions).
Use: adrenocortical insufficiency esp Addison's disease[1], neuropathic postural ↓BP (unlicensed)[2].
CI/Caution/Interactions: 100 micrograms fludrocortisone has glucocorticoid equivalent to ~1 mg hydrocortisone but mineralocorticoid equivalent to ~10 mg hydrocortisone.
SE: H_2O/Na^+ retention, ↓K^+ (monitor U&Es). Also can ⇒ immunosuppression (and other SEs of corticosteroids – see Hydrocortisone iv/po).
Dose: 50–300 micrograms/day po[1]; 100–400 micrograms daily[2].

FLUMAZENIL

Benzodiazepine antagonist (competitive).
Use: benzodiazepine od/toxicity only if respiratory depression and ventilatory support not immediately available. In practice, it is rarely given except in specialist circumstances. **Airway support should be prioritised.**
CI: life-threatening conditions controlled by benzodiazepines (e.g. ↑ICP, status epilepticus).
Caution: mixed ods (esp TCAs), benzodiazepine dependence (may ⇒ withdrawal fx), Hx of panic disorder (can ⇒ relapse), head injury, epileptics on long-term benzodiazepine Rx (may ⇒ fits), L/P/B/E.
SE: N&V, dizziness, flushing, rebound anxiety/agitation, transient ↑BP/HR. Very rarely anaphylaxis.
Dose: initially 200 micrograms iv over 15 sec, then, if required, further doses of 100 micrograms at 1 min intervals. *Max total dose 1 mg (2 mg in ITU).* Can also give as ivi at 100–400 micrograms/h

adjusting to response. *NB:* see p. 403 – TOXBASE recommends higher doses.

NB: short $T_{1/2}$ (40–80 min); observe closely after Rx and consider further doses or ivi (at 100–400 micrograms/h adjusted to response).

☠ *Flumazenil is not recommended as a diagnostic test and should not be given routinely in overdoses, as risk of inducing:*

- fits (esp if epileptic, or if co-ingested drugs that predispose to fits)
- withdrawal syndrome (if habituated to benzodiazepines)
- arrhythmias (esp if co-ingested TCA or amphetamine-like drug)

If in any doubt get senior opinion, exclude habituation to benzodiazepines and get ECG before giving unless life-threatening respiratory depression and benzodiazepine known to be cause. ☠

FLUOXETINE/PROZAC
SSRI antidepressant: long $T_{1/2}$ compared with others.
Use: depression[1], bulimia[2], OCD[3].
CI: mania, poorly controlled epilepsy.
Caution: epilepsy, receiving ECT, Hx of mania or bleeding disorder (esp GI), DM†, glaucoma (angle-closure), ↑risk of bleeding, age <18 years, **H**.
Class SE: GI upset, ↓Wt, insomnia, agitation, headache, hypersensitivity. Can ⇒ withdrawal fx when stopped.
Rarely extrapyramidal and antimuscarinic fx, sexual dysfunction, convulsions, ↓Na⁺ (inc SIADH), bleeding disorders, GI bleed, serotonin syndrome and suicidal thoughts/behaviour, ↑risk of bone fracture, glaucoma.
Specific SE: rarely hypoglycaemia†, **vasculitis (rash** may be first sign).
Interactions: ↓P450 ∴ many, but most importantly ↑s levels of TCAs, benzodiazepines, clozapine and haloperidol. ↑s lithium

toxicity and ⇒ HTN and ↑CNS fx with sele-/rasagiline (and other dopaminergics). ↑risk of CNS toxicity (serotonin syndrome; see p. 410) with drugs that ↑5-HT (e.g. tramadol, sibutramine, sumatriptan, St John's wort). Risk of bleeding with anticoagulants, aspirin and NSAIDs. Levels ↑ by ritonavir. Antagonises antiseizure medications (but ↑s levels of carbamazepine and phenytoin). Avoid with artemether/lumefantrine and tamoxifen. ☠ **Never give with, or ≤2 wks after, MAOIs; do not give MAOIs within 5 wks of stopping fluoxetine. (Mild W+.)** ☠

Dose: initially, 20 mg od[1,3] ↑ to max 60 mg od or divided doses; 60 mg od[2] – give mane, as can ↓sleep. *NB:* **long half-life.** ↓**dose in LF.**

FLUPENTIXOL/FLUANXOL

Typical antipsychotic: D_1/D_2 dopamine receptor antagonist; weak 5-HT_2 antagonist.

Use: psychosis[1], depression[2].

CI: CNS depression, overactivity, phaeo, circulatory collapse.

Caution: as for other antipsychotics, and agitated states, thyroid disease, E.

Class SE: EPSE, ↑prolactin and assoc Sx, sedation, ↑Wt, QT prolongation, VTE, blood dyscrasias, ↓seizure threshold, NMS.

Specific SE: ↑salivation, appetite changes, impaired glucose tolerance, urinary disorder.

Warn: photosensitivity at higher doses.

Monitor: as for all antipsychotics – baseline ECG, BMI, FBC, lipids, HbA1c, prolactin; frequently at the start of treatment and at least annually when stable.

Interactions: ↑risk of QT prolongation with 5-HT_3 antagonists and TCAs; ↑risk of lithium toxicity and NMS with lithium; ↓fx of amantadine, apomorphine, bromocriptine, cabergoline, pergolide, pramipexole, quinagolide, ropinirole, rotigotine.

Dose: 18–65 years: 3–9 mg od/bd, up to max 18 mg/day[1]; >65 years: 0.75–4.5 mg od/bd, up to max 18 mg/day[2]. ≥18 years: 1 mg mane, ↑ to max 3 mg in divided doses at wkly intervals, stop if no benefit; last dose to be given before 4 p.m.

FLUPENTIXOL DECANOATE/DEPIXOL

As flupentixol. Long-acting injection ($t_{1/2}$ ~ 21 days).
Use: maintenance treatment psychosis for patients stabilised on oral therapy.
CI/Caution/SE/Warn/Monitor/Interactions: as for flupentixol.
Dose: initial test dose 20 mg im (administered into upper outer buttock/lateral thigh), then 20–40 mg after 7 days, and 20–40 mg every 2–4 wks, doses above 80 mg every 4 wks should rarely be exceeded, ↓dose in elderly.

FLUPHENAZINE DECANOATE/MODECATE

Discontinued in UK and many other countries.

FLUTICASONE/FLIXOTIDE (various delivery devices available[BNF])

Inhaled corticosteroid for asthma: see Beclometasone.
Dose: 100–2000 micrograms/day inh (or 500 micrograms–2 mg bd as nebs).

1 microgram equivalent to 2 micrograms of beclometasone or budesonide.

FLUVOXAMINE

SSRI antidepressant; potent P450 enzyme inhibitor.
Use: depression[1], obsessive-compulsive disorder[2].
CI: poorly controlled epilepsy, mania.
Caution: ECT, DM, epilepsy, bleeding disorders, Hx mania, glaucoma (angle-closure) H/P/B.
Class SE: GI upset, ↓Wt, insomnia, agitation, headache, hypersensitivity. Can ⇒ withdrawal fx when stopped ∴ *stop slowly*. Rarely extrapyramidal and antimuscarinic fx, sexual dysfunction, convulsions, ↓Na⁺ (inc SIADH), bleeding disorders, GI bleed, serotonin syndrome and suicidal thoughts/behaviour, ↑risk of fracture, glaucoma.

Specific SE: impaired liver function.

Warn: withdrawal fx may occur within 5 days of stopping treatment, worse after regular administration for 8 wks+; ↓dose gradually over 4 wks+.

Interactions: ↓**P450** ∴ ↓fx of clopidogrel; ↑levels of drugs primarily metabolised by CYP1A2/2C19 (e.g. caffeine, some TCAs, some antipsychotics, some benzodiazepines, ropinirole, propranolol, **W+**); ☠ ↑**levels of drugs with narrow TI** (e.g. warfarin, tacrine, theophylline, methadone, phenytoin, carbamazepine and ciclosporin; can increase clozapine levels by 10×)☠; ↑**risk of bleeding** with anticoagulants, antiplatelets, fibrinolytics; ↑risk of serotonin syndrome with drugs that ↑5-HT; **never give with, or ≤2 wks after, MAOIs;** do not give MAOIs within 1 wk of stopping fluvoxamine.

Dose: 50–100 mg in evening, ↑dose gradually if necessary to 300 mg[1,2]; maintenance dose: 100 mg[1], 100–300 mg[2]; if daily dose >150 mg, give in 2–3 divided doses.

> ☠Poisoning by SSRIs causes N&V, agitation, tremor, nystagmus, drowsiness, seizure, ↑HR. Severe poisoning may result in serotonin syndrome.☠

FOLIC ACID (= FOLATE)

Vitamin: building block of nucleic acids. Essential co-factor for DNA synthesis ⇒ normal erythropoiesis.

Use: folate-deficient megaloblastic ↓Hb Rx/Px if haemolysis/dialysis[1] (or GI malabsorption where ↑doses may be needed), Px against neural-tube dfx in pregnancy[2] (esp if on antiseizure medications), Px of methotrexate-induced side effects such as mucositis and GI upset (do not give folic acid on same day as methotrexate)[3].

CI: malignancy (unless megaloblastic ↓Hb due to ↓folate is an important complication).

Caution: undiagnosed megaloblastic ↓Hb (i.e. ↓B_{12}, as found in pernicious anaemia) – never give alone if *B_{12} deficiency, as can precipitate subacute combined degeneration of spinal cord.*

SE: GI disturbance (rare).

Dose: 5 mg od[1] (in maintenance, ↓frequency of dose, often to wkly); 400 micrograms od from before conception until wk 12 of pregnancy[2] (unless mother has neural-tube defect herself or has previously had or has risk of a child with a neural-tube defect, when 5 mg od needed[BNF]); 5 mg once wkly[3].

FOMEPIZOLE Antidote for ethylene glycol and methanol.[BNF]

FONDAPARINUX/ARIXTRA
Synthetic anticoagulant; activated factor X inhibitor.
Use: ACS (UA, NSTEMI or STEMI), Px of VTE, Rx of DVT/PE.
CI: active bleeding, bacterial endocarditis, **B**.
Caution: bleeding disorders, active PU, other drugs that ↑risk of bleeding, recent intracranial haemorrhage, recent brain/ophthalmic/spinal surgery, spinal/epidural anaesthesia (avoid Rx doses), Wt <50 kg. **R** (avoid or ↓dose according to indication and creatinine clearance[SPC/BNF]), **L/P/E**.
SE: bleeding, ↓Hb, ↓(or ↑)Pt, coagulopathy, purpura, oedema, LFT Δs, GI upset. Rarely ↓K+, ↓BP, hypersensitivity.
Dose: UA/NSTEMI/Px of VTE 2.5 mg sc od (start 6 h post-op); STEMI 2.5 mg iv/ivi od for first day then sc; Rx of PE/DVT by Wt (<50 kg = 5 mg sc od, 50–100 kg = 7.5 mg sc od, >100 kg = 10 mg sc od). *NB:* length of Rx depends on indication[SPC/BNF], timing of doses post-op critical if Wt <50 kg or elderly. Consider **↓dose in RF**.

Specialist use only: get senior advice or contact on-call cardiology/haematology.

FORMOTEROL (= EFORMOTEROL)/FORADIL, OXIS, ATIMOS
Long-acting β₂ agonist 'LABA'; as Salmeterol plus **L**.
Dose: 6–48 micrograms daily (mostly BD regime)[SPC/BNF] inh (min/max doses vary with preparations[SPC/BNF]).

FOSTAIR

Combination asthma inhaler: each puff contains 100 or 200*
micrograms beclometasone (steroid) + 6 micrograms formoterol
(long-acting β_2-agonist) in a metered dose inhaler.
Dose: 1–2 puffs bd inh. Specify inhaler strength (100 or 200).*

FUROSEMIDE (previously FRUSEMIDE)

Loop diuretic: inhibits Na^+/K^+ co-transport in ascending loop of
Henle $\Rightarrow$ $\downarrow$reabsorption and $\therefore$ $\uparrow$loss of $Na^+/K^+/Cl/H_2O$.
Use: LVF (esp in acute pulmonary oedema, but also in chronic
LVF/CCF or as Px during blood transfusion), resistant HTN,
oliguria secondary to AKI (after correcting hypovolaemia first).
CI: $\downarrow\downarrow K^+$, $\downarrow Na^+$, Addison's, cirrhosis (if pre-comatose or comatose),
R (if anuria).
Caution: $\downarrow$BP, $\uparrow$prostate, porphyria, diabetes, **L/P/B**.
SE: $\downarrow$BP (inc postural), $\downarrow K^+$, $\downarrow Na^+$, $\downarrow Ca^{2+}$, $\downarrow Mg^{2+}$, $\downarrow$Cl alkalosis,
$\downarrow$proteinaemia. Also $\uparrow$urate/gout, GI upset, $\uparrow$glucose/impaired
glucose tolerance, $\uparrow$cholesterol/TGs (temporary). Rarely **BM**
suppression (stop drug), RF, skin reactions, pancreatitis, tinnitus/
deafness (if $\uparrow$doses or RF or rapid administration: reversible).
Monitor: U&Es, glucose; if $\downarrow K^+$, add po K^+ supplements/
K^+-sparing diuretic or change to combination tablet (e.g.
co-amilofruse).
Interactions: $\uparrow$s toxicity of digoxin, flecainide, sotalol, NSAIDs,
vancomycin, gentamicin and lithium. $\downarrow$s fx of antidiabetics.
NSAIDs may $\downarrow$diuretic response.
Dose: usually 20–80 mg po/im/iv daily in divided doses (higher if
specialist care). $\uparrow$doses used in acute LVF and oliguria. If HF or RF,
ivi (max 4 mg/min) can $\Rightarrow$ smoother control of fluid balance.[SPC/BNF]
For blood transfusions, a rough guide is to give 20 mg with every
unit if *existing LVF*, and with every second unit if *at risk of LVF*.
NB: **may need $\uparrow$dose in RF**.
Give iv if severe oedema, as bowel oedema $\Rightarrow$ $\downarrow$po absorption.

FUSIDIC ACID/FUCIDIN

Antibiotic; good bone penetration and activity against *S. aureus*.

Use: consult local antibiotic prescribing guidelines. Often used for osteomyelitis, endocarditis (2° to penicillin-resistant staphylococci) – needs second antibiotic to prevent resistance. Also available as a cream (± steroids) for superficial staph infections.

Caution: biliary disease or obstruction ($\Rightarrow$ ↓elimination), **L/P/B**.

SE: GI upset, hepatitis*. Rarely skin/blood disorders, AKI.

Monitor: LFTs* (esp if chronic Rx, ↑doses or LF).

Interactions: statins (rhabdomyolysis) in systemic therapy.

Dose: 500 mg tds po (equivalent to 750 mg tds if using suspension) – in severe infection ↑ to 1 g tds po. Skin infection: 250 mg bd.
NB: ↓dose in LF.

GABAPENTIN

Antiepileptic: binds to voltage-gated Ca^{2+} channels in the CNS; modulates GABA and glutamate synthesis. Abuse potential: (schedule 3) controlled drug.

Use: neuropathic pain, epilepsy (adjunctive Rx of focal seizures ± 2° generalisation).

Caution: Hx psychosis or DM, mixed seizures.

SE: fatigue/somnolence, **dizziness, cerebellar fx** (esp ataxia), dipl-/amblyopia, headache, rhinitis, ↓**WCC**, GI upset, arthra-/myalgia, skin reactions, suicidal ideation. Rarely $\Rightarrow$ severe respiratory depression, substance misuse. Can $\Rightarrow$ abuse.

Interactions: fx ↓ by antidepressants and antimalarials (esp mefloquine). Antipsychotics ↓seizure threshold. Combination with other sedative drugs $\Rightarrow$ high respiratory depression risk.

Dose: initially 300 mg od, ↑ing by 300 mg/day to max 3.6 g daily in three divided doses (*NB: stop drug over ≥1 wk*).[BNF] *NB: ↓dose in RF.*[BNF]

Can give false-positive urinary dipstick results for proteinuria.

GALANTAMINE

Acetylcholinesterase inhibitor (reversible); also ↑fx of ACh at nicotinic receptors.

Use: mild-to-moderate Alzheimer's disease.

CI: GI obstruction/post-GI surgery, urinary obstruction/post-bladder surgery, **R** (CrCl < 9 mL/min), **L** (if severe, Child-Pugh > 9).

Caution: as for donepezil, and electrolyte disturbances, Hx of seizures, lower respiratory tract infection, **H**.

SE: as for Donepezil, and asthenia.

Warn: take with food. Stop if rash appears.

Interactions: metab by P450; ↑levels with CYP2D6/3A4 inhibitors, e.g. bupropion, cinacalcet, clarithromycin, cobicistat, darunavir, fluoxetine, itra-/ketoconazole, paroxetine; ↓fx of neuromuscular blocking agents (atracurium, cisatracurium, mivacurium, pancuronium) and anticholinergic agents (atropine, procyclidine, trihexyphenidyl); ↑risk of bradycardia with amiodarone, β-blockers, diltiazem, digoxin, ivabradine.

Dose: immediate-release: initially 4 mg bd for 4 wks, ↑ to 8 mg bd for 4 wks+, maintenance 8–12 mg bd; modified-release: initially 8 mg od for 4 wks, ↑ to 16 mg od for 4 wks+, maintenance 16–24 mg od; halve dose in moderate LF.

> ☠Serious skin hypersensitivity may occur (inc SJS and acute generalised exanthematous pustulosis).☠

GAVISCON Alginate raft-forming oral suspension for acid reflux. Multiple other alginate-based antacids available (e.g. Acidex, Peptac).

Dose: 10–20 mL after meals and at bedtime.

(*NB:* 2.3 mmol Na^+ and 1 mmol K^+/5 mL and 2.25 mmol Na^+ and 1 mmol K^+/tablet.)

> Ensure good hydration, esp if elderly, GI narrowing or ↓GI motility.

GENTAMICIN

Aminoglycoside: broad-spectrum 'cidal' antibiotic; inhibits ribosomal 30S subunit. Good Gram –ve aerobe/staphylococci

cover; other organisms often need concurrent penicillin ±
metronidazole.

G

Use: consult local antibiotic prescribing guidelines.

CI: MG*.

Caution: obesity, **R/P/B/E**.

SE: ototoxic, nephrotoxic (dose and Rx length dependent),
hypersensitivity, rash. Rarely AAC, N&V, seizures,
encephalopathy, blood disorders, myasthenia-like syndrome* (at
↑doses; reversible), ↓Mg^{2+} (if prolonged Rx).

Monitor: U&Es before and during Rx; serum levels** after three
or four doses of multiple daily dosing, or 48 h of once-daily dosing
or after dose change (earlier if RF).

Interactions: fx (esp toxicity) ↑ by loop diuretics (esp
furosemide), cephalosporins, vancomycin, amphotericin,
ciclosporin, tacrolimus and cytotoxics; if these drugs must be given,
space doses as far from time of gentamicin dose as possible. ↑s fx of
muscle relaxants and anticholinesterases, **W+**.

Dose: refer to local protocol if available, otherwise: once-daily
regimen: initially, 5–7 mg/kg ivi (ideal Wt for Ht) adjusting to levels
(*NB:* consult local protocol; od regimen not suitable if endocarditis,
>20% total body surface burns or creatinine clearance <20 mL/
min). Multiple daily regimen: 3–5 mg/kg/day in three divided doses
im/iv/ivi (if endocarditis, give 1 mg/kg bd iv).

NB: ↓doses if RF (and consider if elderly or ↑↑BMI), otherwise adjust
according to serum levels*: call microbiology department if unsure.**

**Gentamicin levels: Measure peak at 1 h post-dose (ideally =
5–10 mg/L) and trough immediately pre-dose (multi-dosing
≤2 mg/L; od dosing <1 mg/L). Halve ideal peak levels if for
endocarditis. If levels high, can ↑*spacing* of doses (as well
as ↓ing *amount* of dose); as ⇒ ↑risk of ototoxicity, monitor
auditory/vestibular function. *NB: od regimens usually only
require *pre-dose* level. **Consult local protocols.**

GLICLAZIDE

Oral antidiabetic (short-acting sulphonylurea).

Use: T2DM; requires endogenous insulin to work.

CI: ketoacidosis, porphyria, L/R (if either severe, otherwise caution), P/B.

Caution: may need to replace with insulin during intercurrent illness/surgery, porphyria, G6PD deficiency, E.

SE: hypoglycaemia (esp in elderly), GI upset, ↑Wt. Rarely hypersensitivity (inc skin) reactions, blood disorders, hepatotoxicity and transient visual Δs (esp initially).

Interactions: fx ↑d by chloramphenicol.

Dose: initially 40–80 mg mane (with breakfast), ↑ing as necessary (max 320 mg/day); doses higher than 160 mg should be divided into bd. MR tablets available (Diamicron MR, also Vitile XL, Dacadis MR) of which 30 mg has equivalent effect to 80 mg of normal release (dose initially is 30 mg od, ↑ing if necessary to max 120 mg od). *NB:* ↓dose in RF or severe LF.

GLIMEPIRIDE

Oral antidiabetic (short-acting sulphonylurea).

Use/CI/Caution/SE/Interactions: as gliclazide, (also SE: ↓Na⁺).
Manufacturer recommends monitoring of FBC and LFTs. CI in severe LF and ketoacidosis. Not CI in acute porphyria. May need to substitute with insulin; seek specialist advice.

Dose: initially 1 mg mane with food, ↑ as necessary[BNF] (max 6 mg/day).

GLIPIZIDE

Oral antidiabetic (short-acting sulphonylurea).

Use/CI/Caution/SE/Interactions: as gliclazide, plus avoid if both L and R. Not CI in acute porphyria. CI in ketoacidosis.

Dose: initially 2.5–5 mg mane (with food), ↑ing as necessary (max single dose 15 mg; max daily dose 20 mg). *NB:* ↓dose in severe LF and RF.

G

GLUCAGON

Polypeptide hormone: $\uparrow$s hepatic glycogen conversion to glucose.

Use: hypoglycaemia: if acute and severe or unable to take po glucose, esp if no IV access or if 2° to xs insulin (see p. 430).

CI: phaeo.

Caution: glucagonomas/insulinomas. Will not work if hypoglycaemia is chronic (inc starvation) or 2° to adrenal insufficiency.

SE: N&V, $\downarrow$ or $\uparrow$BP, $\downarrow$K$^+$, $\uparrow$HR, rarely hypersensitivity, **W+**.

Dose: 1 mg (= 1 unit) im (or SC/IV)$^{SPC/BNF}$; if no response in 10 min, iv glucose must be given.

> Often stocked in cardiac arrest ('crash') trolleys. Good option in psych units, where iv access often limited.

GLYCEROL (= GLYCERIN) SUPPOSITORIES

Rectal irritant bowel stimulant (rapid-acting).

Use: constipation: first-line suppository if oral methods such as lactulose and senna fail.

CI: GI obstruction/blockage.

Dose: <1 year 1 g; 1–12 years 2 g; >12 years and adult 4 g pr prn.

GTN (= GLYCERYL TRINITRATE)

Nitrate: $\Rightarrow$ coronary artery + systemic vein dilation $\Rightarrow$ $\uparrow$O$_2$ supply to myocardium and $\downarrow$preload, $\therefore$ $\downarrow$O$_2$ demand of myocardium.

Use: angina[1], unstable angina/acute MI[2], HF[2], anal fissure[3].

CI: $\downarrow$BP, $\downarrow\downarrow$Hb, aortic/mitral stenosis, constrictive pericarditis, tamponade, HOCM, hypovolaemia, $\uparrow$ICP, toxic pulmonary oedema.

Caution: recent MI, $\downarrow$T$_4$, hypothermia, head trauma, cerebral haemorrhage, malnutrition, glaucoma (closed-angle), **L/R** (if either severe).

SE: $\downarrow$BP (inc postural), headache, dizziness, flushing, $\uparrow$HR.

Warn: may develop tolerance with $\downarrow$therapeutic effect (esp if long-term transdermal patch use); consider removing patches at night to reduce tolerance; do not stop abruptly.

Interactions: ☠ sildenafil, tadalafil and vardenafil (are CI as ⇒ ↓↓BP). ☠ ↓s fx of heparins (if given iv).

Dose: 1–2 sprays or 1–2 tablets sl prn (also available as transdermal SR patches[SPC/BNF])[1]. 10–200 micrograms/min ivi, titrating to clinical response and BP max 400 micrograms/min ivi[2]. 2.5 cm of ointment pr bd for up to 8 wks[3].

▼ GUANFACINE/INTUNIV

α_2-adrenergic receptor agonist ⇒ ↓noradrenaline release.

Use: ADHD in children if stimulants not suitable (initiated under specialist).

CI: hypersensitivity.

Caution: ↓HR/HB/↓K+ (↑risk of torsade de pointes), Hx CVD/↑QTc, lactose intolerance.

SE: sedation, ↓BP, ↓HR, headache, GI upset, fatigue, ↓appetite, Δ mood, anxiety, ↓sleep, dizziness, rash, enuresis, ↑Wt.

Warn: avoid missing doses, if >1 dose missed, inform prescriber ⇒ consider re-titration. On discontinuation, rebound ↑BP/HR. Should not take with high-fat meal (↑absorption and ↑SEs).

Monitor: assess at baseline to identify cardiac status (risks of ↓BP/HR, ↑QTc, arrhythmias), BMI and potential for sedation. Monitor wkly during titration, 3-monthly in first year, then 6-monthly. Check BP/HR when weaning down and after cessation.

Interactions: metab by P450; ↑levels with CYP3A4/3A5 inhibitors (e.g. ketoconazole, clarithromycin, indinavir), ↓levels with CYP3A4 inducers (e.g. rifampicin, carbamazepine, phenobarbital, phenytoin); also ↑levels of valproic acid; ↑risks of hypotension/syncope with antihypertensives; ↑risks of sedation/somnolence with CNS depressants.

Dose: 6–12 years (≥25 kg): initially 1 mg po od, adjusted by 1 mg/wk, maintenance 0.05–0.12 mg/kg od (max 4 mg); 13–17 years (34–41.4 kg): same as previous; 13–17 years (41.5–49.4 kg): same as previous – max 5 mg; 13–17 years (49.5–58.4 kg): same as previous – max 6 mg; 13–17 years (≥58.5 kg): same as previous – max 7 mg).

NB: ↓dose by half with concurrent use of moderate/potent CYP3A4 inhibitors; ↑dose up to max 7 mg od with concurrent use of potent CYP3A4 inducers.

☠ Overdose ⇒ ↑ then ↓BP, ↓HR, resp depression, lethargy. If lethargy develops, observe for up to 24 h. ☠

HALOPERIDOL/HALDOL

Typical antipsychotic: D_2 dopamine receptor antagonist.

Use: schizophrenia and schizoaffective disorder[1], mania in bipolar disorder[2], acute agitation[3]; where other treatments have failed: delirium, tic disorders, Huntington's; in palliative care: N&V, restlessness, confusion.

CI: CNS depression, ↑QTc, Hx ventricular arrhythmia, recent acute MI, ↓K^+, Parkinson's and related disorders, **H.**

Caution: as for other antipsychotics with high likelihood of EPSEs, **baseline and follow-up ECG needed, L.**

Class SE: EPSE, ↑prolactin and assoc Sx, sedation, ↑QTc, VTE, blood dyscrasias, ↓seizure threshold, NMS.

Interactions: metab by P450; levels ↑ by fluoxetine, venlafaxine, quinidine, buspirone and ritonavir. Levels ↓ by carbamazepine, phenytoin, rifampicin. ↑risk of arrhythmias with amiodarone and ↓s fx of anticonvulsants.

Dose: 2–10 mg po daily in one to two divided doses (max 20 mg/day, although 10 mg likely to be sufficient)[1]; 2–10 mg po daily in one to two divided doses (max 15 mg/day)[2]; 5–10 mg po, repeated after 12 h if necessary (max 20 mg/day) or 5 mg im, repeated hrly if necessary (max 12 mg but some sources, e.g. BNF and some SPCs, give max dose as 20 mg im)[3]; use quarter to half adult doses in elderly; bioavailability varies by route: 5 mg po = 3 mg im.

☠ Start at bottom of dose range if naive to antipsychotics, esp if elderly. See p. 393. ☠

HALOPERIDOL DECANOATE/HALDOL DECANOATE

Typical antipsychotic: D_2 dopamine receptor antagonist. Long-acting injection ($T_{1/2}$ ~ 21 days).

Use: maintenance treatment of schizophrenia and schizoaffective disorder in patients stabilised on po haloperidol.

CI/Caution/SE/Warn/Monitor: as for haloperidol.

Interactions: metab by P450; levels ↑ by fluoxetine, venlafaxine, quinidine, buspirone and ritonavir. Levels ↓ by carbamazepine, phenytoin, rifampicin. ↑risk of arrhythmias with amiodarone and ↓s fx of anticonvulsants.

Dose: 10–15 times the daily dose of po haloperidol given every 4 wks im (administered into upper outer buttock/lateral thigh), adjusted if necessary in steps of 50 mg every 4 wks; usual maintenance dose 50–200 mg every 4 wks, max 300 mg every 4 wks; frequency can be up to every 2 wks (halve dose; max 150 mg/2 wks). Elderly: initially 12.5–25 mg every 4 wks; usual maintenance dose 25–75 mg every 4 wks, max 75 mg every 4 wks.

HUMALOG short-acting recombinant insulin. Also available as biphasic preparations (Mix 25, Mix 50), are combined with longer-acting isophane suspension.

HUMULIN Recombinant insulin available in various forms:

1 HUMULIN S soluble, short-acting for iv/acute use.
2 HUMULIN I isophane (with protamine), intermediate acting.
3 HUMULIN M 'biphasic' preparations, combination of short-acting (S) and intermediate-acting (I) forms to give smoother control throughout the day. Numbers denote 1/10% of soluble insulin (i.e. M3 = 30% soluble insulin).

HYDROCORTISONE BUTYRATE CREAM (0.1%)

Potent-strength topical corticosteroid. *NB:* much stronger than 'standard' (i.e. non-butyrate) hydrocortisone cream; see next entry.

HYDROCORTISONE CREAM/OINTMENT (1%)

Mild-strength topical corticosteroid (rarely used as weaker 0.5%, 0.25% and 0.1% preparations).

Use: inflammatory skin conditions, in particular, eczema.

CI: untreated infection, rosacea, acne.

SE: rare compared to more potent steroids: skin atrophy, worsening of infections, acne.

Dose: apply thinly to affected area(s) one or two times per day.

HYDROCORTISONE IV/PO

Glucocorticoid (with significant mineralocorticoid activity: not for use as immunosuppresant).

Use: acute hypersensitivity (esp anaphylaxis, angioedema), Addisonian crisis, asthma, COPD, $\downarrow T_4$ (and $\uparrow T_4$), IBD. Also used po in chronic adrenocortical insufficiency.

CI: systemic infection (unless appropriate antibiotics prescribed), live vaccines, cerebral oedema due to head injury/CVA.

Caution: DM, epilepsy, HTN, glaucoma, osteoporosis, PU, TB, severe mood disorders, **L/R**.

SE: $\uparrow$infections, metabolic (fluid retention, $\uparrow$lipids, $\uparrow$Wt, DM, $\uparrow Na^+$, $\downarrow K^+$), adrenal suppression, bruising, cardiac (HTN, CCF, myocardial rupture post-MI, TE), musculoskeletal (proximal myopathy, osteoporosis), worsening of seizures, Ψ fx (anxiety, depression, psychosis), ocular (cataract, glaucoma, corneal/scleral thinning), GI (peptic/duodenal ulcer – give PPI if on $\uparrow$doses, pancreatitis).

Warn: avoid contact with chickenpox if not infected previously. ☠Risk of Addisonian crisis if abrupt withdrawal – must $\downarrow$ slowly if >3 wks Rx. ☠

Interactions: fx can be $\downarrow$d by rifampicin, carbamazepine, phenytoin and phenobarbital. fx (and risk of adrenal suppression) can be $\uparrow$d by erythromycin, ritonavir, ketoconazole, itraconazole and ciclosporin (whose own fx are $\uparrow$d by methylprednisolone). $\uparrow$risk of $\downarrow K^+$ with amphotericin and digoxin. Risk of $\uparrow$ or $\downarrow$anticoagulant effect of coumarins.

Dose: *acutely:* 100–500 mg im or slowly iv up to qds if required. Exact dose recommendations vary: consult local protocol if unsure. *Chronic replacement:* usually 20–30 mg po daily in divided doses (usually 2/3 in morning and 1/3 nocte), often together with fludrocortisone.

HYDROXOCOBALAMIN

Vit B$_{12}$ replacement.
Use: pernicious anaemia (also macrocytic anaemias with neurological involvement, tobacco amblyopia, Leber's optic atrophy). Cyanide poisoning.
SE: skin reactions, nausea, flu-like symptoms, ↓K$^+$(initially), rarely anaphylaxis.
Interactions: fx ↓ by OCP and chloramphenicol.
Dose: 1 mg im injection: 3×/wk for 2 wks$^{SPC/BNF}$ until no further improvement, then ↓frequency (to once every 1–3 months, see SPC/BNF for maintenance. For cyanide poisoning, see BNF.

HYOSCINE BUTYLBROMIDE/BUSCOPAN

Antimuscarinic: ↓s GI motility. Does not cross blood-brain barrier (unlike hyoscine *hydrobromide*): less sedative.
Use: GI (or GU) smooth-muscle spasm; esp biliary colic, diverticulitis and IBS. Also xs respiratory secretions and rarely dysmenorrhoea.
CI: glaucoma (closed-angle), MG, megacolon, ↑prostate.
Caution: GI obstruction, ↑prostate/urinary retention, ↑HR (inc ↑T$_4$), H/P/E.
SE: antimuscarinic fx (see p. 387), drowsiness, confusion.
Interactions: ↓s fx of metoclopramide (and vice versa) and sublingual nitrates. ↑s tachycardic fx of β-agonists.
Dose: 20 mg qds po (for IBS, start at 10 mg tds) or 20 mg im/iv (repeating once after 30 min, if necessary; max 100 mg/day).

Do not confuse with hyoscine *hydrobromide*: different fx and doses.

HYOSCINE HYDROBROMIDE (= SCOPOLAMINE)

Antimuscarinic: predominant fx on CNS (↓s vestibular activity[1]). Also ↓s respiratory/oral secretions[2,3].

Use: motion sickness[1], terminal care/chronic ↓swallow[2] (e.g. CVA), hypersalivation 2° to antipsychotics[3] (unlicensed use).

CI: GI obstruction, severe UC, pyloric stenosis, ↑prostate/urinary retention, glaucoma (closed-angle).

Caution: cardiovascular disease, HTN, porphyria, Down syndrome, MG, diarrhoea, GORD, UC, ↑thyroid, glaucoma, fever **L/R/P/B/E**.

SE: antimuscarinic fx, generally sedative (although rarely ⇒ paradoxical agitation when given as sc infusion).

Interactions: ↓s fx of sublingual nitrates (e.g. GTN).

Dose: 150–300 micrograms 6-hrly po (max 900 micrograms/24 h)[1] (or as transdermal patches; release 1 mg over 72 h); 600 micrograms–2.4 mg/24 h as sc infusion[2]; 300 micrograms bd po[3] (can ↑ to tds).

Do not confuse with hyoscine butylbromide with different fx and doses.

HYPROMELLOSE 0.3% EYE DROPS

Artificial tears for treatment of dry eyes.

Dose: 1 drop prn.

IBUPROFEN

Mild-to-moderate strength NSAID. Non-selective COX inhibitor; analgesic, anti-inflammatory and antipyrexial[†] properties.

Use: mild-to-moderate pain[1] (inc MSK, headache, migraine, dysmenorrhoea, dental, post-op; not first choice for gout/RA, as ↓anti-inflammatory fx cf other NSAIDs), mild local inflammation[2]. Most CIs, cautions, SEs and interactions are not significant for topical ibuprofen unless used to excess (see BNF).

CI: Hx of hypersensitivity to aspirin or any other NSAID (inc asthma/angioedema/urticaria/rhinitis). **Active/Hx of PU/GI bleeding/perforation, L/R/H** (if any of these three are severe)**/P** (third trimester). Topical: do not use on broken skin.

Caution: asthma, allergic disorders, uncontrolled HTN, IHD, PVD, cerebrovascular disease, cardiovascular risk factors, connective tissue disorders, coagulopathy, IBD. *Can mask signs of infection*[†] **L/R/H/P** (first/second trimester: preferably avoid)/**B/E**.

SE: GI upset/bleeding/PU (*less than other NSAIDs*). AKI, hypersensitivity reactions (esp bronchospasm and skin reactions, inc, very rarely, SJS/TEN), fluid retention/oedema, headache, dizziness, nervousness, depression, drowsiness, insomnia, tinnitus, photosensitivity, haematuria. >1.2 g/day ⇒ small ↑risk of thrombotic events. Reversible ↓female fertility if long-term use. Very rarely, blood disorders, ↑BP, ↑K⁺.

Interactions: leading cause of lithium toxicity, ↑risk GI bleeding with aspirin, clopidogrel, anti-coagulants, corticosteroids, SSRIs, venlafaxine and erlotinib. ↑s (toxic) fx of digoxin, quinolones, lithium, phenytoin, baclofen, methotrexate, zidovudine and sulphonylureas. ↑risk of RF with ACE-i, ARB, diuretics, tacrolimus and ciclosporin. ↑risk of ↑K⁺ with K-sparing diuretics and aldosterone antagonists. ↓s fx of antihypertensives and diuretics. ↑levels with ritonavir and triazoles. Mild **W+**.

Dose: initially 200–400 mg tds po[1] (max 2.4 g/day); topically as gel: apply to affected areas up to tds[2].

NB: avoid/↓dose in RF and consider gastroprotective Rx.

IMIPRAMINE

TCA: blocks reuptake of NA and 5-HT.

Use: depression[1], nocturnal enuresis in children, ADHD in children (unlicensed, consult specialist literature for dosing).

CI: as for amitriptyline, **L/H**.

Caution: as for amitriptyline, **L/H/P/E**.

Class SE: antimuscarinic fx (constipation, dry mouth, blurred vision), **cardiac fx** (arrhythmias, HB, ↑HR, postural ↓BP, dizziness, syncope: **dangerous in od**), ↑Wt, sedation (often ⇒ 'hangover'), seizures, Δ LFTs, ↓Na⁺ (esp in elderly), agitation, confusion, NMS.

Warn: may cause discontinuation symptoms if stopped abruptly.

Monitor: elderly patients for cardiac and psychiatric SE and electrolytes.

Interactions: ☠ never give with, or ≤3 wks after, MAOIs; do not give MAOIs within 3 wks of stopping imipramine. ☠

Dose: initially 75 mg po in divided doses, increasing to 150–200 mg daily; determine maintenance dose (usually 50–100 mg) once in remission[1].^{SPC} See BNF/SPC for dosing for nocturnal enuresis.

> ☠ Overdose is associated with high rate of fatality. TCA overdose ⇒ dilated pupils, arrhythmias, ↓BP, hypothermia, hyperreflexia, extensor plantar responses, seizures, respiratory depression and coma. ☠

INDAPAMIDE

Thiazide derivative diuretic; see Bendroflumethiazide.

Use: HTN.

CI: Hx of sulphonamide derivative allergy, ↓K⁺, ↓Na⁺, ↑Ca²⁺, **L/R** (if either severe).

Caution: ↑PTH (stop if ↑Ca²⁺), ↑aldosterone, gout, nephrotic syndrome, porphyria, previous photosensitivity with other thiazide and related diuretics, **R/P/B/E**.

SE: as bendroflumethiazide, but reportedly fewer metabolic disturbances (esp less hyperglycaemia).

Monitor: U&Es, urate.

Interactions: as bendroflumethiazide (*NB:* ↑s lithium levels).

Dose: 2.5 mg od mane (or 1.5 mg od of MR preparation).

INFLIXIMAB

Monoclonal Ab against TNF-α (inflammatory cytokine).

Use: Crohn's/UC^{NICE}, RA^{NICE}, psoriasis (for skin or arthritis)^{NICE} or ankylosing spondylitis.^{NICE}

CI: TB or other severe infections, **H** (unless mild when only caution), **P/B**.

Caution: infections, demyelinating CNS disorders, malignancy (inc Hx of), hepatitis B, **L/R/P/B**.

SE: severe infections, TB (inc extrapulmonary), **CCF** (exac of), **CNS demyelination.** Also GI upset, flu-like symptoms, cough, fatigue, headache. ↑incidence of hypersensitivity (esp transfusion) reactions.
Dose: specialist use only. Often prescribed concurrently with methotrexate.

INSULATARD Intermediate-acting (isophane) insulin, either recombinant human or porcine/bovine.

INSULIN See under brand name.

IPRATROPIUM

Inh short-acting muscarinic antagonist; bronchodilator and ↓s bronchial secretions.
Use: chronic[1] and acute[2] bronchospasm (COPD>asthma). Used topically for rhinitis.
SE: antimuscarinic fx (see p. 387), usually minimal.
Caution: glaucoma (angle-closure only; protect patient's eyes from drug, esp if giving nebs: use tight-fitting mask), bladder outflow obstruction (e.g. ↑prostate), cystic fibrosis, **P/B.**
Dose: 20–40 micrograms tds/qds inh[1] (max 80 micrograms qds); 250–500 micrograms qds neb[2] (↑ing up to 4 hrly if severe, max 2 mg/day).

IRBESARTAN

Angiotensin II antagonist.
Use: HTN, type 2 DM nephropathy.
Caution/SE/Interactions: see Losartan.
Dose: initially 150 mg od, ↑ing to 300 mg od if required (halve initial dose if age >75 years or on haemodialysis).

IRON TABLETS see Ferrous sulfate/fumarate/gluconate.

ISOCARBOXAZID

MAOI; non-selective and irreversible inhibitor of monoamine oxidase, ↑5-HT, NA and DA in CNS.

Use: depression.

CI: cerebrovascular disease, mania, phaeo, severe CVD.

Caution: L, porphyria, agitation, blood disorders, concurrent ECT, DM, epilepsy, severe hypertensive reaction, surgery, CVD, **E**.

SE: postural ↓BP, hypertensive responses, arrhythmia, oedema, dizziness, dry mouth, GI upset (N&V&C), ↓sleep, blurred vision, drowsiness.

Warn: Avoid tyramine-/dopa-rich food/drinks during Rx/for 2–3 wks after stopping MAOI, withdrawal fx may occur within 5 days of stopping treatment, ↑symptoms after regular administration for 8 wks+, dose reduction gradually over 4 wks+.

Monitor: BP (↑risk of postural hypotension and hypertensive responses).

Interactions: ☠ ↑**risk of severe toxic reaction** with serotonergics, dopaminergics and noradrenergics: SSRIs, SNRIs, NARIs, TCAs (and related drugs), other MAOIs (inc for Parkinson's disease), carbamazepine, linezolid, triptans, pethidine, tramadol. ☠

- Do not start isocarboxazid until these drugs have been stopped and they have cleared: 5 wks for fluoxetine, 3 wks for clomipramine/imipramine, at least 7–14 days for other drugs.
- Wait 2 wks after stopping isocarboxazid before starting any of these medicines.

↑**risk of hypertensive crisis** with sympathomimetics, dopamine agonists, CNS stimulants, buspirone. ↑fx of CNS depressants, antimuscarinics, antidiabetics, antihypertensives.

Dose: initially 30 mg po od, in single/divided doses, ↑ after 4 wks to 60 mg od for 4–6 wks, then ↓ to maintenance dose 10–20 mg od up to 40 mg od. Elderly dosing: 5–10 mg.

☠ Hypertensive crisis may develop if taken with food high in tyramine or DOPA. See p. 223. ☠

ISOSORBIDE MONONITRATE (ISMN)

Nitrate; as GTN, but po rather than sl delivery. GTN usually treatment, but ISMN generally prophylaxis.

Use/CI/Caution/SE/Interactions: as GTN, but ⇒ ↓headache.
Dose: 10–40 mg bd po (od MR preparations available[SPC/BNF]).

ISPHAGHULA HUSK (FYBOGEL)

Laxative: bulking agent (ispaghula husk) for constipation (inc IBS).
CI: ↓swallow, GI obstruction, faecal impaction, colonic atony.
Dose: 1 sachet after meals with water.

IVABRADINE

↓s HR by selective cardiac pacemaker I_f channel current blockade
⇒ ↓SAN myocyte Na^+ and K^+ entry.
Use: angina[1], HF[2] (if sinus rhythm and β-blockers CI/not tolerated
or β-blocker alone inadequate), HF[2].
CI: ↓HR (do not start if <70 bpm[1] or <75 bpm[2]; stop if HR <50 bpm
during treatment) or ↓BP, cardiogenic shock, ACS (inc acute MI),
acute CVA, second- or third-degree HB, SSS, pacemaker dependent,
SAN block congenital ↑QT syndrome, strong **P450 3A4** inhibitors/
diltiazem/verapamil**, **L** (if severe)/**H** (if moderate/severe)/**P/B**.
Caution: retinitis pigmentosa, galactose intolerance*/Lapp lactase
deficiency*/glucose-galactose malabsorption*, **R**.
SE: visual Δs (esp luminous phenomena*), ↓HR, HB, ectopics, VF,
headaches, dizziness. Less commonly GI upset, cramps, dyspnoea,
↑EØ, ↑uric acid, ↓GFR.
Warn: tablets contain lactose*, may ↓vision if night driving/using
machinery with rapid light intensity Δs.
Monitor: HR (maintain resting ventricular rate >50 bpm) and
rhythm, BP.
Interactions: ☠ metab by **P450 3A4**; inhibitors ↑levels and
strong inhibitors** (clari-/ery-/telithromycin, itra-/ketoconazole,
ritonavir, nefazodone) are CI but ↓doses can be given with
fluconazole. Inducers ↓levels (inc rifampicin, barbiturates,
phenytoin, St John's wort). Levels also ↑ by diltiazem and verapamil.
↑risk of VF with drugs that ↑QTc (inc amiodarone, disopyramide,
mefloquine, pentamidine, pimozide, sertindole, sotalol). ☠

Dose: initially 5 mg bd po; ↑ing if required after 3–4 wks[1] or 2 wks[2] to max 7.5 mg bd po. Take with food. *NB:* consider ↓dose if not tolerated, elderly or severe RF.[SPC/BNF]

KAY-CEE-L

KCl syrup (1 mmol/mL) for ↓K⁺; see Sando-K.

Dose: according to serum K⁺: average 25–50 mL/day in divided doses if diet normal. Caution if taking other drugs that ↑K⁺. Give after food. *NB:* ↓dose if **RF**.

KETAMINE

Dissociative anaesthetic via NMDA antagonism.

Use: induction of anaesthesia for short procedures; minimal effect on respiratory drive. Unconfirmed antidepressant effect. Need anaesthetist with appropriate airway support (although ↓respiratory depression than other general anaesthetics).

CI: porphyria, pre-eclampsia, head trauma, HTN, ↑ICP, severe CVD.

Caution: shock, dehydration/hypovolaemia, CVD (particularly valvular disease), ↑CSF pressure, intracranial lesions, Hx of seizures, ↑IOP, upper/lower RTI, thyroid ↓/↑, psychosis, Hx of hallucinations or nightmares, **E**.

SE: anxiety, confusion, hallucination, sleep disorders, diplopia, nystagmus, ↑muscle tone, nausea/vomiting, skin reactions, tonic-clonic movements. Uncommon: ↓appetite, arrhythmias, hypotension, respiratory disorders. Rare: apnoea, (haemorrhagic) cystitis, delirium, dysphoria, flashbacks, hypersalivation.

Interactions: ergotamine, memantine, any drug which could ↓BP.

Dose: varies by weight and indication, ~4 mg/kg iv/im for anaesthesia; subanaesthetic doses (~0.5 mg/kg) used off-label for severe depression.

LACRI-LUBE

Ocular lubricant for dry eyes.

SE: blurred vision ∴ usually used at bedtime (or if vision secondary consideration, e.g. Bell's palsy or blind eye).

Dose: one application prn.

LACTULOSE

Osmotic laxative[1]. Also $\downarrow$s growth of NH_4-producing bacteria[2].

Use: constipation[1], hepatic encephalopathy[2].

CI: GI obstruction, digestive perforation (or risk of) or galactosaemia.

Caution: lactose intolerance.

SE: flatulence, distension, abdo pains.

Dose: 15 mL od/bd[1]/tds ($\uparrow$dose according to response; *NB: can take 2 days to work*); 30–50 mL tds-qds[2]. *Take with plenty of water.*

LAMOTRIGINE

Antiepileptic: $\downarrow$s release of excitatory amino acids (esp glutamate) via action on voltage-sensitive Na^+ channels.

Use: epilepsy (esp focal and 1° or 2° generalised tonic-clonic), Px depressive episode in bipolar disorder.

Caution: avoid abrupt withdrawal† (rebound seizure risk; taper off over ≥2 wks unless stopping due to serious skin reaction). Myoclonic seizures and Parkinson's can be exacerbated. L/R/P/B.

SE: cerebellar symptoms, skin reactions (often severe, e.g. SJS, TEN, lupus, esp in children, if on valproate, or high initial doses), blood disorders ($\downarrow$Hb, $\downarrow$WCC, $\downarrow$Pt), N&V. Rarely, $\downarrow$memory, sedation, aggression, irritability, sleep Δ, pretibial ulcers, alopecia, worsening of seizures, poly-/anuria, hepatotoxicity.

Warn: report rash plus any flu-like symptoms, signs of infection/$\downarrow$Hb or bruising. Do not stop tablets suddenly†. Risk of suicidal ideation.

Monitor: U&Es, FBC, LFTs, clotting.

Interactions: fx are $\downarrow$d by OCP, phenytoin, carbamazepine; fx $\uparrow$d by valproate.

Dose: 25–500 mg daily; $\uparrow$dose slowly to $\downarrow$risk of skin reactions (also need to restart at low dose; repeat dose titration if >5 days missed); standard titration in bipolar disorder: 25 mg od for 14 days, then 50 mg in 1–2 divided doses for 14 days, then 100 mg in 1–2 divided doses for 7 days, then 200 mg maintenance in 1–2 divided doses; titration speed and final dose need adjustment if co-prescribed with valproate or enzyme inducers[BNF,SPC]. *NB: $\downarrow$dose in LF.*

LANSOPRAZOLE

PPI. As omeprazole, but ↓interactions.
Dose: 15–30 mg od po (↓ to 15 mg od for maintenance). For *H. pylori* eradication: 30 mg bd for 7 days.

LATANOPROST 0.005%

Topical PG analogue: ↑s uveoscleral outflow.
Use: ↑IOP in glaucoma and *ocular* HTN (first-line agent).
CI: herpetic keratitis (inc recurrent Hx of).
Caution: asthma (if severe), aphakia, pseudophakia, uveitis, macular oedema, P/B.
SE: iris colour Δ* (can ⇒ permanent ↑brown pigmentation, esp if uniocular use), blurred vision, local reactions (e.g. conjunctival hyperaemia in up to 30% initially). Also darkening of periocular skin and ↑eyelash length (both reversible). Rarely cystoid macular oedema (if aphakia), uveitis, angina.
Warn: can Δ iris colour*.
Dose: 1 drop od (preferably in the evening).

LEVETIRACETAM/KEPPRA

Antiepileptic: Δs intraneuronal Ca^{2+} levels/inhibits pre-synaptic Ca^{2+} channels. Binds to synaptic vesicle glycoprotein 2A.
Use: focal seizures, myoclonic/tonic-clonic seizures.
Caution: may cause ↑QT, avoid abrupt withdrawal, suicidal ideation, R/P/B/H.
SE: nasopharyngitis, headache, somnolence, anorexia (uncommonly ⇒ ↓Wt), N&V&D, abdo pain, dyspepsia, tremor, dizziness, vertigo, convulsion, lethargy, drowsiness, fatigue, agitation, Ψ disturbance (depression, anxiety, psychosis, hallucinations, confusion, panic attack, mood lability, agitation). Uncommonly visual Δ (blurred/diplopia), thrombocyto-/leukopenia, rash, alopecia, suicidal ideation, confusion, amnesia, paraesthesia, Δ LFTs. Rarely pancreatitis, LF, movement disorders, neutro-/pancytopenia, SJS/TEN.
Warn: to seek medical advice if depression/suicidality develop and not to discontinue drug abruptly against medical advice (risk of withdrawal syndrome).

Monitor: for signs of depression and/or suicidality.

Interactions: levels may be ↑ by probenecid (and other drugs affecting tubular secretion). fx potentially ↓ if taken <1 h after macrogol. Can ↑ methotrexate levels.

Dose: initially 250 mg od to 500 mg bd po/IV, ↑ing slowly[BNF/SPC] to max 1.5 g bd po/iv. *NB: consider ↓dose in elderly or if LF or RF.*[BNF/SPC]

LEVOBUNOLOL

β-blocker eye drops: similar to timolol ⇒ ↓aqueous humour production. *Significant systemic absorption can occur.*
Use: chronic simple (wide-/open-angle) glaucoma.
CI/Caution/Interactions: as propranolol; interactions less likely; corneal disease is caution.
SE: local reactions. Rarely anterior uveitis and anaphylaxis. Can ⇒ systemic fx, esp bronchoconstriction/cardiac fx; see Propranolol.
Dose: 1 drop of 0.5% solution od/bd.

LEVOMEPROMAZINE (= METHOTRIMEPRAZINE)

Phenothiazine antipsychotic; as chlorpromazine, but used in palliative care, as has good antiemetic and sedative fx but little respiratory depression.
Use: refractory N&V or restlessness/distress in the terminally ill; also licensed for schizophrenia.
CI/Caution/SE/Interactions: as chlorpromazine, but ↑risk of postural ↓BP (esp in elderly: do not give if age >50 years and ambulant) and ↑risk of seizures (caution if epilepsy/brain tumour). Also caution if FHx of ↑QTc.
Dose: 6.25–25 mg po/sc/im/iv od/bd (can ↑ to tds/qds), or 25–100 mg/24 h sc infusion. Oral dose is approx 50% bioavailable; for parenteral doses, give half the oral dose iv/im/sc. *NB: max dose for N&V is 25 mg/24 h and for restlessness/confusion >100 mg/24 h (under specialist). ↓Dose in elderly.*

LEVOTHYROXINE (= THYROXINE)

Synthetic T_4.

Use: $\downarrow T_4$ Rx (for maintenance). *NB:* acutely, e.g. myxoedema coma, liothyronine (T_3) often needed.

CI: $\uparrow T_4$, adrenal insufficiency.

Caution: panhypopituitarism/other predisposition to adrenal insufficiency (*corticosteroids needed first*), chronic $\downarrow T_4$, cardiovascular disorders (esp HTN/IHD; can worsen)*, DI, DM, P/B/E.

SE: features of $\uparrow T_4$ (should be minimal unless xs Rx): D&V, tremors, restlessness, headache, flushing, sweating, heat intolerance, angina, arrhythmias, palpitations, $\uparrow$HR, muscle cramps/weakness, $\downarrow$Wt. Also osteoporosis (esp if xs dose given; use min dose necessary).

Interactions: can Δ digoxin and antidiabetic** requirements, $\uparrow$fx of TCAs and $\downarrow$levels of propranolol. **W+**.

Monitor: baseline ECG to help distinguish Δs due to ischaemia or $\downarrow T_4$.

Dose: 25–200 micrograms mane (titrate up slowly, esp if >50 years old/$\downarrow\downarrow T_4$/HTN/IHD*).

LIOTHYRONINE (= L-TRI-IODOTHYRONINE) SODIUM

Synthetic T_3: quicker action than thyroxine (T_4).

Use: hypothyroidism (inc myxoedema coma*)[1]. Treatment-resistant depression (off-license)[2].

CI/Caution/SE/Interactions: see levothyroxine.

Dose: 10–20 micrograms/day, increase to 60 micrograms daily in 2–3 divided doses (iv doses available for myxoedema coma)[1]. 20–50 microgram/day po[2]. *NB:* 20 micrograms liothyronine = 100 micrograms (levo)thyroxine.

Concurrent hydrocortisone iv is often also needed.*

LIRAGLUTIDE/SAXENDA/VICTOZA

GLP-1 receptor agonist. Must be prescribed by brand name.

Use: T2DM[1] or adjunct in weight management if BMI ≥30 kg/m², or if BMI ≥27 kg/m² with ≥1 weight-related co-morbidity.[2]

CI: diabetic gastroparesis, IBD, concomitant use with other meds for weight, obesity 2° to endo or eating disorders, DKA, E/P/R.

Caution: Severe congestive heart failure, thyroid disease, **B/H**.
SE: fatigue, GI disturbance, gallbladder disorders, infection risk, insomnia, skin reactions, altered taste, toothache; pancreatitis, renal impairment, thyroid dysfunction.
Warn: reports of DKA when concomitant insulin is rapidly reduced or discontinued.
Interactions: caution with other meds which can ↓glucose.
Dose: Initially 0.6 mg od sc for at least 1 week, increased to 1.2 mg od for at least 1 week, then increased if necessary to 1.8 mg od[1]; initially 0.6 mg od sc, then increased in at ≥1-weekly steps of 0.6 mg, max maintenance dose 3 mg od. Discontinue if <5% weight loss after 12 wks at max dose.

LISINOPRIL

ACE-i; see Captopril.
Use: HTN[1], HF[2], Px of IHD post-MI[3], DM nephropathy[4].
CI/Caution/SE/Interactions: as captopril.
Dose: initially 10 mg od[1] (2.5–5 mg if RF or used with diuretic), ↑ing if necessary to max 80 mg/day; initially 2.5–5 mg od[2,4] adjusted to response to usual maintenance of 5–20 mg/day (max 35 mg/day[2]). Doses post-MI[3] depend on BP.[SPC/BNF] *NB: ↓dose in LF or RF.*

LITHIUM

Mood stabiliser: modulates intracellular signalling; blocks neuronal Ca^{2+} channels and changes GABA pathways.
Use: mania Rx/Px, bipolar disorder Px. Rarely for recurrent depression Px and aggressive/self-mutilating behaviour Rx.
CI: ↓T_4 (if untreated), Addison's, SSS, dehydration, cardiovascular disease, **R/H/B**.
(*NB:* manufacturers do not agree on definitive list and all CI are relative – decisions should be made in clinical context and expert help sought if unsure.)
Caution: thyroid disease, MG, epilepsy, ↑QTc, psoriasis (risk of exacerbation), **P** (⇒ Ebstein's anomaly: esp in first trimester) **E**.

SE: thirst, polyuria, GI upset ($\uparrow$Wt, N&V&D), *fine* tremor*. (*NB*: in toxicity $\Rightarrow$ *coarse* tremor), tardive dyskinesia, muscular weakness, acne, psoriasis exacerbation, $\uparrow$WCC, $\uparrow$Pt. Rarer but serious: $\downarrow$ (or $\uparrow$) T_4 $\pm$ goitre (esp in females), renal impairment (diabetes insipidus, interstitial nephritis), arrhythmias. Very rarely can $\Rightarrow$ neuroleptic malignant syndrome.

Warn: report symptoms of $\downarrow$$T_4$, avoid dehydration/salt depletion/ abrupt withdrawal.

Monitor: serum levels *12 h post-dose:* keep at 0.6–1 mmol/L (>1.5 mmol/L may $\Rightarrow$ toxicity, esp if elderly), U&Es, TFTs, cardiac function.

Interactions: toxicity ($\pm$ levels) $\uparrow$d by **NSAIDs, diuretics**** (esp thiazides), SSRIs, ACE-i, ARBs, amiodarone, methyldopa, carbamazepine and haloperidol. Theophyllines, caffeine and antacids may $\downarrow$lithium levels.

Dose: see SPC/BNF: two *types* (salts) available with different doses ('carbonate' 200 mg = 'citrate' 509 mg) and bioavailabilities of particular *brands* vary $\therefore$ *must specify salt and brand required*. For 'carbonate', starting dose usually 400 mg nocte (200 mg in elderly), adjusting to plasma levels (maintenance usually 600 mg–1 g nocte). *NB:* $\downarrow$**dose in RF.**

> Consider stopping 24 h before major surgery or ECT; restart once e'lytes return to normal. Discuss with anaesthetist $\pm$ psychiatrist.

Lithium toxicity
Features: D&V, coarse tremor*, cerebellar signs, renal impairment/oliguria, $\downarrow$BP, $\uparrow$reflexes, convulsions, drowsiness $\Rightarrow$ coma, arrhythmia. *Rx:* stop drug, control seizures, correct electrolytes (normally need saline ivi; high risk if $\uparrow$Na$^+$: avoid low-salt diets and diuretics**). Consider haemodialysis if RF.

LOFEPRAMINE
TCA.
Use: depression.
CI/Caution/SE/Warn/Monitor/Interactions: as amitriptyline but

also **R** (if severe). Also ⇒ ↓**sedation** (sometimes alerting – do not give nocte if occurs) and ↓**anticholinergic and cardiac SEs** ∴ ↓*danger in od*.
Dose: 140–210 mg daily in divided (bd/tds) doses (consider ↓dose in elderly).

LOFEXIDINE HYDROCHLORIDE

α_2-adrenergic receptor agonist ⇒ ↓noradrenaline release.
Use: symptomatic relief of opioid withdrawal.
Caution: ↓BP/HR, risk factors for ↑QTc, coronary artery disease, cerebrovascular disease, depression, metabolic Δs.
SE: drowsiness, cardiac fx (↓BP, ↓HR), mucosal dryness, ↑QTc.
Warn: withdraw gradually over 2–4 days+ to ↓risk of rebound HTN.
Monitor: pulse, BP at initiation, for at least 72 h/until stable dose achieved, and on discontinuation.
Interactions: ↑risk of ↑QTc with amifampridine, amiodarone, amisulpride, apomorphine, clari-/erythromycin, clopamide, (es)citalopram, fluconazole, haloperidol; ↑risk of ↓K⁺ (↑risk of torsade de pointes) with aminophylline, corticosteroids, bendroflumethiazide, fludrocortisone, furosemide, ↑CNS depressive fx of alcohol, barbiturates, other sedatives; ↑fx of antihypertensives; ↓fx with TCA.
Dose: initially 800 microgram po od in divided doses, ↑ in steps of 400–800 microgram od, max 800 microgram per dose, max 2.4 mg od, duration of 7–10 days if no opioid use.

LOPERAMIDE

Antimotility agent: synthetic opioid analogue; binds to receptors in GI muscle ⇒ ↓peristalsis, ↑transit time, ↑H_2O/electrolyte resorption, ↓gut secretions, ↑sphincter tone. Extensive first-pass metabolism ⇒ minimal systemic opioid fx.
Use: acute diarrhoea[1], chronic diarrhoea[2], pain in bowel colic in palliative care[3].
CI: constipation, ileus, megacolon, bacterial enterocolitis 2° to invasive organisms (e.g. salmonella, *Shigella, Campylobacter*), abdo distension, active UC/AAC, pseudomembranous colitis.

Caution: in young (can $\Rightarrow$ fluid + electrolyte depletion). *Reports of serious cardiovascular events (such as $\uparrow QTc$, torsades de pointes, and cardiac arrest), including fatalities, with $\uparrow$ doses of loperamide associated with abuse or misuse.* L/P/B.

SE: headache, constipation, nausea, flatulence, abdo cramps, bloating, dizziness, drowsiness, fatigue. Rarely hypersensitivity (esp skin reactions), paralytic ileus.

Dose: initially 4 mg, then 2 mg after each loose stool (max 16 mg/day for 5 days[1]), 4–8 mg in divided doses, up to 8 mg bd[2], 2–4 mg qds[3]. *NB: can mask serious GI conditions.*

LORATADINE

Non-sedating antihistamine: see Cetirizine.

Caution: L/P/B.

Dose: 10 mg od. Non-proprietary or as Clarityn.

LORAZEPAM

Benzodiazepine, short-acting.

Use: sedation[1] (esp acute behavioural disturbance/Ψ disorders, e.g. acute psychosis), status epilepticus[2]; used off-label for catatonia, anxiety, insomnia, panic attacks, alcohol withdrawal in liver impairment.

CI/Caution/SE/Interactions: see Diazepam. Do not give im within 1 h of im olanzapine.

Dose: 500 micrograms–2 mg po/im/iv prn (bottom of this range if elderly/respiratory disease/naive to benzodiazepines; top of range if young/recent exposure to benzodiazepines; max 4 mg/day)[1]; 4 mg stat, then 4 mg after 5–10 mins if required[2]. *NB: ↓dose in RF/LF.*

☠ Beware respiratory depression if used in combination with other substances which reduce respiratory drive. ☠

LOSARTAN

Angiotensin II receptor antagonist: specifically blocks renin-angiotensin system $\therefore$ does not inhibit bradykinin and $\Rightarrow$ dry cough.

Use: HTN[1], type 2 DM nephropathy[2] (if ACE-i not tolerated*), chronic HF when ACE-i unsuitable/CI[3].

CI: L(if severe)/H (if severe)/P/B, combination with aliskiren in eGFR <60 mL/min/1.73 m² or in DM.

Caution: RAS, HOCM, mitral/aortic stenosis, if taking drugs that ↑K⁺**, 1° hyperaldosteronism (may not benefit), Hx of angioedema, L/R/E.

SE/Interactions: as captopril, but ↓dry cough (major reason for ACE-i intolerance*). As with ACE-i, can ⇒ ↑K⁺ (esp if taking ↑K⁺-sparing diuretics/salt substitutes or if RF).

Dose: initially 25–50 mg od (↑ing to max 100 mg od)[1,2]; 12.5 mg od (↑ing to max 150 mg od)[3]. *NB:* ↓**dose in LF or RF.**

> ☠ ****Beware if on other drugs that ↑K⁺, e.g. amiloride, spironolactone, triamterene, ACE-i and ciclosporin. Do not give with oral K⁺ supplements (inc dietary salt substitutes).** ☠

LOXAPINE

Typical antipsychotic, D_2 and 5-HT$_{2A}$ receptor antagonist. Structurally related to clozapine.

Use: acute agitation in psychosis or mania.

CI: acute respiratory symptoms, asthma, CVD, cerebrovascular disease, COPD, dehydration/hypovolaemia, BPSD, **E**.

Caution: Parkinson's, ↑QTc (although ↓than most antipsychotics), epilepsy, MG, glaucoma (angle-closure), ↑prostate, severe respiratory disease, jaundice, blood disorders, DM, bronchospasm (have bronchodilator to hand), Hx of EPSEs.

SE: agitation, amenorrhoea, arrhythmias, constipation, dizziness/postural hypotension, drowsiness/fatigue, dry mouth; erectile dysfunction, galactorrhoea, gynaecomastia, ↑BM, ↑prolactin, insomnia, neutro/leucopoenia, EPSEs/parkinsonism, rigidity, ↑QT, rash, seizure, urinary retention, vomiting, ↑weight. Uncommon: agranulocytosis, confusion, thrombosis, NMS. Rare: sudden death.

Interactions: drugs with antimuscarinic, hypotensive and/or sedative effects.
Dose: 4.5 or 9.1 mg inhaled, repeat after 2 h prn.

LURASIDONE

Antipsychotic: D_2, D_3, 5-HT$_{2A}$, 5-HT$_7$ antagonist, α_{2C}-antagonist, 5-HT$_{1A}$ partial agonist
Use: Schizophrenia
CI: Co-administration with strong CYP3A4 inhibitors and inducers
Caution: L/R/P/B/E.
Class SE: EPSE, ↑prolactin and assoc Sx, sedation, ↑Wt, ↑QTc, VTE, blood dyscrasias, ↓seizure threshold, NMS.
Specific SE: Anxiety, drooling, GI Sx, MSK Sx, pruritus, disturbed sleep, dysuria, hyperhidrosis, HTN, ↓Na, angioedema, rhabdomyolysis.
Monitoring: BG* (± HbA1C) after 1 month then 4–6 monthly. LFTs, U&Es, FBC, prolactin (CK only if NMS suspected). Wt and lipids every 3 months for 1 year, then at least annually.
Interactions: *must be taken with food (or exposure much lower)*; metab by CYP3A4 ∴ levels ↑d by many, e.g. clarithromycin, ketoconazole; levels ↓d by many, e.g. carbamazepine, phenytoin, St John's wort
Dose: Initially 37 mg od, ↑ up to 148 mg od (halve doses if taken with moderate CYP3A4 inhibitors e.g.
diltiazem, erythromycin, fluconazole, and verapamil).

When co-administered with mild or moderate CYP3A4 inducers, carefully monitor efficacy and adjust doses accordingly.

LYMECYCLINE

Tetracycline, broad-spectrum antibiotic (see Tetracycline).
Use: consult local guidance on antibiotic choice.
CI/Caution/SE/Interactions: as tetracycline.
Dose: 408 mg od for ≥8 wks (can ↑ to bd for other indications, and can be increased to 1.224–1.632 g in severe infections).

MEBEVERINE

Antispasmodic: direct action on GI muscle.
Use: GI smooth-muscle cramps (esp IBS, diverticulitis).
CI: ileus (paralytic).
Caution: porphyria, P/B.
SE: hypersensitivity/skin reactions.
Dose: 135 mg tds (20 min before food) or 200 mg bd of SR preparation.

MEFENAMIC ACID

NSAID; non-selective COX inhibitor.
Use: musculoskeletal pain (RA/osteoarthritis), post-op pain, dysmenorrhoea, menorrhagia.
CI/Caution/SE/Interactions: as ibuprofen, but also CI if IBD, caution if epilepsy or acute porphyria. Can ⇒ severe diarrhoea, skin reactions, stomatitis, paraesthesia, fatigue, haemolytic/aplastic ↓Hb, ↓Pt. Mild **W+**.
Dose: 500 mg tds.

MELATONIN

Tryptophan derivative; binds to melatonin receptors MT_1/MT_2.
Use: insomnia (short-term use).
Caution: autoimmune disease, risk of increased seizure frequency.
SE: arthralgia, ↑risk of infection, pain.
Interactions: ↑levels with fluvoxamine.
Dose: 2 mg po od taken with food 1–2 h before bedtime, for up to 13 wks. In adults with LD: initially 2 mg ON, increased if necessary to 4–6 mg ON; max 10 mg ON.

MEMANTINE

Glutamatergic NMDA receptor antagonist ⇒ ↓prolonged influx of Ca^{2+}, ↓neuronal excitotoxicity.
Use: moderate-to-severe Alzheimer's disease; oscillopsia in MS (unlicensed).
CI: **L**(if severe)/**R** (if eGFR <5 mL/min/1.73 m²).

Caution: seizures, epilepsy risk factors.
SE: dizziness, headache, constipation, somnolence, ↑BP, hypersensitivity, impaired balance, dyspnoea.
Interactions: ↑risk of CNS toxicity/SE with amantadine, ketamine.
Dose: initially 5 mg po od, ↑ in steps of 5 mg every wk, maintenance dose 20 mg od, max 20 mg od; different dosing in MS.

METFORMIN

Oral antidiabetic (biguanide): ⇒ ↑insulin sensitivity without affecting levels (⇒ ↓gluconeogenesis and ↓GI absorption of glucose and ↑peripheral use of glucose). Only active in presence of endogenous insulin (i.e. functional islet cells).
Use: type 2 DM[1]: usually first line if diet and exercise control unsuccessful (esp if obese, as ⇒ less ↑Wt than sulphonylureas). Also used in PCOS[2] (unlicensed; specialist use), antipsychotic-induced weight gain (unlicensed).
CI: DKA, ↑risk of lactic acidosis (e.g. RF, severe dehydration/infection/peripheral vascular disease, shock, major trauma, respiratory failure, alcohol dependence, recent MI*), **L/R/P/B**.
Caution: general anaesthetic** or iodine-containing radiology contrast media*, **H**.
SE: GI upset (esp initially or if ↑doses), taste disturbance. Rarely ↓vit B_{12} absorption, lactic acidosis† (stop drug).
Dose: initially 500 mg mane, ↑ing as required to max 2–3 g/day in divided doses. For MR tablets initially 500 mg daily, ↑ing as required to max 2 g daily in 1 dose[1]. 500 mg od up to 1.5–1.7 g/day in two to three divided doses[2]. *Take with meals.* NB: ↓dose in mild RF, avoid in **severe RF**.

> ☠ *In coronary angiography: stop drug on day of procedure (giving insulin if necessary) and restart 48 h later, having checked that renal function has not deteriorated. Stop on day of surgery ahead of general anaesthetic** and restart when renal function normal. ☠

METHADONE

Opioid agonist: ↓euphoria and long $T_{1/2}$ (⇒ ↓withdrawal symptoms) compared with other opioids.

Use: opioid dependence as aid to withdrawal, cough in palliative care, severe pain.

CI/Caution/SE/Interactions: as morphine, but levels ↓ by ritonavir, but are ↑ by voriconazole and cimetidine, and ↑risk of ventricular arrhythmias with atomoxetine and amisulpride. Can ↑QTc (caution if FHx of sudden death); ECG monitoring if risk factors for ↑QTc or dose >100 mg/day.

Dose: *individual requirements vary widely according to level of previous abuse:* sensible starting dose is 10–20 mg/day po, ↑ing by 10–20 mg every day until no signs or symptoms of withdrawal – which usually stop at 60–120 mg/day. Then aim to wean off gradually. Available as non-proprietary solutions (1 mg/mL) or as Methadose (10 or 20 mg/mL). Can give sc/im for severe pain. *NB:* ↓dose if LF, RF or elderly.

 Do not confuse solutions of different strengths.

METHYLPHENIDATE HYDROCHLORIDE

CNS stimulant; noradrenaline–dopamine reuptake inhibitor

Use: ADHD[1], narcolepsy[2].

CI: cardiac disease (but see p. 249), severe HTN, vasculitis, cerebrovascular disease, ↑thyroid, phaeo, some Ψ disorders (psychosis, severe depression, suicidal ideation, uncontrolled BPAD, anorexia), **H**.

Caution: tic disorder (or FHx), substance misuse, agitation, epilepsy, dysphagia, restricted GI lumen, glaucoma (angle-closure).

SE: ↓sleep, anxiety, headache, nasopharyngitis, ↓appetite, ↓growth in Ht and Wt, agitation, Δ mood, movement disorder, paraesthesia, visual problems, dizziness, **cardiac fx** (arrhythmia, ↑HR, ↑BP), GI upset, ↑LFTs, alopecia, rash, arthralgia, muscle spasm, sexual dysfunction, pyrexia, fatigue.

Warn: discuss with patients regarding 'drug holidays', which are commonly used and safe.

Monitor: pulse, BP, psychiatric symptoms, appetite, Wt and Ht at initiation of therapy, following each dose adjustment and every 6 months thereafter.

Interactions: 💀 ↑risk of hypertensive crisis with MAOIs & linezolid; ↑risk of dyskinesias with risperidone; ↓fx of apraclonidine.

Dose: specify brand on prescription, as MR preparations can have different fx and $t_{1/2}$. Initially 18 mg po od in morning, adjusted at wkly intervals, max 108 mg od[1]; 10–60 mg po od in divided doses; usual dose 20–30 mg od in divided doses before meals[2].

METHYLPREDNISOLONE

Glucocorticoid (mild mineralocorticoid activity).

Use: acute flares of inflammatory diseases (esp rheumatoid arthritis, MS), cerebral oedema, Rx of graft rejection.

CI/Caution/SE/Interactions: see prednisolone.

Dose: wide dose range, 20–500 mg po od; iv dosing also available. Consult BNF.

METOCLOPRAMIDE

Antiemetic: D_2 antagonist: acts on central chemoreceptor trigger zone and directly stimulates GI tract (⇒ ↑motility).

Use: N&V, hiccup in palliative care, acute migraine (indications now restricted due to risk of extrapyramidal fx[BNF/SPC]).

CI: GI obstruction/perforation/haemorrhage (inc 3–4 days post-GI surgery), phaeo, **B**.

Caution: epilepsy, porphyria, asthma, atopy, bradycardia, cardiac condition disturbance, children, Parkinson's disease, electrolyte imbalance, **L/R/P/E**.

SE: extrapyramidal fx (see p. 389 – esp in elderly and young females: reversible if drug stopped within 24 h or with procyclidine), drowsiness, restlessness, GI upset, behavioural/mood Δs, ↑prolactin. Rarely skin reactions, NMS.

Interactions: ↑s risk of extrapyramidal fx of antipsychotics, SSRIs and TCAs.

Dose: 10 mg tds po/im/iv (max 500 micrograms/kg/day in three divided doses if Wt <60 kg* for 5 days). sc infusion: 30–100 mg/24 h. *NB:* ↓dose if RF, LF, 15–19 years old or Wt <60 kg*. Give iv doses over >3 min.

METRONIDAZOLE

Antibiotic, 'cidal': binds DNA of anaerobic (and microaerophilic) bacteria/protozoa.

Use: consult local guidance on antibiotic choice.

Caution: avoid with alcohol: drug metabolised to acetaldehyde and other toxins ⇒ flushing, abdo pain, ↓BP ('disulfiram-like' reaction), acute porphyria, avoid xs sun/UV light, **L/P/B**.

SE: GI upset (esp N&V), taste disturbed, skin reactions, blood disorders, seizures (transient), ataxia, **peripheral and central neuropathy** (if prolonged Rx).

Interactions: can ↑busulfan, lithium, 5-fluorouracil, ciclosporin and phenytoin levels, **W+**.

Dose: 500 mg tds ivi/400 mg tds po. Lower doses can be given po or higher doses pr (1 g bd/tds) according to indication.[SPC/BNF] *NB:* ↓dose in LF.

MIANSERIN HYDROCHLORIDE

Tetracyclic antidepressant; blocks presynaptic α-adrenoceptors, ↑NA release.

Use: depression.

CI: mania, porphyria, **L**.

Caution: some Ψ states (Hx BPAD/psychosis, ↑suicide risk), epilepsy, ↑prostatic/urinary retention, chronic constipation, DM, ↑thyroid, glaucoma (angle-closure)/↑IOP, phaeo, arrhythmia, post-MI, **P/R/H**.

SE: drowsiness, headache, tremor, blood dyscrasias, Ψ fx (Δ mood, psychosis, suicidality), breast abnormalities, postural ↓BP, rash, seizure, sexual dysfunction, withdrawal Sx, oedema, ↓Na⁺, arthralgia, jaundice.

Warn: If signs of infection, obtain urgent medical assistance.

M

Monitor: full blood count every 4 wks during first 3 months of treatment; monitor for signs of infection (e.g. fever, sore throat, stomatitis).

Interactions: ☠↑risk of toxicity with isocarboxazid, moclobemide, phenelzine, tranylcypromine (avoid with/for 14 days after stopping MAOI)☠; ↓fx of ephedrine.

Dose: initially 30–40 mg po od at bedtime/in divided doses; ↑ gradually, usual dose 30–90 mg.

MICONAZOLE

Imidazole antifungal (topical) but *systemic absorption can occur.*

Use: oral fungal infections[1], cutaneous fungal infections[2], fungal nail infections[3], vaginal and vulval candidiasis[4].

CI: L.

Caution: acute porphyria, P/B.

SE: GI upset. Rarely hypersensitivity, hepatotoxicity.

Interactions: as ketoconazole, but less commonly significant. **W+.**

Dose: 2.5 mL qds for >7 days[1]; apply bd for 10 days[2], 1–2 applications/24 h[3], 1 applicator/24 h for 7 days[4].

MIDAZOLAM

Very short-acting benzodiazepine: $GABA_A$ receptor positive allosteric modulator.

Use: sedation for stressful/painful procedures[1] (esp if amnesia desirable), agitation/distress in palliative care[2], status epilepticus[3].

CI/Caution/SE/Warn/Interactions: see diazepam.

Dose: Consult literature for iv doses[1,2]. Buccal midazolam licensed in children, but commonly used for adults and recommended by NICE (10 mg)[3]. *NB:* ↓dose in RF or elderly.

☠ Beware respiratory depression, esp if respiratory disease or given concurrently with other medications which reduce respiratory drive. ☠

MINOCYCLINE

Tetracycline antibiotic: inhibits ribosomal (30S subunit) protein synthesis; broadest spectrum of tetracyclines.

Use: consult local guidance on antibiotic choice.

CI/Caution/SE/Interactions: as tetracycline, but ↓bacterial resistance, although ↑risk of SLE and irreversible skin/body fluid discoloration. Can also use (with caution) in RF. Check hepatic toxicity every 3 months – discontinue if develops.

Dose: 100 mg od po (can ↑ to bd). Use for ≥6 wks in acne.

MIRTAZAPINE/ZISPIN

Antidepressant: noradrenaline and specific serotonergic antagonist (NASSA); specifically stimulates $5-HT_1$ receptors, antagonises $5-HT_{2C}/5-HT_3$ and central presynaptic α_2 receptors.

Use: depression.

CI/Caution/SE: as fluoxetine, but ⇒ ↓**sexual dysfunction**/GI upset, ↑**sedation** (esp during titration) and ↑**appetite/Wt**. Rarely, blood disorders (inc agranulocytosis), Δ LFTs, convulsions, myoclonus, oedema.

Warn: of initial sedation and to report signs of infection (esp sore throat, fever): stop drug and check FBC if concerned.

Interactions: artemether/lumefantrine and methylthioninium. ☠ Never give with, or ≤2 wks after, MAOIs. ☠

Dose: initially 15–30 mg nocte, ↑ing to 30 mg after 1–2 wks (max 45 mg/day). *NB: lower doses may be more sedating than higher doses.*

MOCLOBEMIDE

MAOI; selective, reversible inhibitor of monoamine oxidase A (MAO-A), ↓metabolism of monoamines, ↑NA, DA and 5-HT.

Use: depression[1], social anxiety disorder[2].

CI: delirium, phaeo.

Caution: ↑thyroid state, agitation, BPAD.

SE: Δ sleep, dizziness, headache, GI upset (N&D&C&V), dry mouth, agitation, paraesthesia, cardiac fx (↑QTc, ↓BP), rash. Rarely serotonin syndrome.

Warn: avoid large quantities of tyramine-rich foods (e.g. mature cheese, salami, pickled herring); withdrawal fx, worse if used for 8 wks+; ↓dose gradually over 4 wks+.

Interactions: ↑risk of severe toxic reaction with TCAs and mianserin; ↑risk of severe HTN with bupropion, ephedrine, isometheptene, lisdexamfetamine, methylphenidate, phenylephrine, reboxetine.

Dose: initially 300 mg po od taken after food in divided doses, usual dose 150–600 mg od[1]; initially 300 mg po od for 3 days, ↑ to 600 mg od in two divided doses continued for 8–12 wks[2].

MODAFINIL

Stimulant; dopamine reuptake inhibitor.

Use: excessive daytime sleepiness in narcolepsy, used off-label for fatigue.

CI: arrythmia, cor pulmonale, left ventricular hypertrophy, stimulant-induced mitral valve prolapse, moderate-to-severe HTN (if uncontrolled), **P/B**.

Caution: Hx of substance misuse/psychosis/mania/depression.

SE: headache, ↓appetite, ↓sleep, Ψ Sx (agitation, depression, confusion), paraesthesia, visual problems, cardiac fx (↑HR, arrhythmia, vasodilatation, chest pain), GI upset (N&D&C&abdo pain), ↑LFTs.

Monitor: ECG before initiation; monitor BP & HR if known HTN.

Interactions: ↑P450 (**CYP1A2, CYP3A4, CYP2B6**), ↓P450 (**CYP2C9, CYP2C19**); ↓fx of COCP, desogestrel, etonogestrel, levonorgestrel, norethisterone, ulipristal; ↓levels of bosutinib, voxilaprevir.

Dose: initially 200 mg po od taken in the morning/in two divided doses taken in the morning and at noon, ↑ to 200–400 mg od/in two divided doses.

MOMETASONE FUROATE

Potent corticosteroid. Comes in cream, inhalator and nasal spray forms.

Use: inflammatory skin conditions, esp eczema[1], asthma prophylaxis[2], rhinitis[3].

CI: facial rosacea, acne, skin atrophy, perioral dermatitis, perianal and genital pruritis, untreated bacterial, fungal and viral skin infections, TB, syphilis, plaque psoriasis or post-vaccine reactions.
SE: skin atrophy, worsening of infections, acne.
Dose: apply thinly od top (use 'ointment' in dry skin conditions).

MONTELUKAST

Leukotriene receptor antagonist: ↓s Ag-induced bronchoconstriction.
Use: *non-acute* asthma, esp if large exercise-induced component or assoc seasonal allergic rhinitis.
Caution: acute asthma, eosinophilic granulomatosis with polyangiitis, **P/B**.
SE: headache, GI upset, myalgia, URTI, dry mouth/thirst. Rarely eosinophilic granulomatosis with polyangiitis: asthma (± rhin-/sinusitis) with systemic vasculitis and ↑EØ*.
Monitor: for development of vasculitic (purpuric/non-blanching) rash, peripheral neuropathy, ↑respiratory/cardiac symptoms: all signs of possible eosinophilic granulomatosis with polyangiitis; neuropsychiatric reactions.[SPC]
Dose: 10 mg nocte (↓doses if <15 years old[SPC/BNF]).

MORPHINE (SULPHATE)

Opiate analgesic.
Use: pain (inc post-op)[1], palliative care (pain and cough)[2], AMI[3] and acute LVF[4].
CI: acute respiratory depression, acute severe obstructive airways disease, ↑risk of paralytic ileus, delayed gastric emptying, biliary colic, acute alcoholism, ↑ICP/head injury (respiratory depression ⇒ CO_2 retention and cerebral vasodilation ⇒ ↑ICP), phaeo, **H** (if 2° to chronic lung disease).
Caution: ↓respiratory reserve, obstructive airways disease, ↓BP/shock, acute abdo, biliary tract disorders (*NB:* biliary colic is CI), pancreatitis, bowel obstruction, IBD, ↑prostate/urethral stricture, arrhythmias, ↓T_4, adrenocorticoid insufficiency, MG, **L** (can ⇒ coma), **R/P/B/E**.

SE: N&V (and other GI disturbance), constipation* (can ⇒ ileus), respiratory depression, ↓BP (inc orthostatic. *NB*: rarely ⇒ ↑BP), ↓/↑HR, pulmonary oedema, oedema, bronchospasm, ↓cough reflex, sedation, urinary retention, RF, biliary tract spasm, ↑pancreatitis, Δ LFTs, hypothermia, muscle rigidity/fasciculation/myoclonus, ↑ICP, dry mouth, vertigo, syncope, headache, miosis, sensory disturbance, pruritis, anorexia, allodynia, mood Δs (↑ or ↓), delirium, hallucinations, restlessness, seizures (at ↑doses), rhabdomyolysis, amenorrhoea, ↓libido, dependence. Rarely skin reactions.

Interactions: 💀 MAOIs (do not give within 2 wks of discontinuing). 💀 Levels ↓ by ritonavir and rifampicin. ↓s levels of ciprofloxacin. ↑sedative fx with antihistamines, baclofen, alcohol (also ⇒ ↓BP), TCAs, antipsychotics (also ↓BP), anxiolytics, hypnotics, barbiturates and moclobemide (also ⇒ ↑/↓BP). ↑s fx of sodium oxybate, gabapentin.

Dose: 5–10 mg po or 5–20 mg sc/im 4 hourly[1]; 2.5–15 mg iv up to 4 hourly (2 mg/min)[2]; 5–10 mg iv (1–2 mg/min), repeated if necessary[3]; 5–10 mg iv (2 mg/min)[4]. **Chronic pain:** use po as Oramorph solution or as MST Continus, Morphgesic, MXL, Sevredol or Zomorph tablets. Dose adjustment may be required when switching brands. Also available pr as suppositories of 10, 15, 20 and 30 mg giving 15–30 mg up to 4 hrly. *Unless short-term Rx, always consider laxative Px*.* **Cough in palliative care:** 5 mg po 4 hrly. Can ↑doses and frequency with expert supervision. Always adjust dose to response. *NB*: ↓dose if LF, RF or elderly.

💀 If ↓BMI or elderly, titrate dose up slowly, monitor O_2 sats and have naloxone ± resuscitation trolley at hand. 💀

MST CONTINUS Oral morphine (sulphate), equivalent in efficacy to Oramorph but SR: dose every 12 h. Need to specify if *tablets* (5, 10, 15, 30, 60, 100 or 200 mg) or *suspension* (sachets of 20, 30, 60, 100 or 200 mg to be mixed with water). prn doses for 'breakthrough pain' often needed.

MUPIROCIN/BACTROBAN

Topical antibiotic for bacterial infections (esp eradication of nasal MRSA carriage); available as nasal ointment (applied bd/tds) or as cream/ointment (tds for up to 10 days).

Local MRSA eradication protocols often exist; if not, then a sensible regimen is to give for 5 days and then swab 2 days later, repeating regimen if culture still positive.

NALMEFENE

Inverse agonist of the μ-opioid receptor.

Use: aids slow ↓drinking in alcohol dependence, particularly those w/o risk of physical withdrawal.

CI: Hx of acute alcohol withdrawal, current opioid use.

Caution: use >1 year, seizures.

SE: ↓appetite, weakness/drowsiness, impaired concentration, confusion, diarrhoea, dizziness, drowsiness, dry mouth, headache, hyperhidrosis, ↓ libido, muscle spasms, nausea/vomiting, restlessness, sleep disorders, palpitations, tachycardia, tremor, ↓weight. Frequency unknown: dissociation, hallucinations.

Dose: 18 mg od, preferably 1–2 h before drinking; max 18 mg/day.

NALOXONE

Opioid receptor antagonist for opioid reversal if od or over-Rx.

Caution: CVD, cardiotoxic, physical dependence on opioids, drugs; maternal chronic opioid use (risk of acute withdrawal in newborn); palliative care (risk of returning pain and acute withdrawal); postoperative use (risk of returning pain); **H**.

Dose: 400 micrograms–2 mg IV (or SC/IM), much larger doses may be needed for certain opioids (e.g. tramadol), repeating after 2 min if no response (or ↑ing if severe poisoning). *NB:* may need to start at 100–200 micrograms if risk of acute withdrawal or when continued therapeutic effect is required (e.g. post-op, palliative care); *short-acting:* may need repeating every 2–3 min (to total 10 mg) then review and consider IVI (10 mg made up to 50 mL with iv fluids; useful start rate is 60% of initial dose over 1 h, then adjusted to response).

NALTREXONE
Opioid antagonist: ↓s euphoria of opioids if dependence and ↓s craving and relapse rate in both opioid and alcohol dependence.
Use: opioid and alcohol dependence relapse prevention.
CI: if still taking opioids (can precipitate withdrawal), **L** (inc acute hepatitis), severe **R/B**.
Caution: **P**.
SE: GI upset, hepatotoxicity, sleep and Δ mood.
Warn: patient trying to overcome opiate blockade by overdosing can ⇒ acute intoxication.
Monitor: LFTs.
Dose: initial dose 25 mg od po, thereafter, 50 mg od (or 350 mg per wk split into 2 × 100 mg and 1 × 150 mg doses in opioid use disorder); specialist use only.

NB: also ↓s fx of opioid analgesics.

NAPROXEN
NSAID; non-selective COX inhibitor.
Use: rheumatic disease[1]; acute musculoskeletal pain and dysmenorrhoea[2]; acute gout[3].
CI/Caution/SE/Interactions: as ibuprofen, but somewhat ↑SEs, notably, ↑risk PU/GI bleeds. Lowest thrombotic risk of any NSAID. Probenecid ⇒ ↑serum levels. Mild **W+**.
Dose: 500 mg–1 g daily in one to two divided doses[1]; 500 mg initially then 250 mg 6–8 hrly (max 1.25 g/day)[2]; 750 mg initially then 250 mg 8 hrly until attack passed[3]. *NB*: avoid or ↓dose in RF and consider gastroprotective Rx.

NICOTINE/NICORETTE, NICOTINELL, NIQUITIN
Nicotinic acetylcholine receptor agonist.
Use: nicotine replacement therapy.
Caution: diabetes, **haemodynamically unstable** with CVA/MI/ arrhythmia, uncontrolled ↑thyroid, phaeo; **inhalation:** obstructive airway disease, bronchospasm; **intranasal:** asthma; **oral:** dentures, GORD; **transdermal:** skin disease, avoid placing on damaged skin.

SE: dizziness, headache, GI upset (N, gastritis), skin reactions; **inhalation:** cough, throat irritation, dry mouth; **intranasal:** nasal irritation (short-lived); **oral:** jaw ache, ↑saliva, throat irritation, denture damage (rare); **sublingual:** irritation to mouth/throat; **transdermal:** local skin reactions.

Warn: acidic beverages (coffee, fruit juice) ↓absorption of nicotine through buccal mucosa (avoid for 15 min before use of oral NRT).

Monitor: diabetes – blood glucose when initiating.

Dose: Refer to table on page 335.

NIFEDIPINE

Ca^{2+} channel blocker (dihydropyridine): dilates smooth muscle, esp arteries (inc coronaries). Reflex sympathetic drive ⇒ ↓HR and ↑contractility ∴ ⇒ ↓HF cf other Ca^{2+} channel blockers (e.g. verapamil, and to a lesser degree diltiazem), which ⇒ ↓HR + ↓contractility. Also diuretic fx.

Use: angina Px[1], HTN[2], Raynaud's[3].

CI: cardiogenic shock, clinically significant aortic stenosis, ACS (inc within 1 month of MI), acute/unstable angina, co-Rx with rifampicin (↓fx of nifedipine*).

Caution: angina or LVF can worsen (consider stopping drug), ↓BP, DM, BPH, acute porphyria, **L/H/P/B/E**.

SE: flushing, headache, ankle oedema, dizziness, ↓BP, palpitations, poly-/nocturia, rash/pruritus, GI upset, weakness, myalgia, arthralgia, gum hyperplasia, rhinitis. Rarely PU, hepatotoxicity.

Interactions: metab by **P450 3A4**. ↑s fx of digoxin, theophylline and tacrolimus. ↓s fx of quinidine. Quinu-/dalfopristin, ritonavir and grapefruit juice ↑fx of nifedipine. Rifampicin*, phenytoin and carbamazepine ↓fx of nifedipine. Risk of ↓↓BP with α-blockers, β-blockers or Mg^{2+} iv/im.

Dose: 5–20 mg tds po[3]; 10 mg bd or 20 mg od starting dose[1,2] (extended-release prep can start at 30 mg) titrating to max 90 mg od using long-acting preparations for HTN/angina, as normal-release preparations ⇒ erratic BP control and reflex ↑HR, which can worsen IHD (e.g. Adalat LA or Retard and many others with differing fx and doses[SPC/BNF]). *NB:* ↓dose if severe LF.

L/R/H = Liver, Renal and Heart failure. **E** = elderly. **P** = pregnancy. **B** = breastfeeding.

NITRAZEPAM

Long-acting benzodiazepine.

Use: insomnia (short-term use).

CI: respiratory depression, severe muscle weakness inc unstable MG, sleep apnoea, acute pulmonary insufficiency, chronic psychosis, depression (do not give nitrazepam alone).

Caution: respiratory disease, muscle weakness (inc MG), Hx of drug/alcohol abuse, personality disorder, porphyria, ↓albumin **L/R/P/B/E**. Do not stop suddenly.

Class SE: respiratory depression (rarely apnoea), drowsiness, dependence. Also ataxia, amnesia, headache, vertigo, GI upset, jaundice, ↓BP, ↓HR, visual/libido/urinary disturbances, blood disorders, paradoxical disinhibition in Ψ disorder.

Specific SE: movement disorders.

Warn: ↑fx of alcohol; occasional paradoxical agitation.

Interactions: ↑sedation with alcohol; ↑clearance with rifampicin.

Dose: 5–10 mg po od at bedtime.

☠ Overdose ⇒ **respiratory depression**, sedation and ataxia. ☠

NITROFURANTOIN

Antibiotic: only active in urine (no systemic antibacterial fx).

Use: UTIs (but not pyelonephritis).

CI: G6PD deficiency, acute porphyria, **R** (if eGFR <45 mL/min; also ⇒ ↓activity of drug, as needs concentrating in urine), infants <3 years old, **P/B**.

Caution: DM, lung disease, ↓Hb, ↓vit B, ↓folate, electrolyte imbalance, susceptibility to peripheral neuropathy, **L/E**.

SE: GI upset, pulmonary reactions (inc effusions, fibrosis), peripheral neuropathy, hypersensitivity. Rarely, hepatotoxicity, cholestasis, pancreatitis, arthralgia, alopecia (transient), skin reactions (esp exfoliative dermatitis), blood disorders, BIH.

Dose: 50 mg qds po (↑ to 100 mg if severe chronic recurrent infection) or 100 mg bd (MR preparation); 50–100 mg od nocte if for Px. *Take with food*. Not available iv or im.

NB: can ⇒ false-positive urine dipstick for glucose and discolour urine.

NORETHISTERONE

Progestogen (testosterone analogue).

Use: endometriosis[1], dysfunctional uterine bleeding and menorrhagia[2], dysmenorrhoea[3], postponement of menstruation[4], breast Ca[5], contraception[6].

CI: liver/genital/breast cancers (unless progestogens being used for these conditions), atherosclerosis, undiagnosed vaginal bleeding, acute porphyria, Hx of idiopathic jaundice, severe pruritis, pemphigoid or severe pruritus during pregnancy.

Caution: risk of fluid retention, ↑susceptibility to TE disease, DM, epilepsy, migraine, HTN, depression, acute impairment of vision, L/H/R.

SE: menstrual cycle irregularities, ↑Wt, nausea, headache, dizziness, insomnia, drowsiness, breast tenderness, acne, depression, Δ libido, skin reactions, hirsutism and alopecia.

Interactions: metab by P450. fx ↓ by phenobarbital, phenytoin, carbamazepine, rifampicin, rifabutin, nevirapine, efavirenz, tetracyclines, ampicillin, oxacillin and cotrimoxazole. ↑s levels of ciclosporin.

Dose: 5 mg bd–tds po for ≥4–6 months, commencing on day 5 of cycle (can ↑ to max 25 mg/day if spotting occurs, ↓ing when stops)[1]; 5 mg tds po for 10 days for Rx (for Px: 5 mg bd po from day 19–26 of cycle)[2]; 5 mg tds po from day 5–24 for three to four cycles[3]; 5 mg tds po starting 3 days prior to expected menstruation onset (bleeding will commence 2–3 days after stopping)[4]; 40 mg od po[5]; 200 mg deep im injection within first 5 days of cycle or immediately after parturition *or* 350 micrograms po od at same time each day from day 1 of cycle[6].

NORTRIPTYLINE

TCA: blocks reuptake of NA (and 5-HT).

Use: depression[1], neuropathic pain (unlicensed)[2].

CI: recent MI (within 3 months), arrhythmias (esp HB), mania, L (if severe).

Caution: cardiac/thyroid disease, epilepsy, glaucoma

(angle- closure)/↑IOP, ↑prostate, phaeo, porphyria. Also Hx of mania, psychosis or urinary retention, **H/P/E**.

SE: antimuscarinic fx (see p. 387), **cardiac fx** (arrhythmias, HB, ↑HR, postural ↓BP, dizziness, syncope: **dangerous in od**), ↑**Wt**, **sedation** (often ⇒ 'hangover'), seizures, GI upset, sexual dysfunction. Rarely hypomania, psychosis, fever, blood disorders, hypersensitivity, Δ LFTs, ↓Na⁺ (esp in elderly), agitation, confusion, tinnitus, NMS, alopecia, gynaecomastia, ↑/↓BP, paralytic ileus, fracture, infection, movement disorders, oedema (inc testicular swelling), peripheral neuropathy, paraesthesia, Δ sleep, stroke, tremor.

Warn: withdrawal fx, worse after regular administration for 8 wks+; ↓dose gradually over 4 wks+; ↑fx of alcohol; dangerous in overdose.

Interactions: metab by P450 (CYP2D6); ☠ ↑**risk of severe toxic reaction with MAOIs (avoid with/for 14 days after stopping MAOI);** ☠ theoretical risk of serotonin syndrome with lithium; ↑fx of adrenaline, noradrenaline, phenylephrine; ↑levels with bupropion, cinacalcet, dronedarone, fluoxetine, paroxetine, terbinafine; ↓fx of ephedrine.

Dose: initiated at low dose, ↑ to 75–100 mg po od/in divided doses, max 150 mg od[1]; initially 10 mg po od taken at night, ↑ gradually to 75 mg od[2].

☠ TCA overdose ⇒ dilated pupils, arrhythmias, ↓BP, hypothermia, hyperreflexia, extensor plantar responses, seizures, respiratory depression and coma. ☠

NYSTATIN

Polyene antifungal.

Use: *Candida* infections: topically for skin/mucous membranes (esp mouth/vagina); po for GI infections (not absorbed).

SE: GI upset (at ↑doses), skin reactions.

Dose: po suspension: 100,000 units qds, usually for 1 wk, for Rx. *Give after food.*

OLANZAPINE/ZYPREXA

'Atypical' (second-generation) antipsychotic: D_1, D_2, D_4 and 5-HT$_2$, H_1 (+ mild muscarinic) antagonist.

Use: schizophrenia[NICE], mania, bipolar Px, acute sedation, anorexia nervosa (rarely, for inpatients).

CI: known risk of narrow-angle glaucoma. If giving im, acute MI/ ACS, ↓↓BP/HR, SSS or recent heart surgery.

Caution: as for other antipsychotics, plus BM suppression, ↓ leukocyte/neutrophil count, paralytic ileus, myeloproliferative disease, **H** (esp if Hx of cardiovascular disease/ ↑risk of CVA/ TIA) **B**.

Class SE: EPSE, ↑prolactin and assoc Sx, sedation, ↑Wt, ↑QTc, VTE, blood dyscrasias, ↓seizure threshold, NMS.

Specific SE: high propensity for ↑Wt, lipids, BG*. Anticholinergic fx. Rarely ↓NØ.

Monitor: BG* (± HbA$_{1C}$) after 1 month then 4–6 monthly. LFTs, U&Es, FBC, prolactin (and CK if NMS suspected). Wt and lipids every 3 months for 1 year, then at least annually. If giving im, closely monitor cardiorespiratory function for ≥4 h post-dose, esp if given other antipsychotic or benzodiazepine.

Interactions: metab by P450 (1A2) ∴ many, but most importantly, levels ↓d by carbamazepine and smoking. ↑risk of ↓NØ with valproate. Levels may be ↑d by ciprofloxacin, fluvoxamine. ↑risk of arrhythmias with drugs that ↑QTc. ↑risk of ↓BP with general anaesthetics and antihypertensives. ↓s fx of anticonvulsants.

Dose: 5–20 mg po nocte (consider 2.5 mg in the elderly). Available in 'melt' form if ↓compliance/swallowing (orodispersible). Available in quick-acting form for acute sedation; give 5–10 mg (2.5–5 mg in elderly) repeating 2 h later if necessary to max total daily dose, inc po doses, of 20 mg (max 3 injections/day for 3 days).

NB: avoid im doses concurrently with IM/IV benzodiazepines (↑risk of respiratory depression) which should be given ≥1 h later; if benzodiazepines already given, use with caution and closely monitor cardiorespiratory function.

L/R/H = Liver, Renal and Heart failure. **E** = elderly. **P** = pregnancy. **B** = breastfeeding.

NB: a depot formulation exists (olanzapine embonate) which is administered 2–4 wkly. ≥3 h post-dose monitoring by a HCP under medical supervision is required due to risk of rapid absorption: many organisations cannot facilitate this.

OLMESARTAN

Angiotensin II antagonist: see Losartan.
Use: HTN.
CI: biliary obstruction, **P/B**.
Caution/SE/Interactions: see Losartan.
Dose: initially 10 mg od, ↑ing to max 40 mg (20 mg in LF and RF).

OMEGA-3-ACID ETHYL ESTERS 90

Essential fatty acid combination: 1 g capsule = eicosapentaenoic acid 460 mg and docosahexaenoic acid 380 mg.
Use: adjunct to diet in type IIb and III ↑TG[1] (with statin) or type IV. Added for 2° prevention within 3 months of acute MI[2].
CI: **B**.
Caution: bleeding disorders, anticoagulants (↑bleeding time), **L/P**.
SE: GI upset; rarer: taste disorder, dizziness, hypersensitivity, hepatotoxicity, headache, rash, ↓BP, ↑BG.
Monitor: LFTs, INR.
Dose: Capsules: 2–4 g od[1]; 1 g od[2]. Take with food.

OMEPRAZOLE

PPI: inhibits H^+/K^+-ATPase of parietal cells ⇒ ↓acid secretion.
Use: PU Rx/Px (esp if on NSAIDs), GORD (if symptoms severe or complicated by haemorrhage/ulcers/stricture).[NICE] Also used for *H. pylori* eradication and ZE syndrome.
CI: avoid use with nelfinavir.
Caution: can mask symptoms of gastric Ca, B_{12} deficiency (may ↓absorption), severe ↓Mg^{2+} if Rx for >3 months, ↑risk of hip/wrist/spine fractures with ↑doses and long durations (>1 year),

particularly in elderly or presence of other risk factors, development of SCLE, **L/P/B**.

SE: GI upset, headache, dizziness, arthralgia, weakness, skin reactions. Rarely, hepatotoxicity, blood disorders, hypersensitivity.

Interactions: ↓ (and ↑) **P450** ∴ many, most importantly ↑s phenytoin, cilostazol, diazepam, raltegravir and digoxin levels. ↓s fx clopidogrel with high doses (80 mg/day), ↓s fx of ataza-/nelfi-/tipranavir, mild **W+**.

Dose: 20 mg od po, ↑ing to 40 mg in severe/resistant cases and ↓ing to 10 mg od for maintenance if symptoms stable; 20 mg bd for *H. pylori* eradication regimens. If unable to take po (e.g. perioperatively, ↓GCS, on ITU), give 40 mg iv od either over 5 min or as ivi over 20–30 min. In ZE syndrome: 60 mg od starting, maintenance dose of 20 mg od up to 120 mg/day in divided doses. *NB:* max dose 20 mg if LF.

NB: also specialist use iv for acute bleeds. Contact pharmacy ± GI team for advice on indications and exact dosing regimens.

ONDANSETRON

Antiemetic: 5-HT₃ antagonist: acts on central and GI receptors.

Use: N&V, esp if resistant to other Rx, post-operative or chemotherapy induced.

CI: congenital long QT syndrome.

Caution: GI obstruction (inc subacute), ↑QTc*, avoid if hereditary galactose intolerance (Lapp lactase deficiency or glucose-galactose malabsorption), **L** (unless mild), **P/B**.

SE: constipation, headache, dizziness. Rarely seizures, chest pain, ↓BP, Δ LFTs, rash, hypersensitivity.

Interactions: metab by **P450**. Levels ↓ by rifampicin, carbamazepine and phenytoin. ↓s fx of tramadol. Avoid with drugs that ↑QTc*.

Dose: 8 mg bd po; 16 mg od pr; 4–8 mg 2–8 hrly iv/im. Max 32 mg/day usually (8 mg/day if LF). Can also give as ivi at 1 mg/h for max of 24 h. Exact dose and route depend on indication.[SPC/BNF]

ORAMORPH

Oral morphine solution for severe pain, esp useful for prn or breakthrough pain.

Dose: multiply sc/im morphine dose by 2 to obtain approximately equivalent **Oramorph** dose. *NB:* ↓**dose if LF or RF.**

OXAZEPAM

Medium-acting benzodiazepine.

Use: anxiety (short-term use)[1], insomnia with anxiety[2].

CI: respiratory depression, severe muscle weakness inc unstable MG, sleep apnoea, acute pulmonary insufficiency, chronic psychosis, OCD, phobia, **L** (if severe).

Caution: respiratory disease, muscle weakness (inc MG), Hx of drug/alcohol abuse, personality disorder, porphyria, organic brain disease; liable to abuse, **L/R/P/B/E**.

SE: respiratory depression (rarely apnoea), drowsiness, dependence. Also ataxia, amnesia, headache, vertigo, GI upset, jaundice, cardiac fx (↓BP, ↓HR, syncope), visual/libido/urinary disturbances, blood dyscrasias, fever, oedema, paradoxical disinhibition in Ψ disorder.

Warn: ↑fx of alcohol; occasional paradoxical agitation.

Interactions: ↑sedation with alcohol.

Dose: 15–30 mg po tds/qds[1]; 15–25 mg od at bedtime, max 50 mg od[2].

OXYBUTYNIN

Anticholinergic (selective M3 antagonist); antispasmodic (↓s bladder muscle contractions).

Use: detrusor instability (also neurogenic bladder instability, nocturnal enuresis in paeds).

CI: bladder outflow or GI obstruction, urinary retention, severe UC/toxic megacolon, glaucoma (narrow angle), MG, **B**.

Caution: ↑prostate, Parkinson's, autonomic neuropathy, hiatus hernia (if reflux), ↑T_4, IHD, arrhythmias, porphyria, cognitive disorders, **L/R/H/P/E**.

SE: antimuscarinic fx (see p. 387), GI upset, palpitations/↑HR, skin reactions – mostly dose-related and reportedly less severe in MR preparations*.

Interactions: ↑anticholinergic SEs when co-Rx'd with other anticholinergic drugs, e.g. amantadine and other antiparkinsonian drugs, antihistamines, antipsychotics, TCAs, quinidine, digitalis, atropine.
Dose: initially 5 mg bd/tds po (2.5–3 mg bd if elderly), ↑ing if required to max of 5 mg qds (bd if elderly). Available as MR tablet (5–20 mg od) and transdermal patch (36 mg; releases 3.9 mg/day and lasts 3–4 days).

OXYCODONE (HYDROCHLORIDE)

Opioid for moderate-to-severe pain (esp in palliative care).
CI: acute respiratory depression, coma, head injury, ↑ ICP, acute abdo, delayed gastric emptying, chronic constipation, cor pulmonale, **L** (if moderate/severe).
Caution: ↓BP, respiratory diseases, IBD, MG, obstructive bowel disorders, ↑prostate, shock, urethral stenosis, **P/B**.
SE/Interactions: as morphine.
Dose: 4–6 hrly po/sc/iv or as sc infusion. *NB:* 1 mg iv/ sc = approximately 2 mg po. Available in immediate release (e.g. OxyNorm 4–6 hrly) or MR form as OxyContin (12 hrly). Available with naloxone (works locally to ↓GI SEs) as Targinact (12 hrly). *NB:* ↓dose if LF, RF or elderly.

OXYTETRACYCLINE

Tetracycline antibiotic: inhibits ribosomal protein synthesis.
Use: acne vulgaris (and rosacea).
CI/Caution/SE/Interactions: as tetracycline, plus caution in porphyria.
Dose: 500 mg bd po (1 h before food or on empty stomach).

PABRINEX

Parenteral (IV or IM) vitamins that come as a pair of vials.
Vial 1 contains B_1 (thiamine*), B_2 (riboflavin) and B_6 (pyridoxine).
Vial 2 contains C (ascorbic acid) and nicotinamide and glucose.
Use: acute vitamin deficiencies (esp thiamine*), risk of Wernicke's encephalopathy (e.g. malnourished or unwell)[1], severe depletion at risk of Wernicke's encephalopathy[2], psychosis following drug abuse or ECT, toxicity from acute infections[4], haemodialysis[5].

Caution: rarely ⇒ anaphylaxis (esp if given iv too quickly; should be given over ≥30 min). *Ensure access to resuscitation facilities.*
Dose: 1 pair od for 3–5 days[1,BAP], 2–3 pairs tds[2], 1 pair bd up to 7 days[3,4], 1 pair every 2 wks[5].

---

*See p. 254 for Wernicke's encephalopathy Px/Rx in alcohol withdrawal.

PALIPERIDONE
PO formulation. Active metabolite of risperidone, 9-hydroxyrisperidone; dopamine D_2 and 5-HT_{2A} antagonist with weak H_1 and $α_1/α_2$ antagonism.
Use: schizophrenia, psychotic or manic symptoms of schizoaffective disorder.
CI: R (if creatinine clearance <10 mL/min).
Caution: cataract surgery (risk of intraoperative floppy iris syndrome), GI obstruction risk, prolactin-dependent tumours, Parkinson's/Lewy body dementia, jaundice, ↑prostate, severe respiratory disease, glaucoma (angle-closure), **R/H/E** (with dementia or risk factors for stroke).
SE: EPSE, ↑prolactin, sedation, ↑Wt, ↑QTc, VTE, blood dyscrasias, ↓seizure threshold, NMS, insomnia.
Monitor: prolactin (see p. 186), physical health monitoring (CVD risk including Wt, BG, lipids) at least once/year.
Interactions: ↑risk of QT prolongation with class 1A and III antiarrhythmics (e.g. quinidine, disopyramide, amiodarone, sotalol), antihistamines, antibiotics (e.g. fluoroquinolones), antimalarials (e.g. mefloquine).
Dose: 6 mg po od in the morning, adjusted in steps of 3 mg over at least 5 days, usual dose 3–12 mg od.

PALIPERIDONE PALMITATE/XEPLION, TREVICTA
im formulation of paliperidone.
Use: maintenance of schizophrenia.
CI: R (if creatinine clearance <50 mL/min).

Caution/SE/Monitor/Interactions: see Paliperidone.
Warn: Trevicta detected in plasma up to 18 m after single dose.
Dose: *1-monthly Xeplion pre-filled syringes (for those previously responsive to paliperidone/risperidone):* 150 mg im for 1 dose on day 1, then 100 mg for 1 dose on day 8, administered into deltoid muscle. Maintenance dose 1 month after second loading dose. Dose adjusted at monthly intervals, maintenance normally 75 mg once a month. Following second dose, monthly maintenance doses administered into either deltoid/gluteal muscle.
3-monthly Trevicta pre-filled syringes (for those who are clinically stable on once-monthly im injection): initially 175–525 mg im every 3 months, administered into deltoid/gluteal, dose should be initiated in place of the next scheduled dose of monthly depot. *6-monthly Byannli pre-filled syringes (for those who are stable on 1-monthly or 3-monthly im injection):* 700–1000 mg every 6 months, administered into gluteal, dose should be initiated in place of the next scheduled dose of monthly depot (700 mg if on 100 mg 1-monthly or 250 mg 3-monthly, 1,000 mg if on 150 mg 1-monthly or 525 mg 3-monthly)

Approximate Equivalent Dosing[MPG]

po risperidone	po paliperidone	im fortnightly risperidone depot	im monthly paliperidone palmitate depot	im 3/12ly paliperidone palmitate depot
1 mg	Unclear	No equivalent	25 mg (unavailable in UK)	No equivalent
2 mg	Unclear	25 mg	50 mg	175 mg
3 mg	6 mg	37.5 mg	75 mg	263 mg
4 mg	9 mg	50 mg	100 mg	350 mg
5 mg	Unclear	Not licensed	No equivalent product	No equivalent product
6 mg	12 mg	Not licensed	150 mg	525 mg

L/R/H = Liver, Renal and Heart failure. E = elderly. P = pregnancy. B = breastfeeding.

(DISODIUM) PAMIDRONATE

Bisphosphonate: ↓s osteoclastic bone resorption.

Use: ↑Ca^{2+} (esp metastatic: also ↓s pain)[1], Paget's disease, myeloma.

CI: P/B.

Caution: Hx of thyroid surgery, cardiac disease, **L/R/H**.

SE: flu-like symptoms (inc fever, transient pyrexia), **GI upset** (inc haemorrhage), **dizziness/somnolence** (common post-dose*), ↑ (or ↓) **BP**, seizures, musculoskeletal pain, osteonecrosis of jaw (esp in cancer patients; consider dental examination or preventative Rx – MHRA advice), e'lyte Δs (↓po_4, ↓ or ↑K^+, ↑Na^+, ↓Mg^{2+}), RF, blood disorders.

Warn: not to drive/operate machinery immediately after Rx*.

Monitor: e'lytes (inc U&E before each dose), Ca^{2+}, po_4, before starting biphosphonate consider dental check, as risk of osteonecrosis of the jaw.

Dose: 15–90 mg ivi according to indication (± Ca^{2+} levels[1]). *NB: if RF, max rate of ivi 20 mg/h (unless for life-threatening ↑Ca^{2+}). Never given regularly for sustained periods.*

PANTOPRAZOLE

PPI; as omeprazole, but ↓interactions and can ⇒ ↑TGs.

Dose: 20–80 mg mane po 1 h before food (↓ing to 20 mg maintenance if symptoms allow). If unable to take po (e.g. perioperatively, ↓GCS, on ITU), can give 40 mg iv over ≥2 min (or as ivi) od. ↑doses if ZE syndrome.[SPC/BNF] *NB: ↓dose if RF or LF.*

PARACETAMOL

Antipyretic and mild analgesic. Unlike NSAIDs, *has no anti-inflammatory fx.*

Use: mild pain (or moderate/severe with other Rx), pyrexia.

Caution: alcohol dependence, **L** (CI if severe liver disease), **R**.

SE: *all rare:* rash, blood disorders, hepatic (rarely renal) failure – esp if over-Rx/od (for Mx, see p. 406).

Interactions: may **W+** if prolonged regular use.

Dose: 500 mg–1 g po/pr; 1 g (or 15 mg/kg if <50 kg) ivi. All doses 4–6 hrly, max 4 g/day (except max 3 g/day ivi in LF, dehydration, chronic alcoholism/malnutrition). Minimum iv dosing interval in RF (eGFR <30 mL/min) is 6 hrly.

PAROXETINE/SEROXAT

SSRI antidepressant; as fluoxetine, but $\downarrow\downarrow T_{1/2}$*.

Use: depression[1], social/generalised anxiety disorder[1], PTSD[1], panic disorder[2], OCD[3].

CI/Caution/SE: as fluoxetine, but ↓frequency of agitation/insomnia, although ↑frequency of **antimuscarinic fx**, **extrapyramidal fx** and **withdrawal fx**. Avoid if <18 years old, as may ↑suicide risk and hostility. Stop if patient enters manic phase. **P**.

Interactions: risk of serotonin syndrome with other serotonergic drugs; ↓P450 ∴ ↑levels of drugs primarily metabolised by CYP2D6 (e.g. pimozide, some TCAs, phenothiazine antipsychotics, risperidone, atomoxetine, propafenone, flecainide, metoprolol, **W+**). ↓fx of tamoxifen. ☠ ↑risk of bleeding with anticoagulants, antiplatelets, fibrinolytics. ↑fx of procyclidine.☠ P450 inhibitors may ⇒ ↑paroxetine levels, so ↓paroxetine dose. **Never give with, or ≤2 wks after, MAOIs;** do not give MAOIs within 1 wk of stopping paroxetine.

Dose: initially 20 mg[1,3] (10 mg[2]) mane, ↑ing if required to max 50 mg[1] or 60 mg[2,3]. Max 40 mg in elderly for all indications. *NB:* ↓dose if RF, LF.

> Taper down very slowly, as short $T_{1/2}$ ⇒ ↑risk of withdrawal syndrome.

PEPPERMINT OIL

Antispasmodic: direct relaxant of GI smooth muscle.

Use: GI muscle spasm, distension (esp IBS).

SE: perianal irritation, indigestion. Rarely rash or other allergy.

Dose: 1–2 capsules tds, before meals and with water.

PEPTAC

Alginate raft-forming oral suspension for acid reflux.
Dose: 10–20 mL after meals and at bedtime (*NB*: 3 mmol Na+/5 mL).

PERINDOPRIL ERBUMINE

ACE-i; see Captopril.
Use: HTN, HF, Px of IHD.
CI/Caution/SE/Monitor/Interactions: as captopril, plus can ⇒ mood/sleep Δs.
Dose: 2–8 mg od^{SPC/BNF}, starting at 2–4 mg od. *NB:* **consider ↓dose if RF, elderly, taking a diuretic, cardiac decompensation or volume depletion.**

PETHIDINE

Opioid; less potent than morphine but quicker action ⇒ ↑euphoria + ↑abuse/dependence potential ∴ not for chronic use, e.g. in palliative care.
Use: moderate/severe pain, obstetric and peri-op analgesia.
CI: acute respiratory depression, risk of ileus, ↑ICP/head injury/coma, phaeo.
Caution: any other condition where morphine CI/cautioned.
SE: as morphine, but ↓constipation.
Interactions: as morphine but 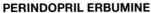 ↑risk of hyperpyrexia/CNS toxicity with **MAOIs**. 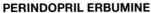 Ritonavir ⇒ ↑levels and ↑s toxic metabolites. May ↑serotonergic effects of duloxetine.
Dose: 25–100 mg up to 4 hrly im/sc (can give 2 hrly post-op or 1–3 hrly in labour with max 400 mg/24 h); 25–50 mg up to 4 hrly slow iv. Rarely used po: 50–150 mg up to 4 hrly. *NB:* ↓**dose if LF, RF or elderly.**

PHENELZINE

MAOI; non-selective and irreversible inhibitor of monoamine oxidase, ↑5-HT, NA and DA in CNS.
Use: depression.

CI: mania, cerebrovascular disease, Δ LFTs, phaeo, **L/H** ☠ interacting medication. ☠

Caution: agitation, blood dyscrasias, current ECT, DM, epilepsy, severe HTN due to drugs/foods, porphyria, surgery, P/B/E.

SE: dizziness, somnolence, fatigue, oedema, GI upset (N&V&C), antimuscarinic fx, postural ↓BP, twitching, ↑reflexes, ↑LFTs, sexual dysfunction, ☠ hypertensive crisis, ☠ mania.

Warn: avoid tyramine- or dopa-rich food/drinks with/for 2–3 wks after stopping MAOI, withdrawal fx may occur within 1–3 days of stopping treatment, ↓dose gradually over 4 wks+.

Monitor: BP (risk of postural ↓BP and HTN).

Interactions: ☠ ↑risk of severe toxic reaction with serotonergics, dopaminergics and noradrenergics: SSRIs, SNRIs, NARIs, TCAs (and related drugs), other MAOIs (inc for Parkinson's disease), carbamazepine, linezolid, triptans, pethidine, tramadol. ☠

- Do not start phenelzine until these drugs have been stopped and they have cleared: 5 wks for fluoxetine, 3 wks for clomipramine/imipramine, at least 7–14 days for other drugs.
- Wait 2 wks after stopping phenelzine before starting any of these medicines.

↑risk of hypertensive crisis with sympathomimetics, dopamine agonists, CNS stimulants, buspirone. ↑fx of CNS depressants, antimuscarinics, antidiabetics, antihypertensives.

Dose: initially 15 mg po tds, respond usually within first wk, ↑ after 2 wks to 15 mg qds (up to 30 mg tds may be used in inpatient); once satisfactory response achieved, ↓dose to lowest maintenance dose.

PHENOXYMETHYLPENICILLIN (= PENICILLIN V)

As benzylpenicillin (penicillin G) but active orally: used for ENT/skin infections (esp erysipelas), Px of rheumatic fever/S. *pneumoniae* infections (esp post-splenectomy).

Dose: 500 mg–1 g qds po (take on empty stomach; ≥1 h before food or ≥2 h after food).

PHENYTOIN

Antiepileptic: blocks Na^+ channels (stabilises neuronal membranes).

P

Use: all forms of epilepsy[1] (except absence seizures) inc status epilepticus[2].

CI: *if giving iv* (do not apply if po), sinus, ↓HR, Stokes-Adams syndrome, SAN block, second-/third-degree HB, acute porphyria.

Caution: porphyria ↓BP, **L/H/P** (⇒ cleft lip/palate, congenital heart disease), **B**.

SE (acute): *dose dependent*: **drowsiness** (also confusion/dizziness), **cerebellar fx, rash** (common cause of intolerance and rarely ⇒ SJS/TEN), N&V, diplopia, dyskinesia (esp orofacial). *If iv, risk of ↓BP, arrhythmias** (esp ↑QTc), **'purple glove syndrome'** (hand damage distal to injection site), CNS/respiratory depression.

SE (chronic): gum hypertrophy, coarse facies, hirsutism, acne, ↓folate (⇒ megaloblastic ↓Hb), Dupuytren's, peripheral neuropathy, osteomalacia. Rarely blood disorders, hepatotoxicity.

Warn: report immediately any rash, mouth ulcers, sore throat, fever, bruising, bleeding.

Monitor: FBC**, keep serum levels at 10–20 mg/L (narrow therapeutic index). ☠ If IV, closely monitor BP and ECG* (esp QTc). ☠

Interactions: metab by and ↑s P450 ∴ many; most importantly ↓s fx of OCP, doxycycline, Ca^{2+} antagonists (esp nifedipine), aripiprazole, mianserin, mirtazapine, paroxetine, TCAs and corticosteroids. fx ↓d by many, inc rifampicin, antipsychotics, TCAs and St John's wort. Levels ↑d by many, inc NSAIDs (esp azapropazone), fluoxetine, mi-/flu-/voriconazole, diltiazem, disulfiram, trimethoprim, cimetidine, omeprazole, amiodarone, metronidazole, chloramphenicol and topiramate (levels of which are also ↓d by phenytoin). Complex interactions with other antiseizure medications.[SPC/BNF] **W−** (or rarely **W+**).

Dose: po[1]: 150–500 mg/day in one to two divided doses.[SPC/BNF] iv[2]: load with 18 mg/kg ivi at max rate of 25–50 mg/min, then maintenance iv doses of approximately 100 mg tds/qds, adjusting to Wt, serum levels and clinical response. If available give iv as *fosphenytoin* (*NB*: doses differ). *NB*: ↓dose if LF.

☠ Stop drug if ↓WCC** is severe, worsening or symptomatic. Also, NHS improvement warning regarding risk of death due to errors with injectable phenytoin, also different bioequivalence of oral preparations, also non-linear pharmacokinetics and accumulation. ☠

PHOSPHATE ENEMA

Laxative enemas; ⇒ osmotic H_2O retention ⇒ ↑evacuation.

Use: severe constipation (unresponsive to other Rx).

CI: acute GI disorders.

Caution: if debilitated or neurological disorder, R/E.

SE: local irritation.

Dose: 1 prn usually no more than once a day.

PIMOZIDE

DA antagonist; antagonises D_2 receptor in CNS.

Use: schizophrenia[1]; delusional disorder, somatic type[2].

CI: arrhythmia, personal Hx/FHx of congenital ↑QTc, drugs that ↑QTc, phaeo, CNS depression.

Caution: Parkinson's, epilepsy, MG, glaucoma (angle-closure), ↑prostate, severe respiratory disease, jaundice, blood disorders, predisposition to postural ↓BP, photosensitivity, H.

SE: EPSE, ↑prolactin, sedation, ↑Wt, ↑QTc*, photosensitisation, VTE, blood dyscrasias, ↓seizure threshold, NMS, ↓appetite, depression, headache, hyperhidrosis, hypersalivation, sebaceous gland overactivity, urinary disorders, blurred vision.

Monitor: ECG before treatment and annually (review if QT prolonged)*.

Interactions: metab by P450 (CYP2D6, CYP3A4); ↑risk of QT prolongation* with drugs that ↑QTc (see p. 184); ↑CNS depression with alcohol, hypnotics, sedatives, strong analgesics; ↓fx of levodopa.

Dose: initially 2 mg po od, ↑ in steps of 2–4 mg at intervals of not <1 wk, usual dose 2–20 mg od[1]; initially 4 mg po od, ↑ in steps of 2–4 mg at intervals of not <1 wk, max 16 mg od[2].

PIOGLITAZONE

Thiazolidinedione (glitazone) antidiabetic; ↓s peripheral insulin resistance (and, to lesser extent, hepatic gluconeogenesis).

Use: type 2 DM (if metformin not tolerated).^{NICE}

CI: previous or active bladder cancer, uninvestigated macroscopic haematuria, **H** (inc Hx of), **L/P/B**.

Caution: concurrent use with insulin^{BNF} and peri-operative use in patients with CVD. **R**.

SE: oedema (esp if HTN/CCF), ↓**Hb**, ↑**Wt**, GI upset (esp diarrhoea), headache, hypoglycaemia (if also taking sulphonylureas), ↑risk of distal fractures, rarely **hepatotoxicity**.

Monitor: LFTs. ☠ *Discontinue if jaundice develops.* ☠ Signs of HF.

Interactions: levels ↓ by rifampicin and ↑ by gemfibrozil. NSAIDs and selective COX-2 inhibitors can ↑ oedema.

Dose: initially 15–30 mg od (max 45 mg od).

PIPOTIAZINE PALMITATE/PIPORTIL

(Not readily available in the UK – requires importing.)

Use: maintenance treatment of schizophrenia or paranoid psychosis.

CI: CNS depression, phaeo, severe cerebral atherosclerosis, **L/R/H**.

Caution: Parkinson's, epilepsy, MG, phaeo, glaucoma (angle-closure), ↑prostate, severe respiratory disease, jaundice, blood disorders, predisposition to postural ↓BP, photosensitivity, alcohol withdrawal, brain damage, severe antipsychotic-induced EPSEs, ↓/↑thyroid.

Class SE: EPSE, ↑prolactin and assoc Sx, sedation, ↑Wt, QT prolongation, VTE, blood dyscrasias, ↓seizure threshold, NMS.

SE: postural ↓BP, insomnia, abnormal LFTs, contact skin sensitisation, visual changes, ↑blood glucose.

Monitor: glucose and ECG monitoring during treatment.

Interactions: ↑risk of arrhythmias with concomitant QT prolonging drugs; ↑fx of alcohol, barbiturates, sedatives; ↑EPSE with tetrabenazine, lithium; ↑CNS toxicity with lithium, ritonavir may ↑levels.

Dose: initially 25 mg im, ↑ by 25–50 mg, administered into gluteal muscle, usual maintenance dose 50–100 mg every 4 wks, max 200 mg every 4 wks.

POTASSIUM TABLETS see Kay-cee-L (syrup 1 mmol/mL), Sando-K (effervescent 12 mmol/tablet). Swallow whole with fluid during meals while sitting or standing.

PRAMIPEXOLE/MIRAPEXIN

Dopamine agonist (non-ergot derived); use in early Parkinson's ⇒ ↓motor complications (e.g. dyskinesias) but ↓motor performance cf L-dopa.

Use: Parkinson's[1], moderate-to-severe restless legs syndrome (RLS)[2].
CI: B
Caution: psychotic disorders, severe cardiovascular disease, R/H/P.
SE: GI upset, sleepiness (inc sudden onset sleep), ↓BP (inc postural, esp initially), Ψ disorders (esp psychosis and impulse control disorders, e.g. gambling and ↑sexuality), amnesia, headache, oedema. **Impulse control disorders.**
Warn: sleepiness and ↓BP may impair skilled tasks (inc driving). Avoid abrupt withdrawal.
Monitor: ophthalmological testing if visual Δs occur.
Interactions: antipsychotics can ↓fx.
Dose: initially 88 micrograms tds[1] (or 88 micrograms nocte for RLS[2]), ↑ing if tolerated/required to max 1.1 mg tds[1] (or 540 micrograms nocte[2]). *NB:* **doses given for BASE (not SALT) and ↓dose if RF.**

PRAVASTATIN

HMG-CoA reductase inhibitor: 'statin'; ↓s cholesterol/LDL (and TG).
Use/CI/Caution/SE/Monitor: see Simvastatin.
Interactions: ↑risk of myositis (± ↑levels) with ☠ fibrates, ☠ nicotinic acid, daptomycin, ciclosporin and ery-/clarithromycin.
Dose: 10–40 mg nocte. *NB:* ↓dose if RF (10 mg if moderate-to-severe RF).

PREDNISOLONE

Glucocorticoid (and mild mineralocorticoid activity).

Use: anti-inflammatory (e.g. rheumatoid arthritis, IBD, asthma, eczema), immunosuppression (e.g. transplant rejection Px, acute leukaemias), glucocorticoid replacement (e.g. Addison's disease, hypopituitarism).

CI: systemic infections (without antibiotic cover).

Caution: DM, epilepsy, HTN, glaucoma, osteoporosis, PU, TB, severe mood disorders, **L/R**.

SE: ↑infections, metabolic (fluid retention, ↑lipids, ↑Wt, DM, ↑Na⁺, ↓K⁺), adrenal suppression, bruising, cardiac (HTN, CCF, myocardial rupture post-MI, TE), musculoskeletal (proximal myopathy, osteoporosis), worsening of seizures, Ψ fx (anxiety, depression, mania, psychosis), ocular (cataract, glaucoma, corneal/scleral thinning), GI (peptic/duodenal ulcer – give PPI if on ↑doses, pancreatitis).

Warn: avoid contact with chickenpox if not infected previously. Carry steroid card. ☠ Risk of Addisonian crisis if abrupt withdrawal – must ↓ slowly if >3 wks Rx. ☠

Interactions: fx can be ↓d by rifampicin, carbamazepine, phenytoin and phenobarbital. fx (and risk of adrenal suppression) can be ↑d by erythromycin, ritonavir, ketoconazole, itraconazole and ciclosporin (whose own fx are ↑d by methylprednisolone). Risk of ↑ or ↓anticoagulant effect of coumarins.

Dose: usually 2.5–15 mg od po for maintenance. In acute/initial stages, 20–60 mg od often needed (depends on cause and often physician preference), e.g. acute asthma (40 mg od), acute COPD (30 mg od), temporal arteritis (40–60 mg daily). Take with food (↓Na⁺, ↑K⁺ diet recommended if on long-term Rx). For other causes, consult^SPC/BNF, pharmacy or local specialist relevant to the disease. Also available as once- or twice-wkly im injection.

☠ Warn patient not to stop tablets suddenly (*can ⇒Addisonian crisis*). Requirements may ↑ if intercurrent illness/surgery, doses often doubled temporarily. Consider Ca/vit D supplements/bisphosphonate to ↓risk of osteoporosis and PPI to ↓risk of GI ulcer. ☠

PREGABALIN/LYRICA

Antiepileptic; GABA analogue.

Use: epilepsy (partial seizures with or without 2° generalisation), neuropathic pain, generalised anxiety disorder.

Caution: substance misuse, avoid abrupt withdrawal, **H** (if severe)/**R**/**P**/**E**.

SE: neuro-Ψ disturbance; esp somnolence/dizziness (↑falls in elderly), confusion, visual Δ (esp blurred vision), mood ↑ or ↓ (and possibly suicidal ideation/behaviour[†]), ↓libido, sexual dysfunction and vertigo. Also respiratory depression, GI upset, ↑appetite/Wt, oedema and dry mouth. Rarely HF (esp if elderly and/or CVS disease). Can ⇒ abuse.

Warn: seek medical advice if ↑suicidality or mood ↓. Do not stop abruptly as can ⇒ withdrawal fx (insomnia, headache, N&D, flu-like symptoms, pain, sweating, dizziness).

Interactions: Combination with other sedative drugs ⇒ high.

Dose: 50–600 mg/day po in two to three divided doses. *NB:* stop over ≥1 wk* and ↓dose if RF.

PROCHLORPERAZINE/STEMETIL

Antiemetic: DA antagonist (phenothiazine ∴ also antipsychotic, but now rarely used for this).

Use: N&V (inc labyrinthine disorders).

CI/Caution/SE/Warn/Monitor/Interactions: as chlorpromazine, but CI are relative and ⇒ ↓sedation. *NB:* can ⇒ extrapyramidal fx (esp if elderly/debilitated); see p. 389.

Dose: *po:* acutely 20 mg, then 10 mg 2 h later (5–10 mg bd/tds for Px and labyrinthine disorders); *im:* 12.5 mg, then po doses 6 h later. Available as quick-dissolving 3 mg tablets to be placed under lip (**Buccastem**); give 1–2 bd. *NB:* ↓dose if RF.

PROCYCLIDINE

Antimuscarinic: ↓s cholinergic to dopaminergic ratio in extrapyramidal syndromes ⇒ ↓tremor/rigidity. No fx on bradykinesia (or tardive dyskinesia; may even worsen).

Use: extrapyramidal symptoms (e.g. parkinsonism), esp if drug induced[1] (e.g. antipsychotics).

CI: urinary retention (if untreated), glaucoma* (angle-closure), GI obstruction, MG.

Caution: ↑prostate, tardive dyskinesia, H/E.

SE: antimuscarinic fx, Ψ disturbances, euphoria (can be drug of abuse), glaucoma*.

Interactions: Combination with other sedative drugs ⇒ high respiratory depression risk.

Dose: 2.5 mg tds po prn[1] (↑ if necessary to max of 10 mg tds); 5–10 mg im/iv if acute dystonia or oculogyric crisis.

NB: do not stop suddenly: can ⇒ rebound antimuscarinic fx.

PROMETHAZINE HYDROCHLORIDE

Sedating antihistamine. Anticholinergic fx.

Use: insomnia[1]. Also used iv/im for anaphylaxis and po for symptom relief in chronic allergies. Used in rapid tranquilisation.

CI: CNS depression/coma, MAOI within 14 days.

Caution: urinary retention, ↑prostate, glaucoma, epilepsy, IHD, asthma, pyloroduodenal obstruction, R (↓dose), L (avoid if severe)/P/B/E (anticholinergic: caution in dementia).

SE: antimuscarinic fx, hangover sedation, headache.

Interactions: ↑s fx of anticholinergics, TCAs and sedatives/hypnotics.

Dose: 25 mg nocte[1] (can ↑dose to 50 mg).

PROPRANOLOL

β-blocker (non-selective): β1 ⇒ ↓HR and ↓contractility, $β_2$ ⇒ vasoconstriction (and bronchoconstriction). Also blocks fx of catecholamines, ↓s renin production, slows SAN/AVN conduction.

Use: HTN[1], IHD (angina Rx[2], MI Px[3]), portal HTN[4] (Px of variceal bleed; *NB: may worsen liver function*), essential tremor[5], Px of migraine[6], anxiety[7], ↑T_4 (symptom relief[8], thyroid storm[9]), arrhythmias[8] (inc severe[9]); also used in Rx of lithium-induced tremor.

CI: asthma/Hx of bronchospasm, peripheral arterial disease (if severe), Prinzmetal's angina, severe ↓HR or ↓BP, SSS, second-/

third-degree HB, cardiogenic shock, metabolic acidosis, phaeo (unless used specifically with α-blockers), **H** (if uncontrolled).

Caution: COPD, first-degree HB, DM*, MG, Hx of hypersensitivity (may ↑ to *all* allergens), **L/R/P/B**.

SE: ↓HR, ↓BP, HF, peripheral vasoconstriction (⇒ cold extremities, worsening of claudication/Raynaud's), fatigue, depression, sleep disturbance (inc nightmares), hyperglycaemia (and ↓sympathetic response to hypoglycaemia*), GI upset. Rarely conduction/blood disorders.

Interactions: ☻ verapamil and diltiazem ⇒ risk of HB and ↓HR ☻. Risk of ↓BP and HF with calcium channel blockers. Risk of ↓BP with α-blockers. ↑s risk of bupiva-/lidocaine toxicity. ↑s risk of AV block, myocardial depression and ↓HR with amiodarone, flecainide. Levels of both drugs can ↑ with chlorpromazine. Risk of ↓BP with moxisylyte. Risk of ↑BP (and ↓HR) with dobutamine, adrenaline and noradrenaline. Risk of withdrawal ↑BP with clonidine (stop β-blocker before slowly ↓ing clonidine).

Dose: 80–160 mg bd po[1]; 40–120 mg bd po[2]; 40 mg qds for 2–3 days, then 80 mg bd po[3] (start 5–21 days post-MI); 40 mg bd po[4] (↑dose if necessary); 40 mg bd/tds po[5,6]; 40 mg od po[7] (↑dose to tds if necessary); 10–40 mg tds/qds[8]; 1 mg iv over 1 min[9] repeating every 2 min if required, to max total 10 mg (or 5 mg in anaesthesia).

NB: ↓po dose in **LF** and ↓initial dose in **RF**. Withdraw slowly (esp in angina); if not can ⇒ rebound ↑ of symptoms.

PYRIDOSTIGMINE

Anticholinesterase: inhibits cholinesterase at neuromuscular junction ⇒ ↑ACh ⇒ ↑neuromuscular transmission.

Use: myasthenia gravis.

CI: GI/urinary obstruction.

Caution: asthma or COPD, recent MI, ↓HR/BP, arrhythmias, vagotonia, ↑T₄, PU, epilepsy, parkinsonism, **R/P/B/E**.

SE: cholinergic fx (see p. 387) – esp if xs Rx/od, where ↓BP, bronchoconstriction and (confusingly) weakness can also occur

(= cholinergic crisis*); ↑secretions (sweat/saliva/tears) and miosis are good clues** of xs ACh.

Interactions: fx ↓d by aminoglycosides (e.g. gentamicin), polymixins, clindamycin, lithium, quinidine, chloroquine, propranolol and procainamide. ↑s fx of suxamethonium. Atropine and hyoscine antagonise the muscarinic fx.

Dose: 30–120 mg po up to qds (can ↑ to max total 1.2 g/24 h; if possible give <450 mg/24 h to avoid receptor downregulation). *NB:* ↓dose if RF.

> 💀 ↑ing weakness can be due to *cholinergic crisis** as well as MG exacerbation; if unsure which is responsible**, get senior help (esp if ↓respiratory function) before giving Rx, as the wrong choice can be fatal! 💀

QUETIAPINE/SEROQUEL

Atypical (second-generation) antipsychotic. 5-HT$_2$ antagonist, α_1 and histamine antagonism. Weak DA antagonism. Some anticholinergic activity.

Use: schizophrenia[1], mania[2], depression in bipolar disorder[3]. Off-licence use for psychosis/behavioural disorders (esp in dementias, but use of antipsychotics in dementia generally not recommended).

CI: B. CYP3A4 inhibitors (e.g clarithromycin, erythromycin).

Caution: Hx of epilepsy, drugs that ↑QTc, **H**.

SE: Sedation (esp initially*), ↑Wt, ↑QTc EPSE, ↑prolactin, VTE, blood dyscrasias, ↓seizure threshold, NMS, ↓BP.

Warn/Monitor/Interactions: as olanzapine, but also levels ↑ by ery-/clarithromycin.

Dose: *needs titration** (*see SPC/BNF*): initially 25 mg bd ↑ing daily to max 750 mg od[1]; initially 50 mg bd ↑ing daily to max 800 mg od[2]; initially 50 mg od ↑ing daily to max 600 mg od[3]. If RF, LF or elderly start at 25 mg od ↑ing less frequently. Available in MR form; initially, 300 mg od then 600 mg od the next day[2], then adjust to response (if giving for depression[3] or if RF, LF or elderly start at 50 mg od then ↑cautiously[SPC/BNF]).

QUININE

Antimalarial: kills bloodborne schizonts.

Use: malaria Rx[1] (esp falciparum), nocturnal leg cramps[2] (efficacy limited, only if sleep regularly disrupted).

CI: optic neuritis, tinnitus, haemoglobinuria, MG.

Caution: **cardiac disease** (inc conduction dfx, AF, HB), G6PD deficiency, H/P/E.

SE: visual Δs (inc temporary blindness, esp in od), **tinnitus** (and vertigo/deafness), **GI upset, headache, rash/flushing, hypersensitivity,** confusion, hypoglycaemia*, seizures. Rarely blood disorders, AKI, cardiovascular fx (arrhythmia). Dose-dependent ↑QTc.

Monitor: blood glucose*, ECG (if elderly) and e'lytes (if given iv).

Interactions: ↑s levels of flecainide and digoxin. ↑s risk of arrhythmias with pimozide, moxifloxacin and amiodarone. ↑risk of seizures and ↑QTc with mefloquine. Avoid artemether/lumefantrine.

Dose: 200–300 mg nocte po as quinine *sulphate*[2]. (*NB:* ↓iv maintenance dose if RF.)

RAMIPRIL/TRITACE

ACE-i; see Captopril.

Use: HTN[1], HF[2], Px post-MI[3]. Also Px of cardiovascular disease (if age >55 years and at risk)[4] and renal disease inc nephropathy.

CI/Caution/SE/Monitor/Interactions: as captopril.

Dose: initially 1.25 mg od (↑ing slowly to max of 10 mg daily)[1,2]; initially 2.5 mg bd then ↑ to 5 mg bd after 3 days[3] (start ≥48 h post-MI), then maintenance 2.5–5 mg bd; initially 2.5 mg od (↑ing to 10 mg)[4]. *NB:* ↓dose if RF.

RANITIDINE/ZANTAC

H_2 antagonist $\Rightarrow$ ↓parietal cell H^+ secretion. Not currently available in UK (withdrawn due to possible impurities).

Use: PU (Px if on long-term high-dose NSAIDs[1], chronic Rx[2], acute Rx[3]), reflux oesophagitis.

Caution: R/P/B. ☠ *May mask symptoms of gastric cancer.* ☠

SE: *all rare:* GI upset (esp diarrhoea), dizziness, confusion, fatigue, blurred vision, headache, Δ LFTs (rarely hepatitis), rash. Very rarely arrhythmias (esp if given iv), hypersensitivity, blood disorders.
Dose: initially 150 mg bd po (or 300 mg nocte)[1,2], ↑ing to 600 mg/day if necessary but try to ↓ to 150 mg nocte or bd for maintenance; 50 mg tds/qds iv[3] (or im/ivi[SPC/BNF]).
NB: ↓**dose if RF.**

R

REBOXETINE
NA reuptake inhibitor; binds to noradrenaline transporter (NAT) > serotonin transporter (SERT).
Use: depression.
Caution: epilepsy, ↑prostate/urinary retention, CVD, BPAD, glaucoma (angle-closure), **H**.
SE: ↓sleep, dizziness, dry mouth, GI upset (C&N&V), ↑sweating, ↓appetite, agitation, headache, paraesthesia, visual disorders, cardiac fx (↑HR, palpitations, ↑/↓BP), rash, urinary disturbance, sexual dysfunction, chills.
Warn: avoid sudden withdrawal.
Interactions: metab by P450 (CYP3A4); 🚱 ↑risk of hypertensive crisis with MAOIs and linezolid. 🚱
Dose: 4 mg po bd for 3–4 wks, ↑ to 10 mg OD in divided doses, max 12 mg OD.

RIFAMPICIN
Rifamycin antibiotic: 'cidal' ⇒ ↓RNA synthesis.
Use: TB Rx, *N. meningitidis* (meningococcal)/*H. influenzae* (type b) meningitis Px. Rarely for *Legionella/Brucella/ Staphylococcus* infections.
CI: jaundice, concurrent saquinavir/ritonavir therapy, acute porphyria.
Caution: L/R/P.
SE: hepatotoxicity, GI upset (inc AAC), headache, fever, flu-like symptoms (esp if intermittent use), orange/red body secretions*, SOB, blood disorders, skin reactions, shock, AKI.
Warn: of symptoms/signs of liver disease; report jaundice/ persistent N&V/malaise immediately. Take 30–60 min before food.

Warn about secretions and can discolour soft contact lenses*.
Monitor: LFTs, FBC (and U&Es if dose >600 mg/day).
Interactions: ↑**P450** ∴ many[SPC/BNF]; most importantly ↓s fx
of OCP**, lamotrigine, phenytoin, sulphonylureas, quinine,
mefloquine, keto-/flu-/itra-/posa-/voriconazole, terbinafine,
antivirals, rivaroxaban, dabigatran, cytotoxics, corticosteroids,
ticagrelor, haloperidol, aripiprazole, eplerenone and Ca^{2+}
antagonists. ↑risk of hepatoxicity with isoniazid, **W–**.
Dose: see SPC/BNF. (*NB:* well-absorbed po; give iv *only* if
↓swallow.) *NB:* ↓**dose if LF or RF.**

Other contraception** needed during Rx.

RISEDRONATE
Bisphosphonate: ↓s osteoclastic bone resorption.
Use: osteoporosis (Px[1]/Rx[2], esp if post-menopausal or steroid
induced), Paget's disease[3].
CI: ↓Ca^{2+}, **R** (if eGFR ≤ 30 mL/min), **P/B**.
Caution: delayed GI transit/emptying (esp oesophageal
abnormalities). Correct Ca^{2+} and other bone/mineral metabolism
Δ (e.g. vit D and PTH function) before Rx, dental procedures in
patients at risk of osteonecrosis of the jaw (e.g. chemotherapy).
SE: GI upset, bone/joint/muscle pain, headache, rash. Rarely iritis,
dry eyes/corneal lesions, oesophageal stricture/inflammation/
ulcer*, osteonecrosis of the jaw and atypical femoral fractures.
Warn: of symptoms of oesophageal irritation and if develop to
stop tablets/seek medical attention. Must swallow tablets whole
with full glass of water on an empty stomach ≥30 min before, and
stay upright until breakfast/other food/oral medications*. Need to
report thigh, hip or groin pain.
Interactions: Ca^{2+}-containing products (inc milk) and antacids
(⇒ ↓absorption) ∴ separate doses as much as possible from
risedronate. Also avoid iron and mineral supplements.
Dose: 5 mg od[1,2] (or 1 × 35 mg tablet/wk as Actonel Once a
Week[2]); 30 mg daily for 2 months[3].

L/R/H = Liver, Renal and Heart failure. **E** = elderly. **P** = pregnancy. **B** = breastfeeding.

RISPERIDONE/RISPERDAL

R

'Atypical' antipsychotic: similar to olanzapine ($\Rightarrow$ ↓extrapyramidal fx cf 'typical' antipsychotics, esp tardive dyskinesia; however, causes more EPSEs than most 'atypical' antipsychotics). DA, 5-HT_2 and α antagonism. Pro-drug: active form paliperidone.

Use: psychosis/schizophrenia (acute and chronic)[NICE], mania and short-term Rx (<6 wks) of persistent aggression unresponsive to non-pharmacological Rx in Alzheimer's.

SE: ↑prolactin, sedation, ↑Wt, EPSE, ↓BP, QT prolongation, VTE, blood dyscrasias, ↓seizure threshold.

Caution: similar to olanzapine, but also caution if dementia with Lewy bodies, prolactin-dependent tumours, dehydration, cataract surgery, acute porphyria.

Interactions: levels may be ↓ by carbamazepine and ↑ by ritonavir, fluoxetine and paroxetine. ↑mortality rate in elderly if taking furosemide. ↑risk of arrhythmias with drugs that ↑QTc and atomoxetine. ↑risk of ↓BP with general anaesthetic. ↓s fx of anticonvulsants.

Dose: initially 2 mg od titrating up if necessary, generally to 4–6 mg od (if elderly, initially 500 micrograms bd titrating up if required to max 2 mg bd po). Also available as liquid or quick dissolving 1, 2, 3 or 4 mg tablets and as long-acting im 2-wkly injections ('**Consta**') for ↑compliance. *NB:* ↓dose if LF or RF.

▼ RIVAROXABAN/XARELTO

Oral anticoagulant; direct inhibitor of activated factor X (factor Xa).

Use: Px of VTE following knee[1] or hip[2] replacement surgery, initial Rx of DVT[3] or PE[3], continued Rx of DVT or PE[4], Px of recurrent DVT or PE[4], Px of stroke and systemic embolism in non-valvular AF and at ≥1 risk factor (e.g. CHF, HT, previous stroke or TIA, symptomatic HF, E ≥75 years of age, DM)[5], Px of atherothrombotic events after ACS with ↑cardiac biomarkers (in combination with aspirin alone or aspirin and clopidogrel)[6].

CI: active bleeding or significant risk of major bleeding[BNF], in ACS– previous stroke, in ACS–TIA, malignant neoplasms, oesophageal varices, recent brain surgery, recent GI ulcer, recent intracranial haemorrhage, ophthalmic surgery or spine surgery, vascular aneurysm, **L** (if coagulopathy present)/ **R**(if severe)/**P/B**.

Caution: ☠ anaesthesia with post-operative indwelling epidural catheter (risk of paralysis), see BNF; bronchiectasis, prosthetic heart valve (efficacy not established), risk of bleeding); ☠ do not use as alternative to unfractionated heparin in patients with PE and haemodynamic instability, or who may receive thrombolysis or pulmonary embolectomy; severe HTN, vascular retinopathy, mild-to-moderate liver impairment.

SE: anaemia, haemorrhage, menorrhagia, ↓BP/dizziness, GI upset, headache, fever, oedema, pain in extremity, renal impairment, skin reactions, wound complications. Less common: allergic oedema, angioedema, dry mouth, hepatic disorders, intracranial haemorrhage, syncope, ↑HR, ↓ or ↑Pt. Rarely vascular pseudoaneurysm.

Dose: To be taken with food[1,2], to be started 6–10 h after surgery – 10 mg bd po for 2 wks[1]; for 5 wks[2]. 15 mg bd po for 21 days, to be taken with food[3]. 20 mg od po (see SPC for duration of treatment and dose[4]), 20 mg od po[5]; 2.5 mg bd po (usual duration 12 months[6]). ↓dose in RF.[BNF] See SPC for how to change from, or to, other anticoagulants.

RIVASTIGMINE/EXELON

Acetylcholinesterase inhibitor that acts centrally (crosses blood-brain barrier): replenishes ACh, which is ↓↓d in certain dementias.
Use: Alzheimer's disease[NICE] and Parkinson's disease dementia.
CI: B.
Caution: conduction defects (esp SSS), PU susceptibility, Hx of COPD/asthma/seizures, bladder outflow obstruction, **R/P/L**.
SE: cholinergic fx, ↓Wt, GI upset (esp nausea initially), headache, dizziness, behavioural/Ψ reactions. Rarely GI haemorrhage, ↓HR, AV block, angina, seizures, rash.
Monitor: Wt, pulse.
Dose: 1.5 mg bd po initially (↑ing slowly to 3–6 mg bd: specialist review needed for clinical response and tolerance). Give with

morning and evening meals. Available as daily transdermal patch releasing 4.6 mg or 9.5 mg/24 h.

NB: If >3 days are missed for any formulation, retitration at the lowest dose is necessary.

ROPINIROLE/REQUIP[1] or ADARTREL[2]

Dopamine agonist (non-ergot derived); use in early Parkinson's ⇒ ↓motor complications (e.g. dyskinesias) but ↓motor performance cf L-dopa. Also adjunctive use in Parkinson's with motor fluctuations.
Use: Parkinson's[1], moderate-to-severe restless legs syndrome (RLS)[2].
CI: P/B/L/R.
Caution: major psychotic disorders, severe cardiovascular disease.
SE: GI upset, sleepiness (inc sudden-onset sleep), ↓BP (inc postural, esp initially), Ψ disorders (esp psychosis and impulse control disorders, e.g. gambling and ↑sexuality), confusion, hallucinations, leg oedema, paradoxical worsening of restless legs syndrome symptoms or early morning rebound (may need to withdraw or reduce dose).
Warn: sleepiness and ↓BP may impair skilled tasks (inc driving). Avoid abrupt withdrawal. Take with food.
Dose: initially 250 micrograms tds[1] (or 250 micrograms nocte for RLS[2]) ↑ing if tolerated/required to max 8 mg tds[1] (or 4 mg nocte for RLS[2]). Available in MR preparation 2–24 mg od[1].

ROSUVASTATIN/CRESTOR

HMG-Co A reductase inhibitor; ↓cholesterol (and TG).
Use/CI/Caution/SE: as simvastatin, but can ⇒ DM and proteinuria (and rarely haematuria). Avoid if severe RF.
Interactions: ↑risk of myositis with ☠ fibrates and ciclosporin ☠, daptomycin, protease inhibitors, fusidic and nicotinic acid. Levels ↓ by antacids, erythromycin. Mild **W+**.
Dose: initially 5–10 mg od. If necessary ↑ to 20 mg after ≥4 wks (if not of Asian origin or risk factors for myopathy/rhabdomyolysis, can ↑ to 40 mg after further 4 wks). *NB: ↓dose if RF, Asian origin or other ↑risk factor for myopathy.*

Significantly higher frequency of Q141K variation of ABCG2 gene (a critical rosuvastatin-efflux pump) in Asian populations. Establishing frequency of Q141K in different Asian subgroups will lead to improved individualised rosuvastatin dosing.

SALBUTAMOL

β_2 agonist, short acting: dilates bronchial smooth muscle (and endometrium). Also inhibits mast-cell mediator release.

Use: chronic[1] and acute[2] asthma. Rarely $\uparrow K^+$(give nebs prn), premature labour (IV).

Caution: cardiovascular disease (esp arrhythmias*, susceptibility to $\uparrow$QTc, HTN), DM (can $\Rightarrow$ DKA, esp if iv $\therefore$ monitor CBGs), $\uparrow T_4$, **P/B**.

SE: *neurological:* fine tremor, headache, nervousness, behavioural/sleep Δs (esp in children); CVS: $\uparrow$**HR**, palpitations/ arrhythmias (esp if IV), $\uparrow$QTc*; *other*: $\downarrow K^+$, muscle cramps. Rarely hypersensitivity, paradoxical bronchospasm. Lactic acidosis with high doses.

Monitor: K^+ and glucose (esp if $\uparrow$ or iv doses).

Dose: 100–200 micrograms (aerosol) or 200 micrograms (powder) inh prn up to qds[1]; 2.5–5 mg QDS 4-hrly neb[2]. If life-threatening (see p. 423), can $\uparrow$nebs to every 15 min or give as ivi (initially 5 micrograms/ min, then up to 20 micrograms/min according to response).

SALMETEROL/SEREVENT

Bronchodilator: long-acting β_2 agonist (LABA).

Use: first choice add-on for asthma Rx[1] (on top of short-acting β_2 agonist and inh steroids). Also COPD[2].

Not for acute Rx.

Caution/SE/Monitor: as salbutamol.

Dose: 50–100 micrograms BD inh[1]; 50 micrograms BD inh[2].

SANDOCAL

Calcium supplement; available as '1000' (1 g calcium = 25 mmol Ca^{2+}) effervescent tablets.

L/R/H = Liver, Renal and Heart failure. **E** = elderly. **P** = pregnancy. **B** = breastfeeding.

SANDO-K
Effervescent oral KCl (12 mmol K+/tablet).
Use: ↓K+.
CI: K+ >5 mmol/L, **R** (if severe, otherwise caution).
Caution: **R**, untreated Addison's, taking other drugs that ↑K+ and cardiac disease.
SE: N&V, GI ulceration, flatulence.
Dose: according to serum K+: start with 2–4 tablets/day if diet normal. Take with food. *NB:* ↓**dose in RF/elderly** (↑ if established ↓K+).

SAXAGLIPTIN

Oral antidiabetic (dipeptidylpeptidase-4 inhibitor): ⇒ ↑insulin secretion and ↓glucagon secretion. Does not appear associated with ↑Wt. ↓incidence of hypoglycaemia than with sulfonylureas.
Use: type 2 DM as monotherapy (if metformin inappropriate), or combined with other antidiabetic drugs (including insulin) if existing Rx fails to achieve glycaemic control.
CI: history of serious hypersensitivity to dipeptidylpeptidase-4 inhibitors. **L** (if severe)/**P/B**.
Caution: history of pancreatitis **L/R/E**.
SE: abdominal pain, constipation, vomiting, dizziness, tiredness, headache, ↑risk of infection, skin reactions. Uncommon: pancreatitis. Rarely angioedema.
Dose: 5 mg od po. Dose of concomitant sulphonylurea or insulin may need to be ↓d. ↓dose in RF.

SEMAGLUTIDE

GLP-1 receptor agonist.
Use: T2DM.
CI: DKA, **P/B/R**.
Caution: diabetic retinopathy, pancreatitis, severe congestive heart failure, **H**.
SE: GI disturbance, cholelithiasis, weight decrease; pancreatitis (rare).
Warn: reports of DKA when concomitant insulin is rapidly reduced or discontinued.

Interactions: caution with other meds which can ↓glucose, levothyroxine.
Dose: po: 3 mg od for 1 month, increased to 7 mg od for 1 month, then if necessary to 14 mg od, take on empty stomach; sc: 0.25 mg OW for 4 wks, increased to 0.5 mg once weekly for 4 wks, then increase if necessary to 1 mg once weekly.

14 mg po od ≈ sc 0.5 mg once weekly. Due to high pharmacokinetic variability of po form, the effect of switching between po and sc semaglutide cannot easily be predicted.

▼ SEMISODIUM VALPROATE/DEPAKOTE
See (Sodium) valproate: semisodium valproate = equimolar amounts of sodium valproate and valproic acid.
Use: treatment of mania[1]; migraine prophylaxis (unlicensed)[2].
CI/Caution/SE/Warn/Monitor/Interactions: see (Sodium) valproate.
Dose: initially 750 mg PO OD in two to three divided doses, ↑ to 1–2 g od, doses >45 mg/kg OD require careful monitoring[1]; initially 250 mg BD, ↑ to 1 g OD in divided doses[2].

NB: semisodium valproate and sodium valproate have the same adverse effects but the severity/frequency may differ slightly due to different times to convert to free valproate.

☠ Anyone of childbearing potential must not be prescribed valproate without being enrolled on a Pregnancy Prevention Programme. ☠

SENNA/SENOKOT
Stimulant laxative; takes 8–12 h to work.
Use: constipation.
CI: GI obstruction.
Caution: P (try bulk-forming or osmotic laxative first).
SE: GI cramps. If chronic use atonic non-functioning colon, ↓K+.
Dose: 2 tablets nocte (can ↑ to 4 tablets nocte). Available as syrup.

S

SERETIDE: combination asthma or COPD inhaler with possible synergistic action: long-acting β_2 agonist (LABA) salmeterol 50 micrograms (Accuhaler) or 25 micrograms (Evohaler) + fluticasone (steroid) in varying quantities (50, 100, 125, 250 or 500 micrograms/puff). Note different devices have different licensed indications.

SERTRALINE/LUSTRAL

SSRI antidepressant; also increases dopamine levels; see Fluoxetine.
Use: depression[1] (also PTSD, OCD, social anxiety disorder and panic disorder). Relatively good safety record in pregnancy and breastfeeding (can use if benefits > risks).
CI/Caution/SE/Warn/Interactions: as fluoxetine, but ↑agitation/insomnia, does not ↑carbamazepine levels, but does ↑phenytoin/pimozide levels (CI with pimozide).
Dose: initially 50 mg OD (25 mg for PTSD and anxiety disorders), ↑ing in 50 mg increments over several weeks to max daily dose 200 mg. *NB:* ↓**dose or frequency if LF.**

SILDENAFIL/VIAGRA

Phosphodiesterase type-5 inhibitor: ↑s local fx of NO ($\Rightarrow$ ↑smooth-muscle relaxation ∴ ↑blood flow into corpus cavernosum).
Use: erectile dysfunction[1], pulmonary artery hypertension[2] (and digital ulceration under specialist supervision).
CI: recent CVA/MI, ↓BP (systolic <90 mm Hg), hereditary degenerative retinal disorders, Hx of non-arteritic anterior ischaemic optic neuropathy and conditions where vasodilation/sexual activity is inadvisable, **L/H** (if either severe).
Caution: cardiovascular disease, LV outflow obstruction, bleeding disorders (inc active PU), anatomical deformation of penis, predisposition to prolonged erection (e.g. multiple myeloma/leukaemias/sickle cell disease), **R/P/B**.
SE: headache, flushing, GI upset, dizziness, visual disturbances, nasal congestion, hypersensitivity reactions. Rarely serious cardiovascular events and priapism.
Interactions: ☠ *Nitrates (e.g. GTN/ISMN/ISDN) and nicorandil can ↓↓BP ∴ never give together.* ☠ Antivirals (esp rito-/ataza-/

indinavir) ↑ its levels. ↑s hypotensive fx of α-blockers; avoid concomitant use. Levels ↑d by keto-/itraconazole and grapefruit juice.

Dose: initially 50 mg PO approximately 1 h before sexual activity[1], adjusting to response (1 dose per 24 h, max 100 mg per dose); 20 mg PO or 10 mg IV TDS[2]. *NB:* ↓**dose if RF or LF.**

SIMVASTATIN

HMG-CoA reductase inhibitor ('statin'): ⇒ ↓cholesterol (↓s synthesis), ↓LDL (↑s uptake), mildly ↓s TG.

Use: ↑cholesterol, Px of atherosclerotic disease: IHD (inc 1° prevention), CVA, PVD.

CI: L (inc active liver disease or Δ LFTs), **P** (contraception required during, and for 1 month after, Rx), **B**. Do not prescribe concurrently with antifungals, macrolides and protease inhibitors.

Caution: ↓T_4, alcohol abuse, Hx of liver disease, **R** (if severe).

SE: hepatitis and myositis* (both rare but important), headache, GI upset, rash. Rarely pancreatitis, hypersensitivity, anaemia, tendinopathy.

Monitor: LFTs (and CK if symptoms develop*).

Interactions: ↑risk of myositis (±↑levels) with ☠ fibrates, ☠ clari-/ery-/telithromycin, itra-/keto-/mi-/posaconazole, ciclosporin, protease inhibitors, nicotinic acid, fusidic acid, colchicine, danazol, amiodarone, dronedarone, verapamil, diltiazem, amlodipine, ranolazine and grapefruit juice, mild **W+**.

Dose: 10–80 mg nocte (usually start at 10–20 mg[SPC/BNF]), ↑ing at intervals ≥4 wks. ↓max dose if significant drug interactions.[SPC/BNF] *NB:* ↓**dose if RF** or other ↑risk factor for myositis*.

> ☠ Myositis* can rarely ⇒ rhabdomyolysis; ↑risk if ↓T_4, RF or taking drugs that ↑levels/risk of myositis (see previous discussion). ☠

▼ (SODIUM) VALPROATE/EPILIM

Antiepileptic and mood stabiliser: potentiates and ↑s GABA levels.

Use: epilepsy[1], mania[2] (and off-licence for other Ψ disorders).

S

CI: acute porphyria, personal or family Hx of severe liver dysfunction, **L** (inc active liver disease); women and girls of childbearing potential unless conditions met of Pregnancy Prevention Programme.[MHRA]

Caution: SLE, ↑bleeding risk*, women of childbearing age **R**, **P** (⇒ neural-tube/craniofacial and other developmental defects**; therefore, give Px folate), **B**.

SE: sedation, **cerebellar fx** (see p. 389; esp tremor, ataxia), **headache**, GI upset, ↑Wt, SOA, alopecia, skin reactions, ↓cognitive/motor function, Ψ disorders, encephalopathy (2° to ↑ammonia). Rarely but seriously **hepatotoxicity**, **blood disorders** (esp ↓Pt*), **pancreatitis** (mostly in first 6 months of Rx).

Warn: of clinical features of pancreatitis and liver/blood disorders. Inform women of childbearing age of teratogenicity/need for contraception**.

Monitor: LFTs, FBC ± serum levels *pre-dose* (therapeutic range 50–100 mg/L; useful for checking compliance but ↓use for efficacy).

Interactions: fx ↓d by antimalarials (esp mefloquine), orlistat, carbapenems, antidepressants (inc St John's wort), antipsychotics and some antiseizure medications.[SPC/BNF] Levels ↑ by cimetidine. ↑s fx of aspirin and primidone. ↑risk of ↓NØ with olanzapine. Mild **W+**.

Dose: initially 300 mg bd, ↑ing to max of 2.5 g/day[1]; initially 750 mg in 1–2 divided doses, ↑ing to usual dose of 1–2 g in 1–2 divided doses[2]. *NB:* ↓**dose if RF.**

Can give false-positive urine dipstick for ketones.

SPIRONOLACTONE

K⁺-sparing diuretic: aldosterone antagonist at distal tubule (also potentiates loop and thiazide diuretics).

Use: ascites (esp 2° to cirrhosis or malignancy), oedema, HF (adjunct to ACE-i and/or another diuretic), nephrotic syndrome, 1° aldosteronism.

CI: ↑K⁺, ↓Na⁺, Addison's, anuria, **P/B**.

Caution: porphyria, **L/R/E**.
SE: ↑K⁺, gynaecomastia, GI upset (inc N&V), impotence, ↓BP, ↓Na⁺, rash, confusion, headache, hepatotoxicity, blood disorders.
Monitor: U&E.
Interactions: ↑s digoxin and lithium levels. ↑s risk of RF with NSAIDs (which also antagonise its diuretic fx).
Dose: 100–400 mg/day po (25 mg od if for HF).

> ☠ Beware if on other drugs that ↑K⁺, e.g. amiloride, triamterene, ACE-i, angiotensin II antagonists and ciclosporin. Do not give with oral K⁺ supplements inc dietary salt substitutes. ☠

ST JOHN'S WORT
Herbal medicinal product – unlicensed.
Use: mild low mood and anxiety. Not recommended.[NICE]
CI: photosensitivity, phototherapy, concomitant use of interacting medications (see Interactions).
SE: GI upset (N&D), abdominal pain, photosensitivity, ↓appetite, dizziness, confusion, fatigue, sedation, restlessness, headache.
Interactions: ↑P450 (CYP3A4, CYP1A2); fx vary between preparations; ↓levels of antiretrovirals, benzodiazepines (e.g. alprazolam, midazolam), COCP, immunosuppressants (e.g. cyclosporine, tacrolimus), antiarrhythmics (e.g. amiodarone, flecainide, mexiletine), β-blockers (e.g. metoprolol, carvedilol), calcium channel blockers (e.g. verapamil, diltiazem, amlodipine, pregabalin), statins (e.g. lovastatin, simvastatin, atorvastatin), digoxin, methadone, omeprazole, phenobarbital, theophylline, warfarin, levodopa, buprenorphine; ↑serotonergic fx with TCA (e.g. amitriptyline, clomipramine), MAOI (e.g. moclobemide), SSRI (e.g. citalopram, escitalopram, fluoxetine, fluvoxamine, paroxetine, sertraline), duloxetine, venlafaxine, anxiolytics (e.g. buspirone), 5-HT agonists (e.g. Sumatriptan).
Dose: preparations vary – see relevant SPC.

> ☠ Multiple drug interactions. ☠

▼ STRONTIUM RANELATE/ARISTO

↑s bone formation and ↓s bone resorption.

Use: osteoporosis[NICE] if at ↑risk and other treatments such as bisphosphonates CI/not tolerated.[SPC/BNF]

CI: VTE (inc Hx of), temporary or prolonged immobilisation, IHD (inc PHx of), peripheral arterial/cerebrovascular disease, uncontrolled HTN, phenylketonuria (contains aspartame), **P/B**.

Caution: ↑risk of VTE (must assess risk if >80 years old), Δs urinary and plasma Ca^{2+} measurements, **R** (avoid if severe).

SE: severe allergic reactions*, GI upset.

Warn: to report any skin rash* and immediately stop drug.

Interactions: absorption ↓ by concomitant ingestion of Ca^{2+} (e.g. milk) and Mg^{2+}. ↓s absorption of quinolones and tetracycline.

Dose: 2 g (1 sachet in water) po od at bedtime.[SPC/BNF] *Avoid food/ milk 2 h before and after taking.* **NB** specialist use only.

> 💀 Rash* can be early DRESS syndrome: Drug Rash, Eosinophilia and Systemic Symptoms (e.g. fever); lymphadenopathy and ↑WCC also seen early. Can ⇒ LF, RF or respiratory failure ± death. 💀

SULPIRIDE

Benzamide, atypical antipsychotic; selective dopamine D_2 antagonist.

Use: schizophrenia, predominantly −ve symptoms[1]; schizophrenia, predominantly +ve symptoms[2].

CI: CNS depression, phaeo, prolactin-elevating tumour, **H**.

Caution: Parkinson's, epilepsy, MG, glaucoma (angle-closure), ↑prostate, severe respiratory disease, jaundice, blood disorders, predisposition to postural ↓BP, photosensitivity, aggression/ agitation (even low doses may ↑symptoms), Hx/FHx of Ca breast (due to ↑prolactin).

SE: ↑prolactin and assoc Sx, ↓sleep, sedation, **EPSEs**, constipation, ↑LFTs, rash, ↑Wt, **cardiac fx** (↑QTc, arrhythmia), **VTE**, blood dyscrasias, **NMS**, ↓seizure threshold.

Warn: EPSEs and withdrawal fx in neonate if used in third trimester, ↑fx of alcohol.

Monitor: ECG may be required, esp if (risk factors for) CVD or inpatient admission; prolactin at start of therapy, 6 months and then yearly; physical health monitoring (CVD risk) at least once/year.

Interactions: ↑risk of ↑QTc/torsade de pointes with β-blockers, calcium channel blockers, diuretics, stimulant laxatives, class 1A and III antiarrhythmics (e.g. quinidine, disopyramide, amiodarone, sotalol), ↑sedative fx of alcohol, ↓fx of levodopa, ropinirole.

Dose: 200–400 mg po bd, max 800 mg od[1]; 200–400 mg po bd, max 2.4 g od[2].

SUMATRIPTAN/IMIGRAN

5-HT$_{1B/1D}$ agonist.

Use: migraine (acute). Also cluster headache (sc route and intranasally).

CI: IHD, coronary vasospasm (inc Prinzmetal's), PVD, HTN (moderate, severe or uncontrolled). Hx of MI, CVA or TIA.

Caution: predisposition to IHD (e.g. cardiac disease), **L/H/P/B/E**.

SE: sensory Δs (tingling, heat, pressure/tightness), dizziness, flushing, fatigue, N&V, seizures, visual Δs and drowsiness.

Interactions: ↑risk of CNS toxicity with SSRIs, MAOIs, moclobemide and St John's wort. ↑risk of vasospasm with ergotamine and methysergide.

Dose: 50 mg po (can repeat after ≥2 h if responded then recurs and can ↑doses, if no **LF**, to 100 mg if required). Max 300 mg/24 h. Available sc or intranasally.[BNF/SPC]

> *NB:* frequent use may ⇒ *x*medication overuse headache.

SYMBICORT

Combination asthma/COPD inhaler: each puff contains *x* microgram budesonide (steroid) + *y* microgram formoterol (long-acting β$_2$ agonist) in the following '*x/y*' strengths; '100/6', '200/6' and '400/12'. *NB:* different strengths have different licenses.

TADALAFIL/CIALIS/ADCIRCA

Phosphodiesterase type-5 inhibitor; see Sildenafil.
CI/Use/Caution/SE/Interactions: as sildenafil plus CI in
moderate HF and uncontrolled HTN/arrhythmias.
Dose (for erectile dysfunction): initially 10 mg ≥30 min
before sexual activity, adjusting to response (1 dose per 24 h, max
20 mg per dose, unless RF or LF when max 10 mg).

TAMOXIFEN

Oestrogen receptor antagonist.
Use: oestrogen receptor-positive Ca breast[1] (as adjuvant Rx: ⇒
↑survival, delays metastasis), anovulatory infertility[2].
CI: P** (exclude pregnancy before starting Rx), history of TE.
Caution: ↑risk of VTE* (if taking cytotoxics), porphyria, B.
SE: hot flushes, GI upset, menstrual/endometrial Δs (🦷 inc Ca: if
Δ vaginal bleeding/discharge or pelvic pain/pressure ⇒ urgent Ix
🦷. Also fluid retention, exac bony metastases pain. Many other
gynaecological/blood/skin/metabolic Δs (esp lipids, LFTs).
Warn: of symptoms of endometrial cancer and VTE* (and to
report calf pain/sudden SOB). If appropriate, advise non-hormonal
contraception**.
Interactions: W+, SSRIs.
Dose: 20 mg od po[1]; for anovulatory infertility[2], see SPC/BNF.

TAMSULOSIN/FLOMAXTRA XL

α-Blocker ⇒ internal urethral sphincter relaxation (∴ ⇒ ↑bladder
outflow) and systemic vasodilation.
Use: BPH.
CI/Caution/SE/Interactions: as doxazosin plus L (if severe).
Dose: 400 micrograms mane (after food).

TELMISARTAN/MICARDIS

Angiotensin II antagonist; see Losartan.
Use: HTN[1]. Px of cardiovascular events if established
atherosclerosis or type 2 DM with organ damage[2].

CI: biliary obstruction, **L** (if severe, otherwise caution), **P/B**.
Caution/SE/Interactions: as losartan, plus ↑s digoxin levels.
Dose: 20–80 mg od[1] (usually 40 mg od); 80 mg od[2]. *NB:* ↓**dose if LF or RF.**

TEMAZEPAM

Benzodiazepine, short-acting.
Use: insomnia (short-term management).
CI/Caution/SE/Interactions: see Diazepam.
Dose: 10 mg nocte (can ↑dose if tolerant to benzodiazepines, but beware respiratory depression) max dose 40 mg od.
NB: **Dependency common: max 4 wks Rx.** *NB:* ↓**dose if LF, severe RF or elderly.**

TERBINAFINE/LAMISIL

Antifungal: oral[1,2] or topical cream[3].
Use: ringworm[1] (*Tinea* spp), dermatophyte nail infections[2], fungal skin infections[3]. *NB:* Ineffective in yeast infections.
Caution: psoriasis (may worsen), autoimmune disease (risk of lupus-like syndrome), **L/R** (neither apply if giving topically), **P/B**.
SE: headache, GI upset, mild rash, joint/muscle pains. Rarely neuro-Ψ disturbances, blood disorders, hepatic dysfunction, serious skin reactions (stop drug if progressive rash).
Dose: 250 mg od po for 2–6 wks[1] or 6 wks–3 months[2]; 1–2 topical applications/day for 1–2 wks[3].

TERBUTALINE/BRICANYL

Inhaled β_2 agonist similar to salbutamol.
Dose: 500 micrograms od-qds inh (powder or aerosol); 5–10 mg up to qds neb. Can also give po/sc/im/iv.[SPC/BNF]

TETRACYCLINE

Tetracycline broad-spectrum antibiotic: inhibits ribosomal (30S subunit) protein synthesis.
Use: acne vulgaris[1] (or rosacea), genital/tropical infections (*NB:* doxycycline often preferred).

CI: age <12 years (stains/deforms teeth), acute porphyria, **R/P/B**.
Caution: may worsen MG or SLE, **L**.
SE: GI upset (rarely AAC), oesophageal irritation, headache, dysphagia. Rarely hepatotoxicity, blood disorders, photosensitivity, hypersensitivity, visual Δs (rarely 2° to BIH; stop drug if suspected).
Interactions: ↓absorption with milk (do not drink 1 h before or 2 h after drug), antacids and Fe/Al/Ca/Mg/Zn salts. ↓s fx of OCP (small risk). ↑risk of BIH with retinoids. Mild **W+**.
Dose: 500 mg bd po[1], otherwise 250–500 mg tds/qds po. *NB:* **max 1 g/24 h in LF.**

NB: swallow tablets whole with plenty of fluid while sitting or standing and take ≥30 min before food.

THIAMINE (= VITAMIN B1)
Use: replacement for nutritional deficiencies (esp in alcoholism).
Dose: 100 mg bd/tds po in severe deficiency (25 mg od if mild/chronic).

For iv preparations, see pabrinex.

TICAGRELOR/BRILIQUE
Antiplatelet agent (P2Y$_{12}$ receptor antagonist): prevents ADP-mediated P2Y$_{12}$-dependent Plt activation and aggregation.
Use: Px of atherothrombotic events in ACS[1] (in combination with aspirin)[NICE], Px of atherothrombotic events if previous AMI and ↑risk of atherothrombotic events[2] (in combination with aspirin).[NICE]
CI: active bleeding; history of intracranial haemorrhage, severe LF, **P/B**.
Caution: asthma, COPD; unless pacemaker fitted – bradycardia, 2° or 3° AV block or SSS; stop 5 days before elective surgery if antiplatelet effect not desirable, history of hyperuricaemia; ↑risk of bleeding[BNF] (unless pacemaker fitted), LF, monitor renal function for 1 month if Rx for ACS.
SE: haemorrhage, GI upset, dizziness/syncope, dyspepsia, dyspnoea; hyperuricaemia/gout/gouty arthritis, headache; skin reactions, angioedema; confusion.

Dose: initially 1 dose of 180 mg po, then 90 mg bd po (usually for ≤12 months)[1]; 60 mg bd po, extended Rx may be started without interruption after initial 12-month therapy for ACS[2]. Rx[2] may also be started <2 years from AMI, ≤1 year after stopping previous ADP receptor inhibitor Rx (limited data on continuing Rx[2] beyond 3 years[BNF]).

TIMOLOL EYE DROPS/TIMOPTOL

β-blocker eye drops; ↓aqueous humour production.

Use: glaucoma (second line), ocular HTN (first line); not useful if on systemic β-blocker.

CI: asthma, ↓HR, HB, **H** (if uncontrolled).

Caution/SE/Interactions: as propranolol plus can ⇒ local irritation.

Dose: 1 drop bd (0.25% or 0.5%). Also available in long-acting od preparations TIMOPTOL LA (0.25% and 0.5%) and NYOGEL/TIOPEX (0.1%). Timolol 0.5% also available in combination with other classes of glaucoma medications; carbonic anhydrase inhibitors (dorzolamide Cosopt, brinzolamide Azarga), PG analogues (latanoprost Xalacom, travoprost DuoTrav, bimatoprost Ganfort), α-agonists (brimonidine Combigan).

☠ Systemic absorption possible despite topical application.☠

TINZAPARIN

Low-molecular-weight heparin.

Use: thromboprophylaxis and treatment of thrombosis.

CI: see enoxaparin.

Caution: see enoxaparin.

SE: see enoxaparin. Common: anaemia. Rare: angioedema, priapism, Steven–Johnson syndrome, thrombocytosis.

Monitoring: see enoxaparin.

Interactions: see enoxaparin.

Dose: varies by indication and patient, usually 40 mg od sc for prophylaxis of DVT/PE.

TIOTROPIUM/SPIRIVA

Long-acting inh muscarinic antagonist for COPD (and asthma as Respimat solution); similar to ipratropium, but only for chronic use and caution in RF. Also caution in arrhythmias, IHD or HF for Respimat.

SE: dry mouth, urinary retention, glaucoma.
Dose: 18 micrograms (Spiriva) or 10 micrograms (Braltus) dry powder inhaler od inh; 5 micrograms by solution inhaler (Respimat) od inh.

TOLBUTAMIDE

Oral antidiabetic (short-acting sulphonylurea).
Use/CI/SE/Interactions: as gliclazide, avoid where possible in acute porphyrias. Can also ⇒ headache and tinnitus.
Caution: G6PD deficiency, can encourage weight gain, E.
Dose: 500 mg–2 g daily in divided doses, with food. *NB:* ↓dose if LF.

TOLTERODINE/DETRUSITOL

Antimuscarinic, antispasmodic.
Use: detrusor instability; urinary incontinence/frequency/urgency.
CI/Caution/SE: as oxybutynin (SEs mostly antimuscarinic fx; see p. 387) plus caution if Hx of, or taking drugs that, ↑QTc, **P/B**.
Interactions: ↑risk of ventricular arrhythmias with amiodarone, disopyramide, flecainide and sotalol.
Dose: can start at 2 mg bd. Reduce to 1 mg bd if not tolerated. MR prep: 4 mg od. *NB:* ↓dose if RF or LF. (MR preparation available as 4 mg od po; not suitable if RF or LF.)

TOPIRAMATE

Anticonvulsant; exact mechanism unknown – acts to stabilise cell membrane via Na^+ or Cl^- channels.
Use: monotherapy for generalised tonic-clonic or focal seizures[1], adjunctive treatment in epilepsy[2], migraine prophylaxis[3].
CI: women of childbearing potential if not on highly effective contraception, **P** (if for migraine).

Caution: risk of renal stones/metabolic acidosis, porphyria, cognitive impairment, ↑ammonia, **B/P**.

SE: nasopharyngitis, Ψ fx (depression, mood Δs, agitation, expressive dysphasia), paraesthesia, somnolence, dizziness, GI upset, fatigue, ↓Wt/appetite, blood dyscrasias, hypersensitivity (rash), impaired cognition, ataxia, visual problems, tinnitus, muscle/joint pain, twitching, renal stones, pyrexia.

Warn: risk of major congenital malformations/need for contraception if given to women of childbearing age. Ensure high fluid intake to avoid renal stones.

Monitor: prenatal monitoring (e.g. fetal growth).

Interactions: ↓fx of COCP, desogestrel, etonogestrel, levonorgestrel, norethisterone, ulipristal; ↑risk of toxicity with valproate (encephalopathy); ↑risk of renal calculi with zonisamide, ↓levels by carbamazepine, phenytoin and primidone.

Dose: initially 25 mg po od at night for 1 wk, ↑ in steps of 25–50 mg every 1–2 wks, usually dose 100–200 mg od in two divided doses, max 500 mg od[1]; initially 25–50 mg po od at night for 1 wk, ↑ in steps of 25–50 mg every 1–2 wks, usual dose 200–400 od in two divided doses, max 400 mg od[2]; initially 25 mg po od at night for 1 wk, ↑ in steps of 25 mg every wk, usual dose 50–100 mg od in two divided doses, max 200 mg od[3].

TRAMADOL

Opioid. Also ↓s pain by ↑ing 5-HT/noradrenergic transmission.

Use: moderate-to-severe pain (esp musculoskeletal).

CI/Caution: as codeine, but also CI in uncontrolled epilepsy, patients taking MAOIs, **P/B**. Not suitable as substitute in opioid-dependent patients.

SE: as morphine, but ↓respiratory depression, ↓constipation, ↓addiction. ↑confusion (esp in elderly) compared to codeine.

Interactions: as codeine; also ↑risk convulsions with SSRIs/TCAs/antipsychotics, ↑risk serotonin syndrome with SSRIs. Carbamazepine and ondansetron ↓ its fx, **W+**.

Dose: initially 100 mg, then 50–100 mg up to 4-hrly po/im/iv, max 400 mg/day. Post-op: initially 100 mg im/iv, then 50 mg every 10–20 min prn (max total dose of 250 mg in first hour), then 50–100 mg 4–6 hrly (max 400 mg/day). *NB:* ↓dose if RF, LF or elderly; see BNF for dosing differences between formulations.

TRANDOLAPRIL/GOPTEN
ACE-i for HTN, HF and LVF post-MI.
CI/Caution/SE/Monitor/Interactions: see Captopril.
Dose: initially 500 micrograms od, ↑ing to 1–2 mg od at intervals of 2–4 wks; maximum 4 mg/day (max 2 mg if RF). ↓doses if given with diuretic. If for LVF post-MI, start ≥3 days after MI.

TRANEXAMIC ACID
Antifibrinolytic: inhibits activation of plasminogen to plasmin.
Use: bleeding: acute bleeds[1] (esp 2° to anticoagulants, thrombolytic/anti-Pt agents, epistaxis, haemophilia), menorrhagia[2], hereditary angioedema[3].
CI: VTE disease, Hx of convulsions, **R** (if severe, otherwise caution).
Caution: gross haematuria (can clot and obstruct ureters), DIC, **P**.
SE: GI upset, colour vision Δs (stop drug), VTE.
Dose: 15–25 mg/kg bd/tds po (if severe, 500 mg–1 g tds iv)[1]; 1 g tds po for 4 days (max 4 g/day)[2]; 1–1.5 g bd/tds po[3]. *NB:* ↓dose if RF.

TRANYLCYPROMINE
MAOI; non-selective and irreversible inhibitor of monoamine oxidase, ↑5-HT, NA and DA in CNS.
Use: depression.
CI: mania, phaeo, cerebrovascular disease, ↑T_4, porphyria, concomitant amphetamine use, **L/H**.
Caution: agitation, concurrent ECT, Hx of dependence, suicidal ideation, blood dyscrasias, DM, epilepsy, surgery, severe hypertensive reactions, **P/B/E**.
SE: insomnia, chest pain, diarrhoea, drug dependence, extrasystole, flushing, hypomania, mydriasis, pain, pallor, photophobia, sleep Δs, headache, liver injury (rare), ☠ **hypertensive crisis.** ☠

Warn: avoid tyramine-rich or dopa-rich food/drinks with/for 2–3 wks after stopping MAOI; withdrawal fx may occur within 5 days of stopping treatment, worse after regular administration for 8 wks+; ↓dose gradually over 4 wks+ (longer if used long term).
Monitor: BP (risk of HTN and postural ↓BP), LFTs.
Interactions: ↓P450 (CYP2A6); ☠ ↑risk of severe toxic reaction with serotonergics, dopaminergics and noradrenergics: SSRIs, SNRIs, NARIs, TCAs (and related drugs), other MAOIs (inc for Parkinson's), carbamazepine, linezolid, triptans, pethidine, tramadol. ☠

- Do not start tranylcypromine until these drugs have been stopped and they have cleared: 5 wks for fluoxetine, 3 wks for clomipramine/imipramine, at least 7–14 days for other drugs.
- Wait 2 wks after stopping tranylcypromine before starting any of these medicines.

↑**risk of hypertensive crisis** with sympathomimetics, dopamine agonists, CNS stimulants, buspirone. ↑fx of CNS depressants, antimuscarinics, antidiabetics, antihypertensives.
Dose: initially 10 mg po bd taken no later than 3 p.m., ↑ after 1 wk to 10 mg in the morning and 20 mg in the afternoon, maintenance 10 mg od, closer supervision if doses >30 mg od.

> ☠ Hypertensive crisis may develop if taken with food high in tyramine or DOPA. See p. 223 ☠.

TRAZODONE HYDROCHLORIDE

Antidepressant and anxiolytic; binds at 5-HT$_2$ receptors and ↓5-HT reuptake, with α-adrenergic and histaminergic blockade (sedative fx).
Use: depression[1], anxiety[2].
CI: arrhythmia (esp HB), mania, post-MI, **L** (if severe).
Caution: acute MI, phaeo, ↑T$_4$, sedative intoxication, chronic constipation, DM, epilepsy, Hx of bipolar disorder/psychosis, ↑intraocular pressure, suicide risk, urinary retention, ↑prostate, glaucoma (angle-closure), **L/R** (if severe).
SE: drowsiness, headache, ↑/↓appetite, cardiac fx (↑QTc, ↑BP, postural ↓BP, arrhythmia, syncope), blood dyscrasias, antimuscarinic

fx (mild; see p. 387), GI upset (C&D&N&V), SOB, ↓Na, sexual
dysfunction, liver disorders, Ψ fx (agitation, confusion, psychosis,
mania, suicidal ideation), amnesia, movement disorder, **paralytic
ileus, serotonin syndrome, seizure**, rash, ↓Wt, sleep Δs, paraesthesia.
Warn: ↑fx of alcohol.
Interactions: metab by P450 (CYP3A4); ☠ ↑risk of
serotonin syndrome with TCA ☠; ↑levels with CYP3A4 inhibitors
(e.g. erythromycin, ritonavir), ↓levels with COCP, phenytoin,
carbamazepine, barbiturates.
Dose: initially 150 mg po od at bedtime/taken after food
in divided doses, ↑ to 300–600 mg od[1]; 75 mg po od, ↑ to 300 mg od[2].

TRIFLUOPERAZINE
Phenothiazine, typical antipsychotic; blocks post-synaptic
dopamine D_1/D_2 receptors.
Use: high dose: psychosis, short-term adjunctive management of
agitated/aggressive behaviour[1]; **low dose:** adjunctive treatment of
severe anxiety[2]; severe N&V[3].
CI: CNS depression, phaeo, **L**.
Caution: Parkinson's, drugs that ↑QTc, epilepsy, MG, glaucoma
(angle-closure), ↑prostate, severe respiratory disease, jaundice,
blood disorders, **H/P/B**.
Class SE: EPSE, ↑prolactin and assoc Sx, sedation, ↑Wt, QT
prolongation, VTE, blood dyscrasias, ↓seizure threshold, NMS.
SE: anxiety, ↓appetite, blood dyscrasia, jaundice, cataract,
weakness, oedema, skin reactions, antimuscarinic fx (see p. 387).
Warn: if used in third trimester, monitor for EPSEs in neonate;
avoid direct sunlight at higher doses (photosensitisation), ↑fx of
alcohol. Gradual withdrawal advised if on high doses – risk of
withdrawal Sx (N&V, insomnia, involuntary movements).
Monitor: ECG may be required, esp if (risk factors for) CVD or
inpatient admission; prolactin concentration at start of therapy,
6 months, then yearly.
Interactions: ☠ ↑risk of neuroleptic malignant syndrome with
MAOIs ☠; ↑risk of neurotoxicity with lithium and reduced levels
by lithium; ↓fx of levodopa.

Dose: initially 5 mg po bd, ↑ by 5 mg after 1 wk, then further ↑ in steps of 5 mg at intervals of 3 days (when satisfactory control achieved, ↓ gradually until effective maintenance level established), max dose in practice 30 mg/day[1]; 2–4 mg po od in divided doses, max 6 mg od.[2,3] In the elderly, initially up to 2.5 mg bd, daily dose may be increased by 5 mg after 1 wk. If necessary, dose may be further increased in steps of 5 mg at intervals of 3 days.

TRI-IODOTHYRONINE
See Liothyronine; synthetic T_3 mostly used in myxoedema coma.

TRIMETHOPRIM
Antifolate antibiotic: inhibits dihydrofolate reductase.
Use: consult local antibiotic prescribing guidelines.
CI: blood disorders (esp megaloblastic ↓Hb).
Caution: ↓folate (or predisposition to), porphyria, **R/P/B/E**.
SE: see Co-trimoxazole (Septrin), but much less frequent and severe (esp BM suppression, skin reactions). Also GI upset, rash, rarely other hypersensitivity.
Warn: those on long-term Rx to look for signs of blood disorder and to report fever, sore throat, rash, mouth ulcers, bruising or bleeding.
Interactions: ↑s phenytoin and digoxin levels. ↑s risk of arrhythmias with amiodarone, antifolate fx with pyrimethamine and toxicity with ciclosporin, azathioprine, mercaptopurine and methotrexate, **W+**.
Dose: 200 mg bd po (100 mg nocte for chronic infections or as Px if at risk; *NB*: risk of ↓folate if long-term Rx). *NB*: ↓**dose if RF**. Refer to local antibiotic guidelines for specific indications/ duration of use.

TRIMIPRAMINE
TCA; antagonises H_1, $5\text{-}HT_{2A}$ and α_1-adrenergic receptors, weak reuptake inhibitor of 5-HT, NA and DA.
Use: depression.
CI: recent MI (within 3 months), arrhythmias (esp HB), mania, porphyria, **H/L** (if severe).

L/R/H = Liver, Renal and Heart failure. E = elderly. P = pregnancy. B = breastfeeding.

Caution: phaeo, $\uparrow T_4$, chronic constipation, DM, epilepsy, Hx of bipolar disorder/psychosis, $\uparrow$intraocular pressure, risks of suicide, urinary retention, $\uparrow$prostate, glaucoma (angle-closure), **L**.

SE: antimuscarinic fx, cardiac fx (arrhythmias, HB, $\uparrow$HR, postural $\downarrow$BP, dizziness, syncope: **dangerous in od**), $\uparrow$**Wt, sedation** (often $\Rightarrow$ 'hangover'), seizures. Rarely mania, fever, blood disorders, hypersensitivity, Δ LFTs, $\downarrow Na^+$ (esp in elderly), agitation, confusion, NMS.

Warn: withdrawal fx within 5 days of stopping treatment, worse after use for 8 wks+; $\downarrow$dose gradually over 4 wks+; $\uparrow$ effects of alcohol.

Interactions: metab by P450; ☠ $\uparrow$risk of serotonin syndrome with MAOI, e.g. isocarboxazid, moclobemide, phenelzine, selegiline, tranylcypromine (**avoid with/for 14 days after stopping MAOI**) ☠; $\uparrow$risk of neurotoxicity with lithium; $\uparrow$levels with bupropion, cinacalcet, dronedarone, fluvoxamine, fluoxetine, paroxetine, terbinafine; $\uparrow$fx of phenylephrine; $\downarrow$fx of adrenaline, ephedrine; some inhaled anaesthetics and sympathomimetics.

Dose: initially 50–75 mg po od at bedtime/in divided doses, $\uparrow$ to 150–300 mg od. Usual maintenance dose 75–150 mg od.

> ☠ Overdose is associated with high rate of fatality. TCA overdose $\Rightarrow$ dilated pupils, arrhythmias, $\downarrow$BP, hypothermia, hyperreflexia, extensor plantar responses, seizures, respiratory depression and coma. ☠

TROPICAMIDE EYE DROPS

Antimuscarinic: mydriatic (lasts approximately 4 h), weak cycloplegic.

Use: dilated retinal examination. See also 'Dilating eye drops'.

CI: untreated acute angle-closure glaucoma.

Caution: $\uparrow$IOP* (inc predisposition to), inflamed eye ($\uparrow$risk of systemic absorption).

SE: transient stinging and blurred vision and $\downarrow$accommodation. Rarely precipitation of acute angle-closure glaucoma ($\uparrow$risk if >60 years, long sighted, FHx).

Warn: unable to drive until can read car number plate at 20 m (approximately 4 h).
Dose: 1 drop 1% solution 15–20 min before examination. 0.5% in children <1 year old. *NB:* rare cause of acute angle-closure glaucoma* (esp if >60 years or hypermetropic).

TRYPTOPHAN

Essential dietary amino acid, precursor of serotonin; ↑inhibitory action of serotonin on amygdaloid nuclei.
Use: treatment-resistant depression (with senior advice).
CI: Hx of eosinophilia myalgia syndrome (EMS).
SE: weakness, headache, dizziness, somnolence, blood dyscrasias, muscle ache, nausea, suicidal ideation, eosinophilia myalgia syndrome.
Monitor: signs of suicidal thoughts, esp on initiation and dose Δs.
Interactions: 💀 ↑risk of serotonin syndrome with MAOI, e.g. isocarboxazid, moclobemide, phenelzine, selegiline, tranylcypromine, and SSRI.💀
Dose: 1 g po tds, max 6 g od.

▼ **VALPROATE** See (Sodium) valproate and Semisodium valproate.

VALSARTAN

Angiotensin II antagonist; see Losartan.
Use: HTN[1], MI with LV failure/dysfunction[2], heart failure[3].
CI: biliary obstruction, cirrhosis, **L** (if severe)/**P/B**.
Caution/SE/Interactions: see Losartan (inc warning about drugs that ↑K+).
Dose: initially 80 mg od[1] (*NB:* give 40 mg if ≥75 years old, LF, RF or ↓intravascular volume), 20 mg bd[2] or 40 mg bd[3], ↑ing every 4 wks if necessary to max 320 mg od[1] or 160 mg bd[2,3].

VANCOMYCIN

Glycopeptide antibiotic. Poor po absorption (unless bowel inflammation*), but still effective against *C. difficile***, as acts 'topically' in GI tract.

Use: serious Gram +ve infections[1] (inc endocarditis Px and systemic MRSA), AAC[2] (give po)**.

Caution: Hx of deafness, IBD* (only if given po), avoid rapid infusions (risk of anaphylaxis), **R/P/B/E**.

SE: nephrotoxicity, ototoxicity (stop if tinnitus develops), blood disorders, rash, hypersensitivity (inc anaphylaxis, severe skin reactions), nausea, fever, phlebitis/irritation at injection site.

Monitor: serum levels: keep pre-dose trough levels 10–15 mg/L; start monitoring after third dose (first dose if RF); *NB:* higher trough often recommended in osteomyelitis, endocarditis. Also monitor U&Es, FBC, urinalysis (and auditory function if elderly/RF).

Interactions: ↑nephrotoxicity with ciclosporin and aminoglycosides. ↑ototoxicity with loop diuretics. ↑s fx of suxamethonium.

Dose: 15–20 mg/kg bd/tds every 8–12 h (max dose 2 g) ivi at 10 mg/min[1]. 125 mg po[2] every 6 h for 10 days; increased if necessary to 500 mg every 6 h for 10 days. Use increased dose if life-threatening or refractory infection. Adjust dose according to plasma concentration. *NB:* ↓dose if RF or elderly.

> *NB:* If ivi given too quickly ⇒ ↑risk of anaphylactoid reactions (e.g. ↓BP, respiratory symptoms, skin reactions).

VARENICLINE

Selective nicotine receptor partial agonist. **Currently withdrawn in the UK.**

Use: smoking cessation aid.

Caution: seizures, CVD, depression.

SE: ↓/↑appetite, ↓/↑stool, GI disorders, fatigue, drowsiness, chest discomfort, dizziness, dry mouth; headache, joint/muscle ache, pain, nausea/vomiting, oral disorders, skin reactions, sleep disorders, ↑weight. Uncommon: allergic rhinitis, anxiety, arrhythmias, abnormal behaviour, burping, conjunctivitis, mood alterations, fever, fungal infection, haemorrhage, hallucination, ↑BM, flu-like Sx, menorrhagia, paraesthesia, palpitations, seizure, sexual dysfunction, suicidal ideation, sweating, tinnitus, tremor, urinary disorders. Rare: angioedema, bradyphrenia, unsteadiness, costochondritis, cyst, DM, dysarthria, eye disorders, glycosuria, ↑tone, polydipsia, psychosis, scleral discolouration, severe cutaneous reactions, snoring, vaginal discharge, eye/vision disorders.

Dose: 500 micrograms od for 3/7, ↑ to 500 micrograms bd for 4/7, then 1 mg bd for 11/52; reduced dose if not tolerated. Start 1–2/52 before target stop date. Course can be repeated in those abstinent to ↓ relapse.

VENLAFAXINE/EFFEXOR

Serotonin and noradrenaline reuptake inhibitor (SNRI): antidepressant with ↓sedative/antimuscarinic fx cf TCAs. ↑danger in od/heart disease than other antidepressants.

Use: depression[1], generalised anxiety disorder, social anxiety disorder, panic disorder ± agoraphobia.

CI: conditions with very high risk of serious cardiac ventricular arrhythmia (e.g. significant LV dysfunction, NYHA class III/IV), uncontrolled HTN.

Caution: Hx of mania, seizures or glaucoma, **L/R** (avoid if either severe), **H/P/B**.

SE: GI upset, ↑BP (dose-related; monitor BP if dose >200 mg/day), withdrawal fx (common even if dose only a few hours late), rash (consider stopping drug, as can be first sign of severe reaction*), insomnia/agitation, dry mouth, sexual dysfunction, Wt Δ, drowsiness, dizziness, SIADH and ↑QTc.

Warn: report rashes*. Do not stop suddenly.

Monitor: BP if heart disease ± ECG.

Interactions: 🐍 *never give with, or ≤2 wks after, MAOIs.* 🐍 ↑s risk of bleeding with aspirin/NSAIDs, dabigatran and CNS toxicity with selegiline. Avoid artemether/lumefantrine and piperaquine/artenimol. Mild **W+**.

Dose: immediate release: 37.5–187.5 mg bd po[1]; start low and ↑dose if required. Max in anxiety 225 mg/day in divided dose.

Effexor XL: MR od preparation available (initial dose 75 mg od; max in MDD 375 mg od, max in anxiety 225 mg od).

NB: Halve dose if moderate LF (PT 14–18 sec) or RF (GFR 10–30 mL/min).

VERAPAMIL

Ca^{2+} channel blocker (rate-limiting type): fx on heart ($\Rightarrow \downarrow$HR, $\downarrow$contractility*) > vasculature (dilates peripheral/coronary arteries); i.e. reverse of the dihydropyridine type (e.g. nifedipine). Only Ca^{2+} channel blocker with useful antiarrhythmic properties (class IV).

Use: HTN[1], angina[2], arrhythmias (SVTs, esp instead of adenosine if asthma)[3].

CI: $\downarrow$BP, $\downarrow$HR (<50 bpm), second-/third-degree HB, $\downarrow$LV function, SAN block, SSS, AF or atrial flutter 2° to WPW, recent treatment with β-blocker, acute, **H** (inc Hx of)*.

Caution: AMI, first-degree HB, **L/P/B**.

SE: constipation (rarely other GI upset), HF, $\downarrow$BP (dose dependent), HB, headache, dizziness, fatigue, ankle oedema, hypersensitivity, skin reactions.

Warn: fx $\uparrow$d by grapefruit juice (avoid).

Interactions: $\uparrow$risk of AV block and HF with ☠ β-blockers ☠ disopyramide, flecainide, dronedarone, colchicine, fingolimod and amiodarone. $\uparrow$s hypotensive fx of antihypertensives (esp α-blockers) and anaesthetics. $\uparrow$s levels/fx of digoxin, theophyllines, carbamazepine, quinidine, ivabradine, dabigatran, tamsulosin and ciclosporin. Levels/fx $\downarrow$ by rifampicin and barbiturates. $\uparrow$risk of myopathy with simvastatin. Sirolimus $\uparrow$s levels of both drugs. Levels may be $\uparrow$ by clari-/erythromycin and ritonavir. Risk of VF with ☠ iv dantrolene.☠

Dose: 240–480 mg daily in 2–3 divided doses po[1]; 80–120 mg tds po[2]; 40–120 mg tds po[3]; 5–10 mg iv (over 2 min [3 min in elderly] with ECG monitoring), followed by additional 5 mg iv if necessary after 5–10 min[3]. MR (od/bd) preparations available.[BNF] *NB:* $\downarrow$oral dose in LF.

VORTIOXETINE

SSRI antidepressant (also 5-HT3 antagonist and 5-HT1A agonist).

Use: Depression

CI: mania, poorly controlled epilepsy.

Caution: epilepsy, receiving ECT, Hx of mania or bleeding disorder (esp GI), glaucoma (angle-closure), ↑risk of bleeding, age <18 years, **L/H/E.**

Class SE: GI upset, ↓Wt, insomnia, agitation, headache, hypersensitivity. Can ⇒ withdrawal fx when stopped. Rarely extrapyramidal and antimuscarinic fx, sexual dysfunction, convulsions, ↓Na+ (inc SIADH), bleeding disorders, GI bleed, serotonin syndrome and suicidal thoughts/behaviour, ↑risk of bone fracture, glaucoma.

Interactions: primarily metab by CYP2D6 levels ↑d by strong CYP2D6 inhibitors (e.g., bupropion, quinidine, fluoxetine, paroxetine); dose adjustment may be considered if co-prescribed with a broad CYP450 inducer (e.g., rifampicin, carbamazepine, phenytoin); ↑risk of CNS toxicity (serotonin syndrome; see p. 410) with drugs that ↑5-HT (e.g. tramadol, sibutramine, sumatriptan, St John's wort). Risk of bleeding with anticoagulants, aspirin and NSAIDs. ☠ **Never give with, or ≤2 wks after, MAOIs; do not give MAOIs ≤2 wks of stopping vortioxetine.** ☠

Dose: Initially 10 mg od, adjust to 5–20 mg od.

WARFARIN

Oral anticoagulant: blocks synthesis of vit K–dependent factors (II, VII, IX, X) and proteins C and S.

Use: Rx/Px of VTE.

CI: severe HTN, PU, severe bleeding, haemorrhagic CVA, **P.**

Caution: recent surgery, bacterial endocarditis, 48 h post-partum, **L/R** (avoid if creatinine clearance <10 mL/min)/**B.**

SE: haemorrhage, rash, fever, diarrhoea. Rarely other GI upset, 'purple-toe syndrome', skin necrosis, hepatotoxicity, hypersensitivity.

Warn: fx are ↑d by alcohol and cranberry juice (avoid); fx with vit K-rich foods (leafy greens).

Dose: refer to specialist for dosing regimen.

☠ *NB:* **W+** and **W–** denote significant interactions throughout this book: take particular care with antibiotics and drugs that affect cytochrome **P450** (see p. 382).☠

ZOLEDRONIC ACID/ZOMETA

Bisphosphonate: ↓s osteoclastic bone resorption.

Use: Px of bone damage[1] in advanced bone malignancy, damage or
Rx of ↑Ca^{2+} in malignancy[2], Rx of Paget's disease of bone[3], Rx of
osteoporosis (post-menopausal or in men)[4].

CI: P/B.

Caution: cardiac disease, dehydration*, øCa^{2+}/po_4^{2-}/Mg^{2+}.
L (if severe)/**R/H**.

SE: flu-like syndrome, fever, bone pain, fatigue, **N&V**. Also arthr-/
myalgia, øCa^{2+}/PO_4^{2-}/Mg^{2+}, pruritus/rash, headache, conjunctivitis,
RF, hypersensitivity, blood disorders (esp ↓Hb), osteonecrosis
(esp of jaw; consider dental examination or preventive Rx before
starting drug) and atypical femur fractures (advise patients to
report thigh/groin pain).

Monitor: Ca^{2+}, PO_4^{2-}, Mg^{2+}, U&E. Ensure patient adequately
hydrated pre-dose* and advise good dental hygiene.

Dose: 4 mg ivi every 3–4 wks[1]; 4 mg ivi as single dose[2]. Also
available as once-yearly preparation 5 mg ivi over ≥15 min[3,4].
Co-prescribe with calcium 500 mg od and vit D 400 units od[1]; at
least 500 mg calcium bd (with vit D) for at least 10 days following
infusion;[2] 50 000–125 000 units of vit D before infusion[4]. *NB:*
↓dose in RF.

ZOLPIDEM (TARTRATE)

'Non-benzodiazepine' hypnotic; see Zopiclone.

Use/CI/Caution/SE/Interactions: as zopiclone but CI in
psychotic illness, **P**.

Dose: 10 mg nocte. *NB:* halve dose if LF (avoid if severe), severe
RF or elderly.

ZOMORPH Morphine sulphate capsules (10, 30, 60, 100 or
200 mg), equivalent in efficacy to Oramorph but SR: 12-hrly doses.

ZOPICLONE

Short-acting hypnotic (cyclopyrrolone): potentiates GABA pathways via same receptors as benzodiazepines (although is not a benzodiazepine): can also ⇒ dependence* and tolerance.

Use: insomnia (not long term*).

CI: respiratory failure, sleep apnoea (severe), marked neuromuscular respiratory weakness (inc MG), **L** (if severe**), **B**.

Caution: Ψ disorders, Hx of drug abuse*, muscle weakness, MG, **R/P/E**.

SE: taste Δs; *rare*: GI upset, behavioural/Ψ disturbances (inc psychosis, aggression), hypersensitivity.

Interactions: levels ↑ by ritonavir, erythromycin and other enzyme inhibitors. Levels ↓ by rifampicin. Sedation ↑d by other sedative medications and alcohol.

Dose: 3.75–7.5 mg nocte, for up to 4 wks. *NB:* halve dose if LF (avoid if severe), severe RF or elderly.

ZUCLOPENTHIXOL ACETATE/CLOPIXOL ACUPHASE

Thioxanthene antipsychotic; antagonises D_1/D_2 receptors, α_1-adrenoceptors and 5-HT_2 receptors.

Use: short-term management of psychosis or mania when an effect of 2–3 days is desirable.

CI: CNS depression, phaeo.

Caution: Parkinson's, ↑QTc, epilepsy, MG, glaucoma (angle-closure), ↑prostate, severe respiratory disease, jaundice, blood disorders, ↑/↓thyroid, NMS, concurrent other antipsychotic prescription, **H**.

Class SE: EPSE, ↑prolactin and assoc Sx, sedation, ↑Wt, QT prolongation, VTE, blood dyscrasias, ↓seizure threshold, NMS.

SE: GI upset (D, discomfort), sexual dysfunction, rash, visual problems, ↓temperature, headaches.

Monitor: ECG may be required, esp if physical examination identifies cardiovascular risk factors/Hx of cardiovascular disease/patient is admitted as inpatient.

Interactions: metab by P450 (CYP2D6, CYP3A4); ↑fx of alcohol, barbiturates, CNS depressants, general anesthetics,

anticoagulants; ↑risk of extrapyramidal effects (e.g. tardive dyskinesia) with metoclopramide, piperazine, antiparkinson medications; ↑risk of neurotoxicity with lithium; ↑risk of ↑QTc with class 1A and III antiarrhythmics (e.g. quinidine, amiodarone, sotalol), antipsychotics (e.g. thioridazine), macrolides (e.g. erythromycin), antihistamines and quinolone antibiotics (e.g. moxifloxacin).
Dose: 50–150 mg im, then 50–150 mg after 2–3 days (one additional dose may be needed 1–2 days after first injection); max 400 mg in 2 wks/max four injections, max duration of treatment 2 wks – change to oral antipsychotic 2–3 days after last injection for maintenance treatment/to a longer-acting antipsychotic depot injection given concomitantly with last injection, administered into gluteal muscle/lateral thigh.

 Do not confuse with zuclopenthixol decanoate.

ZUCLOPENTHIXOL DECANOATE/CLOPIXOL
See Zuclopenthixol acetate.
Use: maintenance in psychosis.
CI: CNS depression, phaeo, children.
Caution/SE/Monitor/Interactions: see Zuclopenthixol acetate.
Dose: test dose 100 mg im, administered into upper outer buttock/lateral thigh, followed by 200–500 mg after at least 7 days, then 200–500 mg every 1–4 wks, higher doses of >500 mg can be used, max 600 mg wkly; max single dose 600 mg at any time.

 Do not confuse with zuclopenthixol acetate.

ZUCLOPENTHIXOL DIHYDROCHLORIDE/CLOPIXOL
See Zuclopenthixol acetate.
Use: psychosis.
CI: CNS depression due to any cause, e.g. alcohol, phaeo, withdrawn states.
Caution/SE/Monitor/Interactions: see Zuclopenthixol acetate.
Dose: initially 20–30 mg po od in divided doses, ↑ to 150 mg od, usual maintenance 20–50 mg od (max single dose 40 mg).

Disorders

PSYCHOSIS

Psychosis is a syndrome defined by three main 'positive' symptoms: delusions, hallucinations and/or thought disorder. There are numerous causes of psychosis and it may be primary or secondary. Secondary psychosis, often with a medical cause ('organic psychosis') can be due to medications, epilepsy or neurodegenerative disease (and many more causes).

In primary psychosis, it is common initially to use the term 'first episode psychosis' (FEP; i.e., 'non-organic psychosis'); this is because it is difficult to determine whether the patient will develop schizophrenia, another psychotic disorder, or experience no enduring mental illness.

Schizophrenia is one example of a primary psychotic disorder. A diagnosis is made when persisting symptoms are accompanied by a broad impairment of function and negative symptoms. The latter are typically a loss of normal behaviours and motivation: affective flattening, alogia, avolition, anhedonia and attentional impairment. Currently, it is impossible to accurately predict who will develop schizophrenia.

The term at-risk mental state (ARMS) describes patients with attenuated psychotic Sx: 20%–30% of cases progress to full psychosis within 2 years. The predictive value of ARMS is challenged and it does not currently seem to have general clinical utility.[BAP] However, it is also clear that patients characterised as being in an ARMS group are at a high risk of many forms of poor psychiatric outcomes aside from psychosis (Beck et al. *Schiz Research* 2019; **203**: 55–61). Other risk and environmental factors (obstetric complications, childhood trauma, urbanicity, migration) should not be ignored (Murray et al. *World Psych* 2021; **20**: 222–223).

Following diagnosis with FEP and appropriate treatment, it is possible to have a complete recovery with no further relapses. However, it is not uncommon for such patients to have residual symptoms and/or to relapse after a recovery. Treatment-resistant schizophrenia is usually defined as a failure to respond to two trials of antipsychotic medications, used at adequate doses for sufficient lengths of time.

Psychosis can also be a feature of mania and severe depression ('affective psychoses'). Delusional disorder is characterised by a persistent delusion without other prominent features of schizophrenia (inappropriate affect, hallucinations, thought disorder).

TYPES OF MEDICATIONS
- First-generation antipsychotics (FGAs, aka 'typicals').
- Second-generation antipsychotics (SGAs, aka 'atypicals').
- Third-generation antipsychotics (TGAs, aka 'atypicals').

Class	Drug name	Route(s) po	im SA	LA	Equiv po dose/ mg[1]	Affinities[2] D_2	5-HT$_2$	Side effects EPSE	Met Syn	Other
FGA	Haloperidol	✔	✔	✔	10	+++	+	+++	+	
	Chlorpromazine	✔			600	+++	+++	++	++	Photosensitivity
	Sulpiride	✔			800	+++	−	+	+	
	Trifluoperazine	✔			20	+++	+	+++	+	
	Flupentixol	✔		✔	10	+++	+	++	+	
	Fluphenazine			✔	12	+++	+	+++	+	
	Zuclopenthixol[3]	✔		✔	50	+++	+	++	+	
SGA	Olanzapine	✔[4]	✔	✔	20	++	+++	+/−	+++	
	Risperidone	✔[4]		✔	6	+++	++	+	++	
	Paliperidone	✔		✔	9	+++	++	+	++	
	Quetiapine	✔			750	+	+	−	++	
	Amisulpride	✔			700	+++	−	+	+	
	Clozapine	✔	✔		400	+	+++	−	+++	See following
	Lurasidone	✔			120[5]	+++	+	+	+	
TGA	Aripiprazole[6]	✔[4]	✔	✔	30	+++	++	+	+	Akathisia

SA = short acting (for acute treatment).

LA = long acting (depot).

[1] Gardner et al., *Am J Psychiatry* 2010.

[2] Richtand et al., *Neuropsychopharmacology* 2007; Correll, *Eur Psychiatry* 2010; PDSP Ki Database (https://pdsp.unc.edu/databases/kidb.php).

[3] Studies on affinities not available; values quoted based on similarity to flupentixol.

[4] Available as quick dissolving/orodispersible preparation.

[5] Leucht & Samara, *Schizophr Bull* 2016. Given available formulations in the UK, this is approximately 111 mg.

[6] Partial agonist at D_2 and 5-HT$_{1A}$. Antagonist at 5-HT$_{2A}$.

All block D_2 receptors to varying degrees (dopamine antagonists); atypicals also antagonise $5-HT_2$ receptors.

Four main DA brain systems account for many effects: nigrostriatal (movement), tuberoinfundibular (prolactin), mesocortical (cognition, emotion) and mesolimbic (motivation, reward).

Efficacy

Apart from clozapine, differences between antipsychotics are small. The following is a comparison of SGAs for overall Sx reduction (Leucht et al., *Lancet* 2013; **382**(9896): 951–62). All medications are compared relative to placebo (symptom reduction of zero).

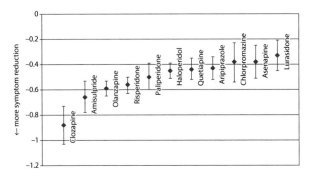

Adherence to antipsychotics

Full adherence rates for oral antipsychotics after discharge from hospital are poor (Leucht & Heres, *J Clin Psychiatry* 2006; **67**(s5): 5–8):

10 days	1 yr	2 yr
75%	50%	25%

- If medication consumption is supervised, orodispersible olanzapine/risperidone/aripiprazole may be an alternative option for improving adherence.

Depot antipsychotics (LAIs)

- Depot antipsychotics (LAIs) can improve adherence, provide consistent bioavailability and give regular contact with a nurse. However, there is a perceived stigma attached to depot injections.
- It is generally appropriate to give a trial of the oral antipsychotic to establish effectiveness and tolerability before initiating a depot.
- Depot injections do not allow rapid adjustments in dose. Ideally, the effective and tolerated doses should be established with oral medications before switching to a depot.
- Paliperidone is 9-hydroxyrisperidone, the active metabolite of risperidone. Patients who have been stabilised on oral risperidone are often switched to paliperidone long-acting injection (LAI), as it has simpler pharmacokinetics than risperidone LAI.
- Depot administration (full training required): See Feetam & White (Eds), *Guidance on the Administration to Adults of Oilbased Depot and Other Long-Acting Intramuscular Antipsychotic Injections*, 6th Edition (2020). Available from https://hull-repository.worktribe.com/output/3632150.
  - Check injection sites and ask Re. SEs.
  - Two registered practitioners to check prescription.
  - Prepare injection according to SPC instructions.
  - Three possible injection sites: deltoid, gluteal, lateral thigh.

Depot	Site	Test dose	Dose range
Arpiprazole (Abilfy Maintena)[1]	Gluteal	Not required/oral	300–400 mg/month
Flupentixol decanoate (Depixol)	Gluteal, thigh	20 mg	50 mg/4 wks – 400 mg/wk
Fluphenazine decanoate (Modecate)	Gluteal	12.5 mg	12.5 mg – 100 mg/ 2 wks
Haloperidol decanoate (Haldol)	Gluteal	25 mg	50–300 mg/4 wks
Olanzapine pamoate[2]	Gluteal	Not required/oral	150 mg/4 wks – 300 mg/2 wks
Paliperidone palmitate (Xeplion, monthly)[1]	Deltoid, gluteal	Not required/oral	50–150 mg/month

Paliperidone palmitate[1] (Trevicta, 3-monthly)[3]	Deltoid, gluteal	Not required/oral	175–525 mg/ 3 months
Pipothiazine palmitate (Piportil)	Gluteal	25 mg	50–200 mg/4 wks
Risperidone (Risperdal Consta)[1]	Deltoid, gluteal	Not required/oral	25–50 mg/2 wks
Risperidone (Okedi)	Deltoid, gluteal	Not required/oral	75–100 mg/4 wks
Zuclopenthixol decanote (Clopixol)	Gluteal, thigh	100 mg	200 mg/3 wks – 600 mg/wk

1. Oral loading required.
2. Risk of post-injection syndrome.
3. Can't start unless completed ≥4 months of monthly paliperidone LAI.

— Gluteal: Expose whole buttock with patient lying on front or side. To avoid sciatic nerve, inject in upper outer quadrant of buttock aiming for gluteus maximus. Aspirate before injecting, and only proceed if no blood.
— Lateral thigh: Inject in the anterolateral aspect of the thigh halfway between the greater trochanter and the later condyle of the femur, aiming for vastus lateralis.
— Avoid injecting into moles/birthmarks, inflammation, oedema or scar tissue.
— To prevent depot leaking back from muscle to subcutaneous tissue, use the **Z-track technique:** Pull the skin sideways before the needle enters. Insert needle at 90°, deep enough to penetrate muscle (this depends on body habitus). Withdraw the needle and then release the skin, preventing tracking of the medication back through the site of needle entry.

CHOOSING A MEDICATION
At-Risk Mental State (ARMS)

- Limited evidence for any intervention preventing the transition from ARMS to FEP; antipsychotic medication should not be used for this indication.[NICE]
- Do not prescribe antipsychotics to prevent transition to FEP.[NICE]

- However, patients with ARMS often have other mental health disorders including anxiety and depression. Prescribing should be appropriate to these individual presentations.

First episode (non-organic) psychosis (FEP)

- No significant difference in efficacy between FGAs and SGAs; a network meta-analysis has shown the superiority of clozapine (Hunn et al., *Lancet*, 2019; 394(10202): 939–951).
- Choose antipsychotic based on[BAP]:
  - Medication's side effect profile (consider using side effect tool at psymatik.com).
  - Patient's propensity for serious side effects (EPSEs, metabolic syndrome).
  - Patient's preference.
  - Relevant medical history.
- Generally recommended to offer oral route first, although depot can be offered first line. Depots should also be offered for maintenance as this is associated with reduction in relapse.[BAP]
- Start at lower end of licensed dose range.[BAP]
- If a FGA is selected, use medium- or low-potency rather than high-potency drugs.[BAP]
  - Potency refers to the quantity of drug required to produce a desired effect.

Managing –ve Sx
- Consider whether –ve Sx might be due to +ve Sx, EPSEs, depression, substance misuse or another medical or psychiatric disorder.
- Treat EPSEs.[BAP]
- Treat depression.[BAP]
- ↑Stimulation in environment.[BAP]
- Consider a selective serotonin reuptake inhibitor (SSRI), even if not depressed,[BAP] but check interactions (p. 382).
- Limited evidence for any antipsychotic medication (including clozapine) in the treatment of negative symptoms.[BAP]
  - Small emerging evidence base suggesting cariprazine may attenuate –ve Sx.

- Specifically warn patients about weight gain before prescribing olanzapine.[NICE]

Relapsed psychosis
- Same principles apply as FEP when choosing an antipsychotic.[BAP]
- Higher doses of antipsychotics are often required, but use the minimum effective dose.[BAP]
- In addition, consider past experience of antipsychotics.[BAP]

Delusional disorder
- Has a reputation for being difficult to treat, partly due to patients' poor insight and late presentation, with longer duration of untreated psychosis (DUP) allowing beliefs to become entrenched.
- Robust evidence significantly lacking; however, some patients may respond to standard antipsychotics +/– cognitive therapy.

Organic psychosis
- Treat the underlying disorder, but antipsychotics may become necessary.
- If medication-induced, consider withdrawal of causative agent. There is evidence for lithium in steroid-induced psychosis.
- If due to epilepsy, control of seizures or withdrawal of the offending anticonvulsant (e.g. levetiracetam, topiramate, zonisamide) is the mainstay of treatment. Benzodiazepines are preferred for psychotic agitation, though antipsychotics are occasionally used. See page 295 for more information.
- If due to dementia, severe and with associated risks, then antipsychotics may be used in low doses. Risperidone is licensed for this use; however, beware ↑stroke risk.
- In Parkinson's or Lewy body dementia, psychosis can be caused by pro-dopaminergic agents. Consider switching these. Otherwise, consider antipsychotic with low propensity for EPSEs, such as clozapine or quetiapine. See page 296 for more information.

- In Huntington's, use atypicals to avoid worsening underlying bradykinesia (Jauhar & Ritchie, *Adv Psychiatr Treat* 2010; **16**(3): 168–75). See page 298 for more information.
- In 22q11.2 deletion syndrome (DiGeorge syndrome), use antipsychotics starting at low doses and titrating slowly. Consider a prophylactic anticonvulsant if treating with clozapine, due to risks of seizures (Fung et al., *Genet Med* 2015; **17**(8): 599–601).

TREATMENT RESISTANCE

- Before diagnosing treatment-resistant schizophrenia, confirm diagnosis (consider e.g. autoimmune encephalitis, substance use and medication concordance).
- Up to one-third of patients respond poorly to antipsychotics, deemed 'treatment resistant'.
- Clozapine has by far the best evidence[BAP] and should be used first line when treatment resistance is established, but response can be slow (see box).

Clozapine response rates (Meltzer, Schizophr Bull *1992; 18(3): 515–542)*		
6 wks	3 months	6 months
30%	50%	60%–70%

- Adequate trial of clozapine is 6 months.[BAP] If clozapine response is poor, optimise therapy as follows:
  - Ensure compliance.
  - Check for ongoing substance misuse.
  - Ensure adequate plasma levels.
- Clozapine non-response (Lally & Gaughran, *Ir J Psychol Med* 2018; **27**: 1–13):
  - Full multidisciplinary team assessment.
  - Reassess primary diagnosis and psychiatric co-morbidities.
  - Look for organic contributors.
  - Minimise other stressors.
  - Optimise clozapine to ensure plasma levels of 0.35–0.5 mg/L.

- Consider trial of clozapine plasma levels of >0.5 mg/L.
- Augment clozapine, e.g. with amisulpride, sulpiride, haloperidol or lamotrigine. If there is an affective component, augment with lithium.[BAP]
- Psychological therapies such as cognitive behavioural therapy for psychosis (CBTp) and family work.
- Antipsychotic (including clozapine)+ECT can be useful if rapid effect required. ECT may be useful in stabilising a patient, such that they are able to tolerate clozapine titration.[BAP]
- High-dose antipsychotics (i.e. above BNF max): no convincing evidence for this strategy and it goes against many guidelines. Risk of sudden cardiac death is higher. Only use as a time-limited tentative trial after other options exhausted and only continue if clear clinical benefit outweighing additional risks. May have a role in fast metabolisers.[BAP]
- Combined antipsychotics (other than with clozapine) → ↑SE, ↑drug interactions, ↓adherence and ↑mortality. Also, hard to work out which drug is having an effect. Only use as a time-limited tentative trial after other options exhausted.[BAP]

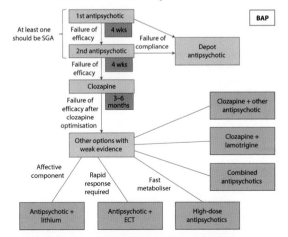

NON-PHARMACOLOGICAL MEASURES

A range of psychosocial interventions can be helpful in psychosis:

- Adherence therapy.
- Behavioural family therapy if presence of high expressed emotion among family members.
- Patient support groups. (Mind, Rethink, Hearing Voices Network)
- Psychoeducation.
- Engagement in education and employment.
- Supported living.
- Care coordination.

CBT for psychosis
- Meta-analysis has shown small effect (pooled effect sizes −0.33). (Jauhar et al., *BJPsych* 2014; **204**(1): 20–9)
- Some evidence in ARMS.
- For established schizophrenia, CBT may be used *in addition* to antipsychotics to ↓ relapse, but is not optimal monotherapy.[NICE]
- Principles:
    - ↓Distress from +ve Sx.
    - ↓Behaviours that may be maintaining factors.
- Techniques:
    - Empathic and supportive stance to overcome paranoia.
    - Avoid both confrontation and collusion.
    - Normalise experiences.
    - Explore evidence for and against beliefs.
    - Teach helpful coping strategies.

STARTING ACUTE MEDICATION

- Do baseline monitoring (see following).
- Generally start in 2° care.[NICE]
- Start at low dose and increase gradually based on clinical response (symptoms and side effects).[BAP]
- For clozapine, start at 12.5 mg od or bd on day 1, then 25 mg od or bd on day 2. If good tolerance, increase daily dose in increments of 25–50 mg, up to daily dose of 300 mg. If further

increase required, increase by 50–100 mg weekly.[SPC] Can titrate
more rapidly if previously tolerated clozapine.

- If considering olanzapine, discuss with the patient the higher risk
  of wt gain, which can occur soon after commencing treatment.[NICE]
- For FGAs, maintenance dose should be 300–600 mg
  chlorpromazine equivalent.[BAP]
- For SGAs, give same maintenance dose as that required during
  acute phase.[BAP]
- Carefully document changes in clinical presentation.[BAP]
- Early response can occur within 24 h of starting antipsychotic.
  Behaviour and emotional preoccupation change before psychotic
  conviction recedes.
- Initial trial of medication for 2–3 wks at effective does, as +ve
  response at 2 wks predicts subsequent response (NPV = 80%). If
  no response at this point, consider increasing doses or changing
  medication.[MPG]
- A full trial is 6 wks of the medication (at least 4 wks of good
  adherence at optimum dose).
- Where no satisfactory response has been achieved, another
  antipsychotic should be trialled.
- Do not use initial loading doses ('rapid neuroleptization').[BAP]
  NB: However, paliperidone long-acting injectable has a
  recommended loading dose to avoid a long time to peak plasma
  concentration.
- Avoid combining antipsychotics (unless cross-titrating).[BAP]

MAINTENANCE THERAPY

- Medication should be selected based on prior treatment
  response, the experience of side effects, level of medication
  adherence and co-morbid physical illness.[BAP]
- Prescription should be within the licensed range.[BAP]
- Dosing should be kept as simple as possible in terms of the
  number of tablets and doses, depots should be considered and,
  ideally, patient–clinician agreement should be sought.
- Any reduction in dosage of antipsychotic medication should be
  cautious and closely monitored, given the increased risk of relapse.

- In long-term prescriptions, SEs should be actively managed.
- Maintenance therapy should be considered for 2 years in the first instance.

SIDE EFFECTS

- As a general rule, FGAs are more likely to cause EPSEs and hyperprolactinaemia, whereas SGAs are more associated with metabolic syndrome. However, this is not exclusive, and there is some overlap.
- Patients may respond differently to different medications.
- An evidence-based tool to rank antipsychotics by side effects balanced against effectiveness can be accessed at psymatik.com.
- For information on how to monitor side effects see section on Monitoring see table on p. 170.

FGAs	SGAs
Dystonia (muscle spasms)	Wt gain
Parkinsonism (rigidity, tremor, bradykinesia)	Dyslipidaemia
Akathisia (restlessness)	Impaired glucose tolerance
Tardive dyskinesia (abnormal movements)	Prolonged QT
↑Prolactin	↑Prolactin
NMS	
Prolonged QT	

Clozapine

Some particular side effects (SEs):

- Neutropenia and agranulocytosis (can be fatal); see below for WBC monitoring guidance
- Myocarditis/cardiomyopathy
- ↑Saliva
- Constipation/gastrointestinal (GI) obstruction (can be fatal if perforates)
- Postural hypotension (common during titration, but often improves)

- Seizures (risk related to plasma levels)
- Pneumonia (also linked to other antipsychotics)

> *Managing clozapine-associated pyrexia and tachycardia*
> *(Mortimer et al. 2018,* BJPsych Adv **17**(4): *256–265)*
> - Pyrexia common in first 3 wks, benign in most cases.
>   Worth clinically excluding rare but serious causes such
>   as myocarditis, infection, neutropenic sepsis and NMS.
>   Antipyretic medication may be given, but most pyrexia
>   resolves spontaneously.
> - Tachycardia can occur in 1/4 patients commenced on
>   clozapine. Worth clinically excluding myocarditis,
>   particularly if other cardiac signs/symptoms. Consider
>   beta-blocker (e.g. atenolol, bisoprolol) or dose reduction if
>   isolated tachycardia. Seek cardiology input if unsure.

Vulnerabilities to side effects

Group	SE vulnerability
Women of reproductive age	↑Prolactin
FEP patients	↑Wt
Young men	Acute dystonia
Elderly	Postural hypotension
	QTc prolongation
	Tardive dyskinesia

Extrapyramidal side effects (EPSEs)

(Saifee & Edwards, *Pract Neurol* 2011; **11**(6): 341–8; Pringsheim
et al., *Can J Psychiatry* 2018; **63**(11): 719–29)

- An umbrella term for a range of iatrogenic side effects. These
  are dose related, usually in response to high-potency FGAs.
- EPSEs can be acute (acute dystonia, parkinsonism, akathisia) or
  chronic (tardive dyskinesia, chronic dystonia).

EPSE	Features	Rx
Parkinsonism	Tremor (3–5 Hz), rigidity, bradykinesia	1. Consider switch or ↓dose
		2. Procyclidine up to 5 mg tds
Akathisia	Subjective restlessness, urge to move, tension when forced to stay still	1. ↓Dose
		2. Consider switch to olanzapine, quetiapine or clozapine
		3. Propranolol 80 mg
		4. Mirtazapine 15 mg
Dystonia (involuntary sustained muscle contraction)	Torticollis (neck), opisthotonus (backward arching), trismus (muscles of mastication), blepharospasm (eyelids forced shut), oculogyric crisis (eyes stuck in upward gaze), laryngeal dystonia (life threatening)	Acute: Procyclidine 5–10 mg im/iv stat; see p. 495 Chronic: Trihexyphenidyl 1 mg, ↑ to 2–4 mg tds or procyclidine, as previously discussed; consider referral for Botox if focal
Tardive dyskinesia	Orofacial dyskinesia (more common): tongue protrusion, lip smacking, sucking, chewing, grimacing Limb/trunk movements (rarer): shoulder shrugging, pelvis rotation, athetosis, choreiform movements	1. Consider switch to clozapine (↓dose of original antipsychotic does not tend to help)
		2. Tetrabenazine 12.5 mg od, ↑slowly to 25–50 mg tds
		3. Consider clonazepam, propranolol or baclofen
NMS	Any two of: mental status change, muscle rigidity, fever, autonomic dysfunction	Stop antipsychotic and give benzodiazepines; see p. 409

- Procyclidine:
  - Often effective as a Rx, but do not prescribe prophylactically.
  - Can add to anticholinergic burden (cognitive impairment, blurred vision, glaucoma, urinary retention, constipation, tachycardia).
  - Some patients request it because of its associated euphoria.

Metabolic syndrome

- Metabolic syndrome consists of obesity, dyslipidaemia, HTN and impaired glucose tolerance.
- It is a common SE of antipsychotics, especially with SGA. Even among SGAs, there is a variation in the propensity to cause metabolic syndrome, with olanzapine and clozapine the worst, and aripiprazole, brexpiprazole, cariprazine, lurasidone and ziprasidone the most benign.
- Certain risk factors have been shown to increase the risk or the degree of metabolic SEs, including personal or family history of metabolic syndrome, increasing age, male sex and non-white ethnicities.
- These factors should be considered when choosing an antipsychotic and weighed against other clinical outcomes.[BAP]

(Pillinger et al. *Lancet Psych* 2020; 7(1): 64–77)

Problem	Diagnosis	Treatment	
Weight gain	BMI >25 or wt gain >5 kg in 3 months	Consider switching antipsychotic (see table on p. 191)	Metformin (off-license) → 3 kg ↓wt and ↑glucose tolerance
Impaired glucose tolerance	Fasting glucose ≥5.6 mmol/L or HbA1c 42–47 mmol/mol		Adding aripiprazole to clozapine/olanzapine → 2 kg ↓wt
Dyslipidaemia	CVD risk of 10% using QRISK3 tool meets NICE threshold for statin	Diet	Atorvastatin 20 mg
HTN	Sys BP >140 or dia BP >90	Exercise	NICE NG136
DM	Fasting glucose ≥7.0 mmol/L, random glucose ≥11.1 mmol/L or HbA1c ≥ 48 mmol/mol	Smoking cessation	NICE NG28

Prolonged QTc

QT interval
- Time from ventricular depolarisation to end of repolarisation.
- Measure in lead II, V5 or V6.
- Measured as distance from start of Q-wave to end of T-wave.
- Corrected QT interval (QTc) can be calculated with *Bazett's formula*:

$$QTc = \frac{QT}{\sqrt{RR \text{ interval}}}$$

- If HR <60 or >100, better to use *Fridericia's formula*:

$$QTc = \frac{QT}{RR^{1/3}}$$

Most antipsychotics have some effect upon the QT interval, increasing the risk of ventricular arrhythmias (especially torsade de pointes) and death. It can also be prolonged by electrolyte abnormalities ($\downarrow K^+$, $\downarrow Ca^{2+}$ or $\downarrow Mg^{2+}$) and congenital long QT syndromes.

Aripiprazole and lurasidone are considered the safest. Risks are increased if other cardiac risk factors are present, or when co-prescribed with other psychotropic or non-psychotropic medication that prolongs the QT interval. If any of these risk factors are present, particular caution should be taken including a more detailed cardiac assessment.[BAP] The following chart offers suggested management.

QTc	Management[MPG]
♂ <440 ms ♀ <470 ms	Normal QTc. No action unless abnormal T-wave morphology.
♂ 440–500 ms ♀ 470–500 ms	Repeat electrocardiogram (ECG). Consider $\downarrow$dose or switching. Check K^+, Ca^{2+}, Mg^{2+}. Consider referral to cardiologist.
>500 ms	Stop drug. Check K^+, Ca^{2+}, Mg^{2+}. Consult cardiologist.
Abnormal T-wave morphology	Consider $\downarrow$dose or switching. Consult cardiologist.

QTc-prolonging drugs (QT interval and drug therapy, Drug Ther Bull *2016*)

- Antipsychotics
- TCAs
- Anti-arrhythmics (e.g. amiodarone, sotalol)
- Macrolides (e.g. clarithromycin, erythromycin, azithromycin)
- Quinolones (e.g. ciprofloxacin, moxifloxacin)
- Triazoles (e.g. fluconazole, ketoconazole)
- Antimalarials (e.g. quinine, chloroquine)
- Antihistamines (e.g. promethazine, hydroxyzine)
- Methadone

Free tool to check drugs at https://crediblemeds.org

↑**Prolactin**

(Gupta et al., *BJPsych Adv* 2017; **23**(40): 278–86)

- Most associated with risperidone, paliperidone, amisulpride, sulpiride and haloperidol. Aripiprazole, clozapine and quetiapine are considered to be prolactin-sparing.[BAP]
- Measure prolactin in low stress environment, ≥2 h after waking and ≥1 h after eating.
- Two forms of prolactin: free prolactin (active) and macroprolactin (inactive).
  - If ↑prolactin, check macroprolactin levels, as this may be causing **pseudohyperprolactinaemia**, which is not clinically significant.
- Often asymptomatic.
- Sequelae include gynaecomastia, galactorrhoea, sexual dysfunction, subfertility and osteoporosis.
- Weigh risks of ↑prolactin against risks of switching antipsychotic.

Prolactin level (mIU/L)	Sx	Management
400–2000	–	If benefits of antipsychotic outweigh risk, continue to monitor prolactin.
2000–3000	+	Consider: ↓dose, switch antipsychotic, add aripiprazole, add DA agonist (cabergoline or bromocriptine) but may worsen psychosis, endocrinology r/f.
	+/–	
>3000 or visual field defect	+/–	Consider other causes of ↑prolactin. Consider magnetic resonance imaging (MRI) pituitary.

Depot side effects

- 15%–20% get inflammation and induration at injection site, causing pain that is usually mild
- → Rx: ↑dose interval

MONITORING

Antipsychotics require the following monitoring.

Test	Baseline	1 month	2 months	3 months	6 months	Annual	Notes
BMI[BAP]	✓	✓		✓	✓	✓	
BP[BAP]	✓	✓		✓	✓	✓	NICE also suggests pulse
ECG[1,BAP]	✓						
Bloods							
HbA1c[BAP]	✓			✓	✓	✓	Consider using plasma glucose to measure immediate effects
Lipids[BAP]	✓			✓	✓	✓	Can use random lipids if fasting not possible
Prolactin (Gupta, *BJPsych Adv* 2017)	✓			✓		✓	Also if symptomatic or considering pregnancy

[1] Perform a baseline ECG if
- First episode of psychosis. [BAP]
- Medication is high risk for QT prolongation (e.g. pimozide, sertindole), high-dose medication used, acute parenteral administration or combination with other QT-prolonging drugs.
- Family history of long QT syndrome.
- Personal history of CVD, electrolyte abnormalities, central nervous system (CNS) disorders or systemic disease.
- Presence of cardiovascular risk factors. [BAP]
- Admitted as inpatient. [NICE]

Perform serial ECGs if
- Abnormality on baseline ECG.
- Sx of CVD (e.g. syncope, palpitations, chest pain).
- High-dose antipsychotics prescribed.
- New-onset symptoms suggestive of arrhythmia (such as syncope) or CVD occur. [BAP]
- Electrolyte abnormalities.

Full blood count (FBC), renal function and liver function tests (LFTs) are also often performed at baseline and annually to assess general health and drug metabolism.

In addition, when reviewing pt, enquire about:

- Efficacy: symptoms, behaviour, cognition
- Compliance
- Side effects: ↑prolactin, EPSEs, anticholinergic
- Substance misuse (alcohol, drugs, smoking)

Clozapine

- Monitor white cell count (WCC) and differential to detect neutropoenia and agranulocytosis[SPC]
  - Baseline
  - Every week for the first 18 wks
  - Every 2 wks between weeks 18 and 52
  - Every 4 wks after 1 yr
  - For 4 wks after stopping clozapine
  - Also, remind patient to immediately seek medical assistance if they have any signs of an infection.
- Acting on WCC:[SPC]

Clozapine and blood dyscrasias
No benign ethnic neutropenia (BEN)

Blood counts (×10⁹/L)	Action
WBC ≥3.5 AND neutrophils ≥2.0	Continue clozapine and usual monitoring
WBC ≥3.0 and <3.5 AND/OR neutrophils ≥1.5 and <2.0	Increase monitoring frequency until levels normalise
WBC <3.0 AND/OR neutrophils <1.5	STOP clozapine treatment immediately

Benign ethnic neutropenia (BEN)

- BEN is a cause of chronic neutropenia, but importantly without an increased risk of infection.
- It is most common in people of African, Middle Eastern and West Indian descent.
- Traditionally because of the risk of neutropenia for clozapine, this has been a potential barrier to its use in people of these ethnic backgrounds.
- Now, different WBC and neutrophil count cut-offs can be used in those with BEN.
- Diagnosis can be made on the basis of genetic testing for the ACKR1 rs2814774 genotype.
- Many clozapine brands have their own in-house haematologist that clinical teams can use.

BEN

Blood counts (×10⁹/L)	Action
WBC ≥3.0 AND neutrophils ≥1.5	Continue clozapine and usual monitoring
WBC ≥2.5 and <3.0 AND/OR neutrophils ≥1.0 and <1.5	Increase monitoring frequency until levels normalise
WBC <2.5 AND/OR neutrophils <1.0	STOP clozapine treatment immediately

(Oloyede et al. *BMC Psychiatry*; 2021 **21**(1): 502)

Plasma levels

- Useful for clozapine. Once titration is complete, measure plasma levels and adjust dose accordingly. Usual range is 350–500 microgram/L, but some respond at lower levels. Norclozapine is a clozapine metabolite, and its levels are also sometimes measured.

— Clozapine:norclozapine ratio is normally ~1.25. A ↓ratio may be caused by enzyme induction (medications or increased smoking), recent non-compliance or incorrect sampling time (>13 hours). An ↑ratio may be due to enzyme inhibition (e.g. reduction or cessation of smoking), incorrect sampling time (<11 hours) or saturation of clozapine metabolism.

- For other antipsychotics, main use is determining concordance, but dose-plasma level relationship is usually not strong enough to determine partial concordance.

STOPPING

- Consensus guidelines recommend continuing an antipsychotic for ≥6 months to 2 yrs after a psychotic episode. Patients should be informed of a high risk of relapse if they stop antipsychotics within 1–2 yr of psychotic episode.[NICE]
- Controversies with some arguing for both longer and shorter durations.

The decision to stop must be assessed on a case-by-case basis, based upon:

- Patient/carer wishes after an informed discussion
- Ongoing psychotic symptoms
- Severity of current adverse effects
- Previous patterns of illness
- Previous response to cessation
- Social circumstances (support and stressors)
- Patient/carer insight into relapse indicators
- Risk of harm to self/others

Withdrawal must be **gradual** (preferably over months) to avoid relapse and discontinuation symptoms of headache, insomnia, nausea, etc. Rebound psychosis is most common with clozapine.

SWAPPING

If intolerable side effects, adverse reactions or poor response, then consider switching to an alternative antipsychotic:

- Consider the risk of destabilisation of illness and adverse effects of the new drug.
- Gradually cross-taper over 2–4 wks.
- Avoid abrupt discontinuation, especially of clozapine (unless for serious adverse effect).
- If switching from oral to depot, gradually reduce oral dose after giving depot.

The following table lists circumstances when a switch may be necessary, with recommended drugs.

Acute EPSEs	Aripiprazole, olanzapine, quetiapine, clozapine
Raised prolactin	Aripiprazole, quetiapine, ziprasidone
Postural hypotension	Amisulpride, aripiprazole, lurasidone
QT prolongation	Aripiprazole, lurasidone
Sedation	Amisulpride, aripiprazole, risperidone, sulpiride
Sexual side effects	Aripiprazole, quetiapine
Tardive dyskinesia	Clozapine
Wt gain	Amisulpride, aripiprazole, haloperidol, lurasidone, ziprasidone
Dyslipidaemia	Aripiprazole, ziprasidone

SPECIAL GROUPS
Children
- Psychosis is less common in children.
- Children are more susceptible to EPSEs and sedation.
- If considering olanzapine, discuss the higher risk of wt gain.[NICE]
- Good options: aripiprazole, olanzapine, risperidone, quetiapine, paliperidone.[MPG]

Elderly
- When antipsychotics have been used in dementia, they have been associated with ↑risk of CVA, so caution is required.
- Lower doses are used.

Pregnancy

Please refer to relevant section on Perinatal Psychiatry (page 312)

Renal impairment[BNF]

- Haloperidol and olanzapine are good options.[MPG]
- Most antipsychotics undergo extensive hepatic metabolism with little unchanged drug being excreted in the urine. Only sulpiride, amisulpride and paliperidone rely heavily on renal excretion. (*NB*: Risperidone is also metabolised to paliperidone.) These are, therefore, best avoided in renal impairment.
- Other antipsychotics are likely to be safe, but check individual monographs.
- Anticholinergic SEs may result in further urinary retention.
- Start with lower doses and titrate more slowly.

Hepatic impairment[BNF]

- Sulpiride, amisulpride and paliperidone are safer, as they undergo negligible hepatic metabolism. Haloperidol has reasonable clinical experience in low doses.[MPG]
- Phenothiazines (chlorpromazine, fluphenazine, trifluoperazine) are hepatotoxic.
- Antipsychotics may precipitate coma in liver failure.
- Clozapine should be avoided.
- Check individual monographs.

Physical health problems

- **Long QT syndrome** (congenital or due to other medications): Avoid antipsychotics that prolong the QT interval. Aripiprazole and lurasidone are safer. See p. 184.
- **Epilepsy**: antipsychotics are generally safe and even clozapine has been used successfully. Titrate slowly and monitor seizure frequency.
- **Diabetes**: SGAs are likely to worsen T2DM. Typicals and aripiprazole are good options.

Persistent aggression

- A trial of clozapine should be considered.[BAP]

- Valproate augmentation of an antipsychotic has some very limited evidence but should be avoided in people of child-bearing potential.[BAP]

Co-morbid depression

(Upthegrove, *Adv Psychiatr Treat* 2009; **15**(5): 372–9)

- Monitor for coexisting mental health problems (including depression, anxiety and substance misuse), especially in early treatment.[NICE]
- Depression is common (40% post-psychotic phase, 80% in longitudinal studies). Strong predictor of suicidal behaviour and poor functional outcome.
- Consider switching antipsychotic if prescribed haloperidol.
- Antidepressant co-prescribing is effective in the treatment of co-morbid major depression: most evidence for SSRIs (Gregory et al., *Br J Psychiatry* 2017; **211**(4): 198–204).
- Generally, good safety evidence for co-prescribing antidepressant with antipsychotic (Tiihonen et al., *Arch Gen Psychiatry* 2012; **69**(5): 476–83) with no higher risk for mortality but significantly decreased risk of completed suicide. Increased QTc monitoring may be needed.
- Avoid citalopram and escitalopram with antipsychotics, as risk of QTc prolongation[MHRA].

Co-morbid substance misuse[BAP]

- Smoking: NRT, bupropion and varenicline all have good evidence. NRT is safest, as there is some controversial evidence about psychological SE (including suicidal ideation) with bupropion and varenicline.
- In alcohol abuse, clozapine has some evidence for reducing substance misuse.

Novel medications – anti-inflammatories

- Accumulating evidence suggests that aberrant innate immune response may be implicated in psychosis.

- Studies have demonstrated higher levels of inflammatory markers in those with psychosis and raised inflammatory markers in childhood are linked to an increased risk of psychosis later in life.
- Potential mechanisms include altered function of glial cells.
- Evidence currently insufficient to recommend the use of anti-inflammatory medications for schizophrenia in clinical practice.[BAP]

FURTHER INFORMATION

Barnes et al. 'Evidence-based guidelines for the pharmacological treatment of schizophrenia: Updated recommendations from the British Association for Psychopharmacology', *J Psychopharmacol* 2020; 34(1): 3–78.

Cooper et al., 'BAP guidelines on the management of weight gain, metabolic disturbances and cardiovascular risk associated with psychosis and antipsychotic drug treatment', *J Psychopharmacol* 2016; 30(8): 717–48.

BIPOLAR AFFECTIVE DISORDER

DIAGNOSIS

BPAD is a relapsing and remitting psychiatric disorder. For a diagnosis to be made, there must be at least one episode of (hypo) mania. **BPAD-I** is characterised by **mania**+depression, whereas **BPAD-II** is characterised by **hypomania**+depression.

Features of mania: **DIG FAST**

- Distractibility
- Impulsive and disinhibited behaviour
- Grandiosity
- Flight of ideas
- Activity ↑
- Sleep ↓
- Talkativeness

Mania can be accompanied by **psychotic features**, usually grandiose delusions, second-person auditory hallucinations or thought disorder. **Hypomania** exhibits the features of mania, but to a mild degree such that there is no severe occupational or social dysfunction. A **mixed episode** has features of both depression and mania.

Differential diagnoses

- **Emotionally unstable personality disorder (EUPD)** (impulsivity, chronic emptiness, emotional instability)
- **Attention deficit hyperactivity disorder (ADHD)** (developmental trajectory, anger, overactivity, mood instability)
- **Cyclothymia** (depression and mild elation not meeting threshold for BPAD)

- **Schizoaffective disorder** (features of schizophrenia and a mood disorder)
- **Depression** (no [hypo]mania)
- **Delirium** (altered consciousness, disorientation, intercurrent illness)

- **Hyperthyroidism** (↑HR, tremor, proptosis, diarrhoea; [Ix]: TFTs)
- **Cushing's disease** (purple striae, facial plethora, buffalo hump, glucose intolerance; Ix: 24 h urinary cortisol, dexamethasone suppression test)
- **Drug-induced psychosis** (especially cocaine, amphetamines, synthetic cannabinoids, anabolic steriods)
- **Prescribed medications** (corticosteroids, antidepressants, DA agonists, anabolic steroids, thyroid hormones, chloroquine)

- **Stroke** (especially R limbic system; vascular RFs, acute onset, unilateral neuro deficits; Ix: computerised tomography [CT] head)
- **MS** (especially orbitofrontal lesions; F>M, diplopia, paraesthesia, asymmetrical upper motor neurone [UMN] signs; Ix: MRI brain)
- **Brain tumour** (especially frontal; subacute, headache worse in mornings/coughing, papilloedema, focal UMN signs; Ix: CT/MRI brain)

Differentiating BPAD and EUPD

BPAD and EUPD are often confused and may be co-morbid, particularly in BPAD-II.

	BPAD	EUPD
Duration of mood episodes	Consistent for a few days or longer	Variability over hours to days
Distinctiveness of episodes	Mood episodes can be distinguished from baseline	Less distinguishable from background
Impulsivity	Present only in (hypo)manic episodes	More frequently present
Triggers for episodes	Often none obvious	Tend to be present
Frequent self-harm	Uncommon	Common

BPAD is treated with 'mood-stabilising' drugs, which is a commonly used but imprecise term.

Clinicians should aim to pick the right treatment for the patient over two intersecting axes:

- Depressive to manic symptoms
- Acute management to long-term prophylaxis

Drugs used in BPAD have varying levels of effectiveness across these two axes.

DRUGS USED IN BPAD

Drug	Pharmacology	Side effects				
		Sedation	GI Sx	↑wt	Stevens–Johnson syndrome (SJS)/ toxic epidermal necrolysis (TEN)	Teratogenicity
Lithium	Modulates multiple cellular signalling cascades	+	+	++	–	Some cardiac risk described but not replicated
Valproate	Inhibits GABA transaminase ⇒ ↑synaptic GABA	++	++	++	–	+++
Lamotrigine	Stabilises sodium channels	–	–	–	++	+
Carbamazepine	Stabilises sodium channels	+	++	++	++	++

– not described, + low risk, ++ medium risk, +++ high risk.
Source: Schmidt & Schachter, *BMJ* 2014; **28**(348): g254.

Oxcarbazepine and eslicarbazepine have a similar mechanism to carbamazepine but are occasionally used for their slightly different SE profile and lower potential for drug–drug interactions.

See Psychosis section for details of antipsychotics.

Formulations

Lithium, valproate and carbamazepine are all available in various formulations. For clarity, the brand should always be prescribed alongside the drug name and formulation, e.g. sodium valproate 500 mg MR tablets (Epilim Chrono).

Lithium

- Lithium is available as two compounds: **lithium carbonate**, as a tablet, and **lithium citrate**, as a liquid.
- The two main brands in use in the United Kingdom are Priadel and Camcolit. Brands should be kept the same where possible, as equivalent bioavailability cannot be guaranteed.
- Priadel may be withdrawn from the market by the manufacturer (for non-medical reasons); however, it is still prescribable at the time of writing.
- For tablets, lithium carbonate can be prescribed as Priadel MR, Camcolit IR or Camcolit MR.
- For liquid, lithium citrate can be prescribed as Priadel liquid or Li-Liquid (both **IR**). There is no liquid MR formulation. State strength of liquid and dose to be taken.
- Lithium citrate and lithium carbonate doses are markedly different – see table below.
- Conversion:

Lithium citrate liquid		Equivalent lithium carbonate tablet dose
Formulation	Dose	
Priadel liquid	520 mg (5 mL)	204 mg (≈200 mg)
Li-liquid*	509 mg (5 mL)	200 mg

* Li-liquid is also available as 1018 mg in 5 mL.

- IR formulations (liquid and tablets) are taken bd.
- MR formulations (tablets) have the advantage of od dosing and ↓nephrotoxicity.

Valproate

Chemical form	Brand	IR formulation	MR formulation	Liquid	License for BPAD	License for epilepsy
Sodium valproate	Epilim	✔	✔	✔		✔
	Episenta		✔		✔	✔
Valproic acid	Convulex	✔				✔
Semisodium valproate	Depakote	✔			✔	

- **Valproate is highly teratogenic. Significant restrictions on prescribing in those of childbearing potential.**
- Valproate is available in three chemical forms:
    - **Sodium valproate** (Epilim and Episenta).
    - **Valproic acid** (Convulex).
    - **Semisodium valproate** (Depakote).
- Semisodium valproate has equimolar quantities of sodium valproate and valproic acid.
- Despite the restricted licenses, Epilim Chrono (the MR) form is often used to improve compliance in BPAD.
- The stated doses on different valproate formulations should be bioequivalent, but monitor response carefully if switching. Available doses of tablets are often different; e.g. Epilim Chrono has 200 mg, 300 mg and 500 mg tablets, whereas Depakote comes as 250 mg and 500 mg tablets.

CHOOSING A MEDICATION

Most evidence is for bipolar I disorder, so caution is required with extrapolation to bipolar II.

Treatment of mania and mixed episodes

Stop antidepressants

Optimise current prophylactic treatment
Increase dose to highest tolerated.
If on lithium, check levels and aim for
upper end of dose range. A recent level
well below the upper limit is a reasonable
ground for ↑ dose.

Start antimanic drug
Antipsychotics > mood stabilisers.
Preferred agents: olanzapine, risperidone,
haloperidol, quetiapine.
Other options: valproate, other
antipsychotics, carbamazepine, lithium.

Combination therapy
Lithium + antipsychotic
or valproate + antipsychotic.

Rx resistance
Clozapine or ECT.

Recovery

Medication reduction
Wait until full remission.
↓ Benzodiazepines as soon as possible.
↓ Any other medications not required for
prophylaxis over ≥4 wks.

Benzodiazepines for tranquillisation and restoring sleep. **Z-drugs** may also be used as hypnotics.

BAP

- Strongly consider inpatient admission[BAP] and ensure a calming environment with reduced stimulation.[NICE]
- If on prophylactic Rx, first optimise with doses up to highest tolerated.
- Medications are necessary; psychotherapy is not an alternative.[BAP]
- Antipsychotics are the preferred option.[NICE] They are not merely sedative and are more effective than anticonvulsants or lithium.[BAP] If the first antipsychotic is poorly tolerated, offer an alternative antipsychotic.[NICE]
- Olanzapine and haloperidol have the advantage of having a short-acting im formulation.[BAP]
- Avoid antipsychotics with a high propensity to EPSEs, as BPAD patients are more sensitive than SZ patients.[BAP]
- Lithium has the advantage that it is the most effective long-term treatment, but titration means that its effect is usually much slower than other agents in mania.[BAP]
- If using ECT, bear in mind that benzodiazepines and anticonvulsants ↑seizure threshold, so ↓dose of medications or higher starting voltages likely to be required.
- Medication should be reduced slowly. There is evidence for benefits from continuing an antipsychotic at 6 months but not at 1 yr.[BAP]
- Mixed episodes should be treated similarly to manic episodes. Antipsychotics may be used. Antidepressants should be avoided. ECT is an option.[BAP]
- There is some evidence that cariprazine is effective at treating manic and depressive episodes.[MPG]

Treatment of depression

- Evidence base is poor with controversies over the use of antidepressants.
- BAP recommend lamotrigine as first-line pharmacotherapy, as shown in algorithm on p. 199, but NICE recommends olanzapine+fluoxetine combination or quetiapine monotherapy as first line.
- Lamotrigine may be added on to existing therapy.[BAP]

- Evidence for lithium is limited, but it is likely to be effective and may be considered.[BAP] If patient already taking lithium, check plasma level and ensure adequate dose.[NICE]

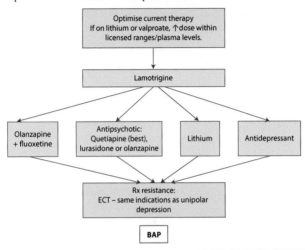

Antidepressants in BPAD
- If antidepressants are used in bipolar I disorder, they should be given with lithium, valproate or an antipsychotic.[BAP]
- Antidepressants are sometimes used as monotherapy in bipolar II disorder, but titration should be slow and patients should be closely monitored for hypomania.[BAP]
- SSRIs seem to be less likely to cause a manic switch than TCAs and SNRIs. When combined with a mood stabiliser, they are unlikely to cause mania.[BAP]
- Bipolar depression can remit more quickly than unipolar depression. Consider tapering down an antidepressant after 12 wks in remission.[BAP]
- Avoid in patients with mixed features, rapid cycling or as monotherapy.[BAP]
- Overall, lamotrigine is a better option.[BAP]

Long-term prophylaxis

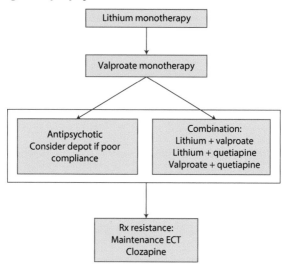

Role of lithium
- Overall, the best option for relapse prevention with strong evidence[BAP, NICE]
- Prevents mania and (to a lesser extent) depression
- Reduces suicide rates
- Early use of lithium $\Rightarrow$ better long-term outcome
- But intermittent lithium Rx can cause rebound mania, so patients must be able to take it consistently for $\geq$2 yr.[BAP]

- A within-patient trial is often used to guide therapy, i.e. if a patient responds well to an acute anti-manic agent, this may be continued long term.[BAP,NICE] This is a valid strategy but results in disproportionate use of antipsychotics over lithium in long term.[BAP]
- Antipsychotics have the advantage that many are available as depots.[BAP] They can also be helpful if there are features of non-affective psychosis. The only depot with randomised controlled trial (RCT) support is risperidone. Since the pharmacokinetics of risperidone LAI make it hard to use, paliperidone palmitate is a good option. Naturalistic studies suggest depot medication prevents re-admission more effectively than oral equivalent.
- In general, there is a hierarchy for preferred medications: lithium > valproate* > olanzapine > lamotrigine > quetiapine > carbamazepine.[BAP]
- However, when considering which agent, consideration should be given to which pole affects the patient most:[BAP]

*But avoid valproate in those of childbearing potential.

Prevention of mania	Prevention of depression
Lithium	Lithium
Olanzapine	Lamotrigine
Quetiapine	Quetiapine
Risperidone LAI	Lurasidone
Valproate	Any treatment that has been effective in acute
Carbamazepine	depression for the patient

Rapid cycling BPAD
- Defined as ≥4 episodes/yr.
- Treat in the same way as BPAD in general.[BAP/NICE]
- Clozapine (with mood stabilisers) may be used in treatment-resistant cases.[BAP]
- Thyroid disorders may contribute. Reduce/discontinue any antidepressants that might be contributing.[BAP]

Early signs of relapse
- Consider acute prescriptions of antipsychotics or benzodiazepines if patient shows early signs of relapse (e.g. insomnia).[BAP]
- With appropriate education and support, some patients can have 'rescue packs' prescribed and dispensed in advance to use if they experience signs of relapse.[BAP]

Rescue packs
- Suitable for patients with a good understanding of their illness.[BAP]
- To be used by patient if they spot warning signs of mania.
- Options:
  - Higher doses of current medications.
  - Benzodiazepines or Z-drugs to assist sleep.
  - Antipsychotics.

- If clozapine has been required in the manic episode, it may be continued as prophylaxis.[BAP]
- If antidepressants are used, they should be combined with a mood stabiliser or antipsychotic.[BAP]
- Valproate should not be offered to women of childbearing potential.

Prophylaxis in BPAD-II
Consider lamotrigine or quetiapine monotherapy.[BAP]

- Because of interactions with carbamazepine, it should be used in combination with caution.[BAP]
- Oxcarbazepine and eslicarbazepine use has been extrapolated from carbamazepine without strong evidence, based on their chemical similarities.[BAP] Their side effect burden sometimes means they are better tolerated.

NON-PHARMACOLOGICAL MANAGEMENT

- Evidence for psychological therapy for bipolar depression is poorer than for unipolar depression. There have been large failed trials using CBT.[BAP]
- The most important non-pharmacological intervention is psychoeducation.[BAP]
  - Can be delivered in a group setting.[BAP]
  - Best early in the illness.[BAP]
  - http://beatingbipolar.org is a good resource.
- Other psychological therapies with some evidence in relapse prevention:
  - Family focussed therapy.
  - CBT (showed initial promise, but no benefit in larger RCTs).
  - Interpersonal social rhythm therapy (relies on ensuring regular sleep and daily activities; good early evidence).
- Group cognitive remediation may improve longer-term cognitive outcomes.[BAP]
- Consider developing an advanced directive with the patient specifying which treatments they would prefer when they are unwell.[BAP]

Psychoeducation: Key points
- Sx: Depression and (hypo)mania
- Medications: SEs, compliance, not stopping suddenly
- Pregnancy: Risks of relapse and medications
- Drugs: Avoid recreational drugs; alcohol only in moderation
- Family and friends: Involve in care if possible
- Relapse indicators: Know yours; sleep disturbance is common
- Sleep hygiene and regular routine: Some apps can help
- Life decisions: Avoid while manic[NICE]

STARTING

- **Lithium:** Start at 400 mg in one or two divided doses and adjust dose every 5–7 days aiming for plasma levels of 0.6–0.8 mmol/L (levels of 0.8–1.0 mmol/L may be more effective but risks are higher if continued in long term). Once levels are stable, switch to *nocte* dosing, as bd may ↑nephrotoxicity.[BAP] MR formulation often preferred. Restart at previous dose after periods of non-adherence, if no evidence of reduced renal function.

- **Valproate:** Sodium valproate has an MR formulation (Epilim Chrono), so may be given once daily (at night). Otherwise, valproate formulations should be prescribed BD. Faster loading may be used in acute mania, although do not use in those of childbearing potential.

- **Lamotrigine:** Titration is very important to avoid SJS/TEN. Rate of titration (see monograph) depends on whether it is being co-prescribed with any enzyme inhibitors (e.g. valproate) or inducers (e.g. carbamazepine). Valproate inhibits lamotrigine metabolism, so if given together lamotrigine dose should be halved.[BAP]
  - If a patient has not been taking lamotrigine for ≥5 half-lives, it should be re-titrated as if starting for the first time. Half-life is 33 h in a healthy person with no other medications, but is higher with enzyme inhibitors and lower with enzyme inducers.[SPC]

- **Carbamazepine:** Potent enzyme inducer, so check interactions carefully (see monograph and p. 383). It also induces its own metabolism, so within a few weeks of Rx clearance can ↑threefold. Dose adjustments are recommended to ensure therapeutic efficacy. Titration is not as essential as with lamotrigine, but it is recommended to reduce the initial sedation.

SIDE EFFECTS

- Prolonged release formulations can ↓some SEs.
- Lithium toxicity can occur as an emergency (see p. 411).

Side effect	Medications	Mx
Hypothyroidism (2%–3%. F > M. Best marker is ↑TSH)	Lithium	• If slightly ↑TSH with normal T_4, monitor. Usually transient. • Treat with levothyroxine if symptomatic, ↓T_4 or TSH > 10. Check thyroid autoantibodies. • r/f to endo if complicated.
Hyperparathyroidism (dyspepsia, renal stones, osteoporosis)	Lithium	• Usually mild and asymptomatic, just monitor PTH and calcium. • If severe or symptomatic, consider withdrawing Li. • If Li needs to be continued, r/f to endo for consideration of cinacalcet or parathyroidectomy.
Postural tremor (*NB:* **cerebellar** tremor on lithium suggests toxicity)	Lithium, valproate	• ↓dose, MR formulation. • Propranolol 30–100 mg/day in divided doses (if not asthmatic).
SJS/TEN	Lamotrigine > carbamazepine	• Patient should contact psychiatrist or GP immediately if any rash. • In early rash, hard to distinguish between serious and benign, so always stop lamotrigine.[BAP] • If rash is trivial and resolves on its own, lamotrigine may be re-introduced at a slower rate.[BAP] • If rash is widespread, mucosal, heavily involving the face or accompanied by fever or sore throat, all possible causative agents should be stopped. Consideration should be given to never retrying lamotrigine, or using extreme caution if it is.[BAP]

(*continued*)

Side effect	Medications	Mx
Nephrogenic diabetes insipidus (polyuria, nocturia, polydipsia)	Lithium	• If no impact on function, monitor. • If impairing, measure 24 h urine volume and osmolality. • Fluid restriction contraindicated.[BAP] • ↓dose, MR formulation or switch. • Consider amiloride, but monitor urea and electrolytes (U&Es).[BAP] • Consider renal r/f.
CKD (20% overall, but CKD 5 only in 1%; risk factors: chronic Rx, Li toxicity, co-morbidities)	Lithium	• Monitor Li levels at ≤2 month intervals. • Keep levels at lower end of range. • Avoid other nephrotoxins. • If eGFR <60, consider stopping Li but balance risks and benefits.
↑LFTs	Valproate	Stop valproate if[NICE]: • 3× upper limit of normal. • Continuing to rise or • Symptomatic.
Haematological abnormalities	Carbamazepine (↓neutrophils), valproate (↓Plt), lamotrigine (↓neutrophils)	Monitor, but more important that clinicians and patients are aware of Sx (neutropoenia → fever, sore throat, rash, mouth ulcers; ↓Plt → bruising). Encourage patient to seek urgent medical attention[BAP] and perform FBC if Sx occur.

Source: Ferrier et al., *BJPsych Adv* 1995; **1**(4): 102–8; Canning et al., *Men Heal Clin* 2012; **1**(7): 174–6; Ferrier et al., *BJPsych Adv* 2006; **12**(4): 256–64; Gupta et al., *BJPsych Adv* 2013; **19**(6): 457–66.

MONITORING

• Many medications used in BPAD are associated with adverse metabolic side effects, but not all of the poor cardiovascular outcomes in BPAD are due to medications.

- If prescribed an antipsychotic, follow guidance in the Psychosis section (p. 169).
- In general, drug plasma levels are taken at trough (i.e. just before the next dose is given). Lithium is the exception: levels are generally taken 12 h post-dose, regardless of the regimen.[MPG] See Drug Monitoring section on page 350.

Drug	Baseline	Follow-up	Annual
All patients (regardless of medications)[BAP]	BP BMI HbA1c/glucose Lipids		BP BMI HbA1c/glucose Lipids
Lithium[1,BAP]	U&Es TFTs Calcium	Li levels: 5–7 days post-dose increase. When stable, 3-monthly intervals for 1 yr, then 6-monthly thereafter.	U&Es TFTs Calcium
Valproate[BAP]	FBC LFTs Pregnancy test (if relevant)	LFTs within 6 months	
Lamotrigine[NICE]	FBC U&Es LFTs		
Carbamazepine[1,BAP]	FBC U&Es LFTs HLA-B1502 genetic screening[2,MHRA]	Rpt FBC, U&Es and LFTs within 2 months	

[1] Can be pro-arrhythmogenic, so some sources also recommend a baseline ECG if any established cardiac disease or risk factors for it.

[2] This predicts SJS/TEN.

Lithium

- More frequent monitoring is necessary if patients are physically unwell or taking drugs that alter lithium levels (e.g. diuretics, ACE-i, NSAIDs).[BAP]
- Toxicity can be present with normal Li levels. Levels >2 mmol/L are associated with life-threatening toxicity.

STOPPING

- Relapse does still occur after years of remission. General advice is for prophylaxis indefinitely.[BAP]
- Discontinuing is safer in patients who meet all of the following criteria[BAP]:
  - Currently completely well
  - No mood episodes for 4 yrs
  - No serious risks in previous depression or mania
  - No rapid cycling
- Before stopping medications, discuss risks and benefits.
- If stopping any medication, ↓dose over ≥4 wks, preferably longer.[BAP]
  - Abrupt lithium discontinuation → 50% risk of mania in 12 wks. Only stop abruptly in medical emergency or overdose.
- Put crisis plan in place for relapse.[BAP]
- Antidepressants should be stopped abruptly in mania, but should otherwise follow the schedules on p. 225. If used in rapid cycling BPAD, a more rapid taper should be used than with unipolar depression.[BAP]

SWAPPING

- Lithium, valproate, lamotrigine and carbamazepine can each be used in combination with the exception of lithium+carbamazepine, which increases neurotoxicity.[BNF] Antipsychotics may also be combined with mood stabilisers. The main SE to be aware of is cumulative sedation.
- Therefore, best practice is usually to titrate up the new drug before reducing the old to minimise risk of relapse.

SPECIAL GROUPS

Children

- Start at lower doses, but be prepared to increase to higher doses relative to body mass.
- Harder to diagnose BPAD. Requires monitoring over a period of time by an experienced clinician.[BAP]
- In mania, use aripiprazole first line.[BAP, NICE] Other options are olanzapine, quetiapine and risperidone.[BAP]
- In bipolar depression, extrapolate from adult guidelines, but bear in mind that antidepressants may more easily induce a switch to mania in children.[BAP] Offer a structured psychological intervention (CBT or IPT) lasting ≥3 months.[NICE]
- Risk of disruption to education and emotional development may incline clinicians towards prophylaxis.[BAP]

Elderly

- 10% of BPAD develops in >50s.
- Carbamazepine and valproate can ↓bone mineral density, resulting in ↑risk of fractures.
- Consider lower doses and slower titration.[BAP]

Pregnancy

Please refer to relevant section on perinatal psychiatry (page 316).

Renal impairment

- If possible, avoid lithium. Enhanced monitoring is necessary.[MPG]
- Valproate, carbamazepine and lamotrigine with slow titration are good options.[MPG]

Hepatic impairment

- Valproate should be avoided due to potential hepatotoxicity.
- Lithium is the best option, but careful monitoring is required.[MPG]

Physical health problems

- Check interactions (p. 383). Carbamazepine is a notorious enzyme inducer. Valproate inhibits metabolism of a few drugs.
- **MS**: Patients might reduce fluid intake due to urethral sphincter disturbance. Lithium requires a good fluid intake, so should be avoided in these patients. Antipsychotics are good options.[MPG]

- **Epilepsy:** Liaise with neurologist to find medications that can treat both disorders. In general, valproate is good for generalised seizures, while lamotrigine and carbamazepine are preferred for focal seizures.
- **HIV:** Avoid carbamazepine due to risk of neutropoenia and potential failure of antiretrovirals.[MPG]

Further information

Goodwin et al., 'Evidence-based guidelines for treating bipolar disorder: revised third edition recommendations from the British Association for Psychopharmacology', *J Psychopharmacol* 2016; 30(6): 495–553.

Baldwn et al. Withdrawal of, and alternatives to, valproate-containing medicines in girls and women of childbearing potential who have a psychiatric illness. 2016. Available from https://www.bap.org.uk/pdfs/PS04-18-December2018.pdf.

DEPRESSION

DIAGNOSIS

- Depression is a syndrome characterised by the following clinical features:
  - Depressed mood
  - Energy low (anergia)
  - Pleasure lost (anhedonia)
  - Retardation or agitation
  - Eating ↑/↓ (appetite or wt)
  - Sleep ↑/↓
  - Suicidal ideation
  - I'm a failure (loss of confidence)
  - Only me to blame (guilt)
  - No concentration
- For a new diagnosis of depression, the following Ix may be appropriate: FBC, U&E, LFTs, bone profile, TFTs. Consider other Ix as previously discussed if suggested by clinical picture.

Differential diagnosis

- BPAD (screen for mania and hypomania; screening Ix: MDQ or HCL-16)
- Anxiety disorders (see p. 229)
- Acute stress reaction (hours-days)
- Adjustment disorder (clearly related to life event)
- EUPD (impulsivity, chronic emptiness, emotional instability)
- Dysthymia (less severe than depression but lasting ≥2 yr)
- Substance misuse (screen for EtOH and drugs)
- Negative symptoms of schizophrenia (screen for psychosis)

- Hypothyroidism (fatigue++, ↓HR, cold intolerance, constipation; Ix: TFTs)
- Anaemia (fatigue, breathlessness, chest pain; Ix: FBC)
- B12/folate deficiency (glossitis, peripheral neuropathy, diarrhoea; Ix: FBC, B12/folate levels)
- Dementia (can be hard to distinguish from depressive pseudodementia; Hx of gradual cognitive decline; Ix: Mini-Mental State Examination [MMSE])
- Obstructive sleep apnoea (OSA) (excessive daytime sleepiness, nocturnal apnoeic episodes; Ix: Epworth Sleepiness Scale)
- Cushing's disease (purple striae, facial plethora, buffalo hump, glucose intolerance; Ix: 24 h urinary cortisol, dexamethasone suppression test)
- Drugs (esp. tetrabenazine, steroids, baclofen, ß-blockers, opioids)
- Addison's (postural hypotension, skin pigmentation, ↓Na$^+$, ↑K$^+$; Ix: serum cortisol, short Synacthen test)
- Parkinson's (tremor, rigidity, bradykinesia)
- Hypercalcaemia (renal stones, abdominal groans, pain in bones)

- Depression may be categorised by severity based on number of symptoms, intensity and functional impairment. The following types of depression may also be considered:
  - Melancholic depression: unreactive mood, diurnal variation (worse in morning), early morning wakening, psychomotor agitation/retardation, ↓wt/appetite.
  - Atypical depression: mood reactivity, ↑wt/appetite, hypersomnia, leaden paralysis, fatigue. F > M.
  - Psychotic depression: severe depression with hallucinations or delusions that are generally mood congruent.

TYPES OF ANTIDEPRESSANT DRUGS[BAP(ADAPTED)]

Class	Drug	Action	Side effects							Lethality in overdose
			Anticho-linergic	Sedation	Insomnia/agitation	Postural ↓BP	Sexual dysfunction[a]	↑Wt	Other	
SSRI	Citalopram	SRI	–	–	+	–	++	–	Nausea, ↑QTc	Low
	Escitalopram	SRI	–	–	+	–	++	–	Nausea, ↑QTc	Low
	Sertraline	SRI	–	–	+	–	++	–	Nausea	Low
	Fluoxetine	SRI	–	–	++	–	++	–	Nausea, rash	Low
	Fluvoxamine	SRI	–	–	+	–	+	–	Nausea	Low
	Paroxetine	SRI	+	+	+	–	+++	+	Nausea	Low
SNRI	Duloxetine	SRI+NRI	–	–	+	–	++	–	Nausea, sweating	?Low
	Venlafaxine	SRI>NRI	–	–	+	–	++	–	Nausea, HTN, sweating	Mod
Tricyclic antidepressant (TCA)	Clomipramine	SRI+NRI	++	++	+	++	++	+	Cardiac fx	Mod
	Amitriptyline	NRI>SRI	++	++	–	++	+	++	Cardiac fx	High
	Dosulepin	NRI>SRI	++	++	–	++	+	++	Cardiac fx	High
	Imipramine	NRI>SRI	++	+	+	++	+	+	Cardiac fx	High
	Nortriptyline	NRI	+	+	+	++	+	–	Cardiac fx	High
	Lofepramine	NRI	+	–	+	+	+	–	Cardiac fx, sweating	Low
	Doxepin	SRI+NRI	++	++	–	++	+	++	Cardiac fx	High
	Trimipramine	SRI+NRI	++	+++	–	++	+	++	Cardiac fx	High

(continued)

Class	Drug	Action	Side effects							Lethality in overdose
			Anticho-linergic	Sedation	Insomnia/ agitation	Postural ↓BP	Sexual dysfunction[a]	↑ wt	Other	
Receptor antagonists	Mirtazapine	5-HT$_2$+5-HT$_3$+α$_2$ ant	–	++	–	–	–	+++		Low
	Mianserin	5-HT$_2$+α$_1$+α$_2$ ant	+	++	–	–	–	–		Low
	Trazodone	5-HT$_2$+α$_1$ ant > SRI	–	++	–	++	–	+	Priapism	Low
Monoamine oxidase inhibitor (MAOI)	Phenelzine	Irreversible MAO-A/B	+	+	++	++	++	++	HTN crisis, oedema	High
	Tranylcy-promine	Irreversible MAO-A/B	+	+	++	++	++	++		High
	Isocarboxazid	Irreversible MAO-A/B	+	+	++	++	++	++		High
	Moclobemide	Reversible MAO-A	–	–	+	–	–	–		Low
Other	Vortioxetine	SRI+5-HT$_{1A}$ ag, 5-HT$_{1B}$ pa, 5-HT$_{1D/3/7}$ ant	–	–	+	–	+/–	–	Nausea	?
	Reboxetine	NRI	+	–	+	–	+	–		Low
	Bupropion	NRI+DRI	–	–	+	–	–	–	↓Seizure threshold	?Mod
	Agomelatine	MT ag and 5-HT$_{2c}$ ant	–	+	+	–	–	–	Monitor LFTs	?Low

Note: ant, angatonist; DRI, dopamine reuptake inhibitor; MAO, monoamine oxidase inhibitor; NRI, noradrenaline reuptake inhibitor; pa, partial agonist; SRI, serotonin reuptake inhibitor.

CHOICE

Depressive episode

- Effect size for antidepressants is greater for more severe and longer-lasting depression.
- First-line antidepressant should usually be an SSRI.[NICE]
- Consider[BAP]:
  - Side effect profile, given patient preferences and co-morbidities.
  - Lethality in overdose, given suicide risk.
  - Drug interactions.
  - Prior response of patient and family members.

Most effective antidepressants[BAP]
- Sertraline
- Escitalopram (20 mg)
- Mirtazapine
- Venlafaxine (≥150 mg)
- Amitriptyline
- Clomipramine
- Vortioxetine*

* Released since guideline publication and included on the basis of expert advice.

- Use SEs to your advantage:
  - Sedating antidepressants for patients with insomnia
  - Activating antidepressants for somnolent patients
  - Antidepressants that ↑Wt for cachectic patients
- If patient also has an anxiety disorder (see p. 229), pick an antidepressant that also treats the anxiety disorder.
- Consider ECT if urgent response required (e.g. depressive stupor, high risk of suicide, extreme distress and ↓fluid intake), psychotic features present or previous good response.[BAP]
- Avoid St John's wort due to potential for interactions and differing preparations.[BAP,NICE]
- Dosulepin should generally be avoided,[NICE] due to very high risk of death in overdose.

Psychotic depression

- Antidepressant+antipsychotic is better than monotherapy with either.[BAP]
- TCAs are possibly more effective than SSRIs.
- ECT is an option.[BAP]

Pseudobulbar affect

(Ahmed & Simmons, *Ther Clin Risk Manag* 2013)

- Affective lability with inappropriate laughter or crying.
- Occurs in MS, MND, dementia and CVA.
- Use low doses of an SSRI or TCA, e.g. fluoxetine 20 mg od, citalopram 20 mg od, sertraline 50 mg od, amitriptyline 20–100 mg ON, nortriptyline 20–100 mg ON.

TREATMENT RESISTANCE

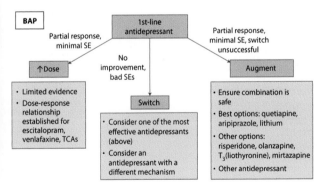

- Assess risks and benefits of further treatment against continued depression.[BAP]
- Address social factors (e.g. occupational issues, financial problems, social isolation, abusive relationships).[BAP]
- Assess for co-morbid disorders, e.g. BPAD or psychosis.[BAP]

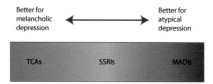

Better for melancholic depression ⟷ Better for atypical depression

| TCAs | SSRIs | MAOIs |

- If a patient discontinues an SSRI due to lack of efficacy, switching to a different class is slightly more effective than switching to another SSRI.[BAP]
- Flupentixol and amisulpride (unlicensed) are antipsychotics with some possible antidepressant actions and are occasionally used.
- Some combinations of antidepressants can be extremely dangerous and risk serotonin syndrome. See 'Possible antidepressant combinations' box on p. 220 for safe options.
- Modafinil may be used in partial responders to SSRIs who are troubled by persistent somnolence or fatigue,[BAP] but it may worsen anxiety.
- Recent meta-analysis suggests CBT, ketamine and atypical antipsychotics may have use in TRD but evidence not firm given low number of studies (Scott et al. *Psychopharm* 2022; 37(3): 268–278).
- For patients who relapse while on an antidepressant, most episodes will be self-limiting within 3 months. ↑Dose of antidepressant is effective in most.[BAP]

Starting an MAOI

- Warn of dietary restrictions (on p. 223).
- Avoid co-prescription with any serotonergic or noradrenergic medications (including antidepressants, sympathomimetics and some opioids). Many other medications are cautioned.
- Advise patient to inform any prescriber that they are taking an MAOI.
- Advise patient to discuss with pharmacist before taking an OTC nasal decongestant.
- If choosing an irreversible MAOI, an initial approach could be to trial phenelzine (better tolerated) and then switch to tranylcypromine (following washout) if there is no remission.[BAP]
- Moclobemide is safer than irreversible MAOIs and requires a less strict diet, but is possibly less efficacious.
- If diet not tolerated, selegiline, mainly an MAO-B inhibitor with some MAO-A inhibition, can be used without dietary restriction at lower doses, although it is not widely available in the United Kingdom.
- Discontinuation rates of MAOIs due to SEs similar to SSRIs/ SNRIs.[BAP]

- Due to their complex interactions, MAOIs should be used with care.
- The combination of venlafaxine + mirtazapine is sometimes termed 'California Rocket Fuel'.

Possible antidepressant combinations

- All combinations risk serotonin syndrome
- None of the evidence for combinations is especially strong

    Evidence for safety

    Evidence for safety and efficacy

= = = = = Evidence for efficacy but caution required. Start MAOI and TCA together at low doses and gradually titrate up.

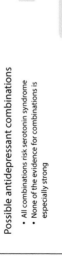
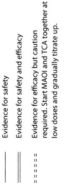

* Beware of pharmacokinetic interactions (see p. 383) (Rojo et al., Acta Psychiatr Scand Suppl 2005; **112**(s428): 25–31. Langan et al., Ther Adv Psychopharmacol 2011; **1**(6): 175–80; Sühs et al., Brain Behav 2015; **5**(4): e00318.)

ECT in depression
- Indications: Urgent response required, psychotic features, previous good response.
- Some antidepressants (especially TCAs) can ↓seizure threshold.
- Acute efficacy +++, but relapse common, so start antidepressant.
- Maintenance ECT only if response >> antidepressants. Regularly assess risks and benefits.

NON-PHARMACOLOGICAL MEASURES
- CBT and antidepressants are similarly efficacious in acute Rx, but CBT may better prevent relapse.
- CBT, IPT and behavioural activation can all be used as monotherapy in mild-moderate depression. For severe depression, do not use psychotherapy monotherapy.[BAP]

CBT for depression
1 Collaborative formulation with patient using five areas: situation, thoughts, moods, behaviour, biology. Emphasise connections.
2 Behavioural activation: Monitor activities with diary and demonstrate how lack of pleasurable activities → ↓mood. Schedule new activities that give pleasure and sense of achievement.
3 Cognitive reformulation: Identify automatic thoughts. Discuss evidence for and against thoughts. Develop modified perspectives.

STARTING
- Prescribe antidepressant if depression is moderate-severe or any severity that lasts ≥2 yr.[BAP]
  - Consider antidepressant if depression with previous history of moderate-severe episode or current episode lasts ≥2–3 months.[BAP]
- Rule out BPAD by screening for mania/hypomania.

- Patient education: Nature of disorder, time to efficacy, possibility of suicidal thoughts on starting Rx, SEs, duration of Rx and problems with discontinuing.
- If ↑risk of suicide, consider providing prescriptions weekly or fortnightly. Instalment prescriptions can also be provided.
- If titrating up (e.g. TCAs), increase dose every 3–7 days.
- 35% of improvement occurs within first week, but very dramatic response suggests placebo and may not be sustained.[BAP]
- If augmenting with an antipsychotic, doses are usually lower than for treatment of psychosis (see individual monographs). However, lithium augmentation should still aim for plasma levels >0.6 mmol/L.[BAP]

> **Are antidepressants addictive?**
> - Antidepressants can cause a withdrawal syndrome *but* they are not addictive.
> - There is no tolerance, craving, compulsion or euphoria.

SIDE EFFECTS

- Cardiac arrhythmias:
  - Citalopram and escitalopram prolong the QTc. These should be avoided in patients with congenital long QT syndrome or in those taking other medications that prolong the QTc (see p. 184).
  - TCAs prolong the PR interval, QRS complex and QT interval. They are unsuitable for those with pre-existing cardiac disease.
- Serotonin syndrome is an acute and potentially life-threatening reaction to antidepressants involving autonomic dysfunction, neuromuscular disturbance and altered mental status (see p. 410).
- SSRIs can ↑risk of bleeding by inhibiting platelet aggregation. See under special groups for appropriate actions.

- General management of SEs:
  - Dose reduction +/– slower retitration
  - Switch to drug with lower propensity to this SE
  - Lifestyle modifications (e.g. sleep hygiene, diet, exercise)
- Specific management:

Side effect	Rx
Dry mouth	Sipping water regularly, sugar-free gum, OTC saliva substitutes (e.g. BioXtra, Salivese, Xerotin).
Drowsiness	Distinguish from hypersomnolence of depression. Dose sedating drugs in evening or at night. Consider modafinil,[BAP] but beware worsening co-morbid anxiety.
Nausea	Usually transient. Provide reassurance.[BAP]
Paradoxical anxiety/agitation in first 1–2 wks of Rx	Explanation and reassurance. Consider short course of benzodiazepine[BAP] (e.g. diazepam 2 mg tds for 7–10 days).
Male sexual dysfunction	For erectile dysfunction, consider sildenafil or tadalafil.[BAP]
Female sexual dysfunction	Bupropion or sildenafil.[BAP]
Hyponatraemia • Early features: headache, fatigue, loss of appetite, insomnia, muscle cramps • Late features: N&V, confusion, seizures, coma, death	If asymptomatic and Na⁺ ≥130 mmol/L, monitor. Otherwise, try to discontinue antidepressant. If euvolaemic, fluid-restrict (e.g. 1–1.5 L/day). If dehydrated, may need iv hypertonic saline. If antidepressant needs to be continued, consider demeclocycline or tolvaptan with endocrinology input.

MAOI tyramine ('cheese') effect

- Causes a hypertensive crisis.
- Occurs in patients on MAOIs in combination with foods high in tyramine.
- Risk is lower on moclobemide.
- Effect can also occur in patients who take the OTC nasal decongestants pseudoephedrine and phenylephrine with an MAOI.

> *Food to avoid with MAOIs*
> - **A**lcohol (especially beer)
> - **B**eans
> - **C**heese
> - **Y**east extracts (Marmite)
> - **P**rocessed meat
>
> *For details, see the Sunnybrook MAOI Diet*

MONITORING

- After starting an antidepressant, arrange a follow-up appointment in 1–2 wks. (This in itself may be therapeutic.)
- Thereafter, assess as clinically indicated.
- Assess:
  - Rx response
  - SE
  - Suicide risk
- Agomelatine has been associated with hepatotoxicity, but no fatalities. LFTs should be measured before starting (or increasing the dose) and then at 3 wks, 6 wks, 3 months and 6 months.[SPC]
- Plasma level monitoring is *rarely* used, but has the following roles[BAP]:
  - Detecting non-concordance.
  - Finding fast metabolisers.
  - Determining effects of interactions.
  - Supporting diagnosis of TCA toxicity.

STOPPING

- Highest risk of relapse is in 6 months after stopping antidepressant.
- For a single episode of depression, continue for 6–9 months after remission.[BAP]
- If multiple episodes, continue for ≥1 yr. If high risk of relapse, consider long-term Rx.[BAP]
- Continuing an antidepressant at treatment doses reduces relapse risk from 56% to 39% at 1 yr. (Lewis et al., *NEJM* 2021; 385(14): 1257–67).

- Speed of discontinuation[BAP]:

Situation	Rate of discontinuation
Serious adverse effect	Abrupt or rapid
Mild adverse effect	4 wks
Planned withdrawal after long-term prophylaxis	Several months

---

Risk of relapse
The following are associated with high risk of relapse on stopping an antidepressant:

- Short time from previous episode
- Chronic depression
- Severe episode
- Rx resistance
- Psychosis
- Physical co-morbidity

Antidepressant withdrawal syndrome

- Can occur following withdrawal from any antidepressant
- Significant variability in degree of withdrawal symptoms: some suffer considerably, many have none
- For more information, see 'Tapering' section

Risk factors	Features	Rx
- Abrupt discontinuation - Short half-lives (e.g. venlafaxine, paroxetine, fluvoxamine), but agomelatine has very low rates - High doses - Rx ≥ 9 wks	**FINISH** - **F**lu-like Sx - **I**nsomnia (with vivid dreams) - **N**ausea - **I**mbalance - **S**ensory disturbances (tingling, electric shocks) - **H**yperarousal (irritability, anxiety)	- Explanation and reassurance (usually effective) - Re-start antidepressant and slowly taper down - For SSRIs/SNRIs, can switch to fluoxetine (long half-life); continue fluoxetine until Sx subside, then stop abruptly

SWAPPING

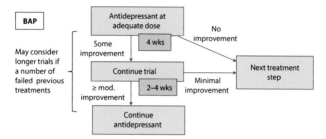

- If switching to a drug of the same class (usually to another SSRI) or one that would be compatible in a combination, switch abruptly. This simplifies the process for the patient and avoids discontinuation Sx.[BAP]
- To avoid pharmacodynamic interactions, when switching to/ from an MAOI, taper down and then leave 2–3 wks before starting the new drug.[MPG]
- Fluoxetine has a long half-life. If switching from fluoxetine to an MAOI, leave 5–6 wks drug free before starting the MAOI. If switching from fluoxetine to another antidepressant, usually leave 4–7 days drug free. Cautious cross-tapering may be performed when switching from fluoxetine to agomelatine, mirtazapine or trazodone.[MPG]

SPECIAL GROUPS

Children

- If depression is mild, use watchful waiting for 4 wks before starting treatment.[NICE]
- Antidepressants are not first line. Consider if severe or recurrent.[BAP, NICE] Only offer with concurrent psychological therapy (e.g. CBT/IPT[BAP]).[NICE]

- Antidepressants may be associated with ↑suicidal ideation and behaviours. To avoid agitation on initiation of medications, titrate slowly and monitor carefully.
- SSRIs are the only antidepressants that should generally be used.[BAP] Fluoxetine appears to be most effective. Its long half-life can compensate for slightly erratic compliance.
- If age <13 yr, antidepressant effect is small and not statistically significant, compared to a high placebo response. Evidence is not established, but use of fluoxetine may be considered.[NICE]
- Start with low doses based on age and weight and titrate up. However, children have faster metabolisms, so often require higher final doses relative to their weight than adults.
- Monitor carefully after starting an antidepressant, e.g. weekly contact for first 4 wks.[NICE]

Elderly
- Drug clearance can be lower, so lower doses are often required.
- Response can take longer, and a longer duration of treatment may be required to prevent relapse.
- In Rx-resistant depression, best evidence is for augmenting with lithium. Some evidence for venlafaxine and selegiline.[BAP]
- Often at risk of falls, so try to avoid drugs that cause postural hypotension.
- If sedation is required, mirtazapine is a good option.
- SSRI-induced hyponatraemia is more common.
- Consider bleeding risk with SSRIs, particularly if on anticoagulants or antiplatelets.

Pregnancy
Please refer to relevant section on perinatal psychiatry (page 317).

Renal impairment
- Citalopram and sertraline are reasonable choices.[MPG]
- TCAs can usually be given at normal doses, except dosulepin.
- ↑QTc prolongation is common in renal failure, so monitor carefully if citalopram or TCAs are used.
- Doses often require reduction (see individual monographs).

Hepatic impairment

- Prescribe fewest number of medications possible, starting at low doses and increasing slowly. Avoid medications with extensive metabolism and those with prominent sedation.
- Sertraline and mirtazapine are good options, but reduce dose.[MPG] See individual monographs.
- SSRIs can be used at low doses, but avoid fluoxetine due to long half-life.[MPG]
- Anticholinergic SEs of TCAs can worsen hepatic encephalopathy.
- MAOIs can be hepatotoxic, so should be avoided.

Physical health problems

- Depression more common in presence of medical disorders, but antidepressants may be less effective.
- SSRIs are usually first line, as better tolerated.[BAP]
- Check interactions (p. 341). Citalopram and escitalopram are least prone to interactions.
- **Cardiac failure or arrhythmia:** Avoid TCAs as proarrhythmogenic and ↑risk of MI. Check QTc before prescribing citalopram/escitalopram.[BAP]
- **Acute coronary syndrome:** Best evidence for SSRIs (especially sertraline), mirtazapine and bupropion.[BAP]
- **Bleeding disorders:** Avoid SSRIs.[BAP]
- **Patients on aspirin, NSAIDs or anticoagulants:** Either avoid SSRIs or add in a PPI to reduce risk of GI bleed.[BAP]
- **Diabetes:** SSRIs are preferred. Fluoxetine is useful for T2DM, as it is associated with Wt loss.
- **Epilepsy:** SSRIs are generally considered safe (and may actually be protective) but should be titrated more slowly. Other options are mirtazapine, venlafaxine and moclobemide. Avoid clomipramine and bupropion, as they ↓seizure threshold. Check interactions with anticonvulsants.
- **Stroke:** Due to their effect on Pt aggregation, SSRIs can be protective post-ischaemic stroke, but ↑bleeding risk

post-haemorrhagic stroke. If ischaemic, SSRIs may be used. Otherwise, there is evidence for nortriptyline.

Further information

Cleare et al., 'Evidence-based guidelines for treating depressive disorders with antidepressants: a revision of the 2008 British Association for Psychopharmacology guidelines', *J Psychopharmacol* 2015; **29**(5): 459–525.

ANXIETY DISORDERS

DIAGNOSIS

The drugs in this chapter have substantial overlap with those used in depression, so this chapter should be read in conjunction with the previous section.

Anxiety disorders are common and varied. The algorithm that follows shows a diagnostic screening approach.

- Causes to consider:
  - Drug use (caffeine, amphetamines, cocaine, β-agonists, theophylline)
  - Drug withdrawal (alcohol, benzodiazepines, gabapentinoids)
  - Cardiac arrhythmia (FHx, IHD, syncope, Sx with exercise; Ix: ECG, 7-day Holter monitor)
  - ↑thyroid (↑HR, tremor, proptosis, diarrhoea; Ix: TFTs)
  - Phaeo (palpitations, HTN, headaches; Ix: 24 h urinary metanephrines)
  - ↓Ca^{2+} (muscle spasms, seizures, arrhythmia; Ix: bone profile)
  - Porphyria (rash, blisters, red urine, abdominal pain, vomiting; Ix: urinary porphobilinogen is good screen)
- For a new diagnosis of an anxiety disorder, the following Ix are often appropriate: FBC, U&E, LFTs (including γ-GT), bone profile, TFTs. Consider other Ix if suggested by clinical picture.

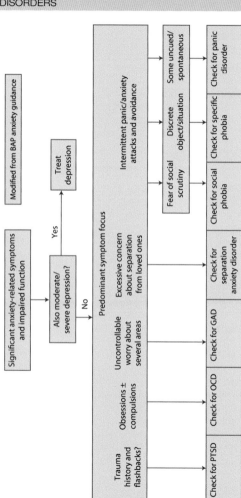

Source: Diagnosis algorithm reprinted from Baldwin et al. *J Psychopharm* 2014; 28(5): 403–439.

TYPES OF ANXIOLYTIC DRUGS

Most drugs used for anxiety disorders are also used in depression and are listed with their SEs on p. 214.

Class	Drug	Side effects					Lethality in overdose
		Sedation	Insomnia/ agitation	Postural ↓BP	↑wt	Other	
Gabapentinoids	Gabapentin	+	−	−	+	Nausea	Low
	Pregabalin	++	−	+	+	Dizziness, nausea, ankle swelling	Low
Other	Buspirone	−	++	−	−	Nausea	?Mod

MEDICATIONS LICENSED FOR ANXIETY DISORDERS[BNF]

	GAD	Panic disorder	Specific phobia	Social anxiety disorder	PTSD	OCD
Citalopram		✓				
Escitalopram	✓	✓		✓		✓
Sertraline		✓		✓	✓	✓
Fluoxetine						✓
Fluvoxamine						✓
Paroxetine	✓	✓		✓	✓	✓
Duloxetine	✓					
Venlafaxine	✓			✓		
Clomipramine			✓			✓
Trazodone	✓					
Moclobemide				✓		
Pregabalin	✓					
Buspirone	✓					
Chlordiazepoxide[1]	✓					
Clonazepam[1]		✓				
Lorazepam[1]	✓	✓				
Oxazepam[1]	✓					

[1] Benzodiazepines are not generally recommended treatments for anxiety[NICE]: they do provide short-term relief, but tend to be ineffective in the long term and cause dependence. Benzodiazepines are covered in more detail on p. 280.

CHOOSING A MEDICATION

> *Recreational drugs*
> - Many people with anxiety symptoms and disorders 'self-medicate'.
> - Ask Re. use of alcohol, cannabis and street benzodiazepines.
> - Consider dual diagnosis with a substance misuse disorder.
> - Pregabalin is now a Class C drug in the UK.

Some recommended medications for anxiety disorders are not licensed for these purposes – for example, sertraline in GAD – despite good evidence from randomised placebo-controlled trials. They can be prescribed off-label.

- For mild disorders, supportive care with patient education and support groups (e.g. Anxiety UK, Obsessive Action) may be sufficient.
- If moderate-severe depression is also present, treat the depression first.[BAP] Anxiety may improve with resolution of depression.
- Pharmacological and psychological therapy are probably similarly effective in acute illness, but should usually be offered separately in the initial stages of treatment.[BAP]
- SSRIs should be considered first-line therapy.[BAP, NICE]
- SNRIs are effective but are somewhat less well tolerated than SSRIs.
- Benzodiazepines should generally be avoided or limited to short-term use ('crisis management').[BAP] Avoid in PTSD, as they tend to be ineffective and risks outweigh benefits.
- Antipsychotics have efficacy in some conditions (e.g. quetiapine in GAD), but their SE profile limits their role. They are usually prescribed in low doses, except in PTSD.
- Propranolol and atenolol are often prescribed in primary care for somatic Sx of anxiety, but there is little evidence to support their use.[BAP]
- Pregabalin has evidence for a dose-response relationship. Response may be seen within the first wk.
- General principles of Rx resistance[BAP]:
  - ↑Dose is a good strategy with pregabalin, but evidence with SSRIs/SNRIs is inconsistent.

- In OCD, consider high doses of SSRIs (even beyond licensed maximums).
- Switch to an alternative Rx.
- Augment SSRI/SNRI with pregabalin or antipsychotic (but depends on disorder).

- Some herbal remedies have evidence for efficacy (lavender oil, Kava/*Piper methysticum*, *Passiflora* extracts, L-lysine and L-arginine), but they are less efficacious than standard Rx and Kava can be hepatotoxic. Overall, they are not recommended.[BAP]
- Clomipramine seems to be the most effective TCA for anxiety disorders, possibly due to its high serotonin reuptake inhibition.

BAP guidance summary

Disorder[BAP]	First line	Second line	Other
PTSD	Some SSRIs (paroxetine, sertraline)[2] Trauma-focused CBT EMDR	Venlafaxine	Augment with olanzapine, risperidone or prazosin; consider phenelzine
OCD	All SSRIs CBT Exposure therapy Cognitive therapy	Clomipramine	Augment SSRI/clomipramine with risperidone, olanzapine, aripiprazole, quetiapine (or ondansetron) Augment SSRI with ondansetron or topiramate
GAD	Some SSRIs (escitalopram, paroxetine, sertraline) CBT Applied relaxation	SNRI Pregabalin	Agomelatine, quetiapine, imipramine, buspirone, hydroxyzine, trazodone Benzodiazepines in patients who prove resistant to multiple pharmacological and psychological treatment approaches and who remain significantly distressed by impairing anxiety symptoms

(continued)

Disorder[BAP]	First line	Second line	Other
Social anxiety disorder	Some SSRIs (escitalopram, fluoxetine, fluvoxamine, paroxetine, sertraline) CBT with exposure	Venlafaxine, phenelzine, moclobemide, gabapentin, pregabalin, olanzapine Augment SSRI with buspirone Benzodiazepines in patients who prove resistant to multiple treatment approaches and who remain significantly distressed by impairing anxiety symptoms	
Specific phobia	Exposure-based psychological Rx[1]	SSRI (paroxetine, escitalopram)	
Panic disorder	All SSRIs CBT	Some TCAs[3] (clomipramine, imipramine, lofepramine), venlafaxine, reboxetine	Gabapentin, valproate Benzodiazepines in patients who prove resistant to multiple treatment approaches and who remain significantly distressed by impairing anxiety symptoms
Health anxiety	(Mindfulness-based) CBT, stress management[1]		

[1]   There is evidence for some forms of psychotherapy for all of the anxiety disorders listed here, but for these disorders it is generally preferred to pharmacotherapy.

[2]   NICE recommends venlafaxine or an SSRI first-line treatment for PTSD.

[3]   NICE recommends SNRIs as second-line treatment for panic and pregabalin as third-line treatment.

NON-PHARMACOLOGICAL MEASURES

Psychological therapy is very important in anxiety disorders. Most evidence-based treatments focus on a broadly cognitive-behavioural model, but it is adapted to individual disorders. For an overview of CBT and other psychotherapy techniques, see p. 359.

In anxiety disorders, CBT-based interventions typically include some of the following elements. These can be adapted and extended in specific disorders.

1 'Objectifying' thoughts (they are just thoughts, not facts).
2 Gradual exposure to anxiety-provoking situations and response prevention.
3 Divide worries into problems that you can change and those you cannot.
4 For problems that you can change, come up with a plan to deal with them. For those that cannot be changed, do not worry about them, as there is nothing you can do.
5 Relaxation and mindfulness techniques.

In specific phobias, these techniques are used with an emphasis on **graded exposure**, in which the feared stimulus is gradually introduced in a supportive environment. In OCD, a similar technique called **exposure and response prevention** (**ERP**) is used; in this the person is exposed to the anxiety-provoking situation until they can do it without a compulsion developing.

Routine 'psychological debriefing' after exposure to traumatic events is not helpful in preventing PTSD.[BAP]

Relaxation exercise
Use this acutely to calm down a very anxious patient or teach them to do this on their own.

1 Take slow deep breaths in and out.
2 Tense the muscles in your legs. Hold for 5 sec. Release. Notice the relaxation.
3 Tense the muscles in your arms. Hold for 5 sec. Release.
4 Tense the muscles in your face. Hold for 5 sec. Release.
5 Feel the release of muscle tension all over your body.

STARTING

- Medications for anxiety (particularly antidepressants) can often worsen nervousness and agitation in the first 1–2 wks before they start to have an effect, so warn patients about this and see them more frequently during this period.[BAP] Consider adding short course of benzodiazepine (e.g. diazepam 2 mg tds for 7–10 days).

- Due to heightened anxiety when starting antidepressants, patients with anxiety disorders may benefit from slower titration, but balance this against a delay in reaching a therapeutic dose.
- Pregabalin should be titrated steadily, towards an initial target dosage of 150 mg/day. If required, it can be increased in steps of 150 mg after 7 days up to 600 mg daily total. However, many patients will benefit from more gradual dose titration.
- Gabapentin requires more complex titration. Day 1: 300 mg od. Day 2: 300 mg bd. Day 3: 300 mg tds.

MONITORING

Routine care: clinical efficacy and SEs. See p. 224.

SIDE EFFECTS

- Heightened anxiety when starting antidepressants is common.
- Gabapentinoids can cause euphoria and dependence. They can be misused or diverted. Those who have a history of substance misuse are at particular risk. They became classified as controlled drugs in 2019. To avoid misuse:
  - If drug is ineffective for target Sx, stop it.
  - If dependence suspected, control access to medication (limited amount prescribed, no replacement prescriptions). Consider planned withdrawal.
- Gabapentinoids can cause respiratory depression, especially in those with RFs (e.g. COPD, concurrent use of opioids).

STOPPING

- For anxiety disorders, there is evidence for benefit of continuing the medication for 6–18 months following remission. Beyond this, evidence is unclear.[BAP]
- ↓Dose over 3 months to ↓ discontinuation or rebound Sx.[BAP]
- For gabapentinoids, gradual discontinuation is preferred:
  - Gabapentin: ↓daily dose by up to 300 mg every 4 days.
  - Pregabalin: ↓daily dose by 50–100 mg/wk.

SWAPPING

- In anxiety disorders, response can take longer and may require up to 12 wks (though usually onset of effect is seen within 4 wks).[BAP]
- For more guidance, see p. 226.

SPECIAL GROUPS

Children

- Diagnosis can be difficult, as fear and worry can be part of normal development, but anxiety disorders are also common in CAMHS. Less research, so therapeutic options are less certain.
- Psychological Rx should be first line.[BAP]
- Use medications for non-responders with much caution and careful monitoring.[BAP]
- SSRI therapy can be effective in GAD, social anxiety, separation anxiety and OCD. Fluoxetine is a good option.[BAP] Benzodiazepines are not recommended.
- NICE does not recommend pharmacological treatment for PTSD in children.
- The balance of risks and benefits favours SSRIs for anxiety more than for depression.[BAP]

Elderly

- Use same treatment options as with younger adults, but be aware of renal and hepatic impairment, co-morbidity, cognitive impairment, risk of falls, risk of bleeding, hypotension and sedative effects.[BAP]

Pregnancy

Please refer to relevant section on Perinatal Psychiatry (page 318).

Renal impairment

- Gabapentinoids are renally excreted with negligible metabolism.
- Therefore, ↓dose in renal impairment.

Hepatic impairment

- Metabolism of gabapentinoids is not expected to be altered.[SPC]

Physical health problems

- **Epilepsy:** Gabapentinoids have anticonvulsant properties (licensed for focal seizures), so may safely be used in epilepsy. However, they should be withdrawn slowly to avoid precipitating seizures.

Further information

Baldwin et al., 'Evidence-based pharmacological treatment of anxiety disorders, post-traumatic stress disorder and obsessive-compulsive disorder: a revision of the 2005 guidelines from the British Association for Psychopharmacology', *J Psychopharmacol* 2014; **28**(5): 1–37.

Baldwin DS. 'Clinical management of withdrawal from benzodiazepine anxiolytic and hypnotic medications', *Addiction* 2022; **117**(5): 1472–1482.

Baldwin DS, Masdrakis VG. 'Non-prescribed use of gabapentinoids: mechanisms, predisposing factors, associated hazards and clinical management', *Eur Neuropsychopharmacol* 2022; **63**: 6–8.

ATTENTION DEFICIT HYPERACTIVITY DISORDER (ADHD)

DIAGNOSIS

ADHD is a **neurodevelopmental** disorder that starts in childhood, although in 20%–40% it persists to adulthood and is sometimes not diagnosed until this point, particularly when co-morbid with mood, anxiety and substance misuse disorders. It may also be missed in the older adult population. The core symptoms of ADHD are **hyperactivity, impulsivity** and **inattentiveness**. These must be persistent and impairing with difficulties demonstrated across at least **two settings** (e.g. school, home, work), so history should be obtained from multiple sources.

ADHD may present as predominantly inattentive, predominantly hyperactive-impulsive or combined (meeting criteria for both).

It is associated with several organic developmental syndromes: Turner's syndrome, fragile X syndrome, Williams' syndrome, PKU and fetal alcohol syndrome. There is a wide differential diagnosis, but special Ix are not indicated unless there is a particular suspicion of another disorder. Rates of co-morbidity are particularly high for anxiety disorders, substance misuse and autism spectrum disorders.

Differential diagnosis[1]:

- **Anxiety** (hyperactivity is driven by psychomotor agitation, exaggerated startle response, anxious cognitions)
- **Substance misuse** (must assess in absence of recreational drugs; Ix: urine drug screen)
- **Depression** (low mood driving poor engagement)
- **EUPD** (impulsivity, chronic emptiness, emotional instability)
- **Conduct disorder** (persistent rule breaking involving aggression, property damage, lying or theft)
- **Oppositional defiant disorder** (similar to conduct disorder but milder)
- **BPAD** (distinct episodes of qualitatively different manic behaviour)
- **Autism** (FHx, stereotyped behaviours/interests, impaired social skills, rigid routines)

- **Learning disability** (Ix: neuropsychological testing shows impaired IQ rather than inattention)
- **Lead toxicity** (old furnishings or upbringing in developing world, peripheral motor neuropathy, bradycardia; Ix: serum lead)
- **Iron deficiency anaemia** (irritability + classic signs of pallor, koilonychia, angular stomatitis; Ix: FBC, iron studies)
- **Hyperthyroidism** ($\uparrow$HR, tremor, proptosis, diarrhoea; Ix: TFTs)
- **Sensory impairment** (auditory or visual; Ix: hearing and eye tests)
- **Absence seizures** (distinct episodes of staring lasting 10–20 sec, sometimes accompanied by eyelid flickering)
- **Medications** (especially ß-agonists, antihistamines, antiseizure medications)
- **Frontal lobe injury** (traumatic brain injury, SOL or degenerative disease resulting in disinhibition, poor executive function and primitive reflexes; Ix: Frontal Assessment Battery)

[1] These may also be co-morbid with ADHD.

TYPES OF MEDICATIONS

	Drug	Mechanism	T$_{1/2}$ (h)	SEs	
Stimulants	Methylphenidate	DARI, NARI	IR: 2.5 MR: 3.5	Abuse potential, insomnia	↑HR, ↑BP, N&V, abdominal pain, ↓appetite, ↓wt, ↓growth
	Dexamfetamine	DARI, NARI	11		
	Lisdexamfetamine	DARI, NARI	1+11[1]		
Other	Modafinil (specialist only)	DARI (weak)	14	Insomnia	
	Atomoxetine	NARI [2]	5	Somnolence, suicidal ideation	
	Bupropion (specialist only)	NDRI	14	Insomnia, GI Sx, agitation, anxiety, tremor	
	Guanfacine MR	α$_2$ agonist	17	↓HR, ↓BP, somnolence, nausea, ↑wt	
	Clonidine	α$_2$ agonist	4		

[1] 1 hr as an inactive form before being converted to dexamfetamine.

[2] Causes ↑DA in prefrontal cortex.

METHYLPHENIDATE FORMULATIONS

Methylphenidate may be prescribed in XL forms, which contain varying ratios of IR and MR drug:

	IR (%)	MR (%)
Concerta XL	22	78
Equasym XL	30	70
Medikinet XL	50	50

Not all the methylphenidate in Concerta XL is bioavailable; hence, 18 mg Concerta XL ≈ 15 mg methylphenidate. The IR portion gives a rapid effect, while the MR continues this over a longer period of time. If switching from an IR form, be aware that an 'equivalent' dose might result in less effectiveness in the morning; e.g. switching from methylphenidate IR 5 mg tds to Concerta XL 18 mg mane (which contains only 4 mg methylphenidate IR) would effectively underdose a patient by 20% in the morning.

CHOOSING A MEDICATION

- Consider the preferences of patient (+/− carers) when considering which interventions to provide.[BAP]
- Consider factors such as schools (which may not keep medication for daytime use).
- These medicines may affect driving, and stimulants are controlled substances for which there are severe penalties for impaired driving.
- Effect sizes in adults are smaller than those in children.
- In adults and children, environmental modifications should be implemented and reviewed before medications are considered.[NICE]
  - If there is little improvement, consider medications.[BAP]
- For adults, lisdexamfetamine or methylphenidate may be given as first-line medications.[NICE] Lisdexamfetamine is licensed in adults; not all other products are licensed in adults.
- **MR** methylphenidate is less liable to be abused than **IR**, is easier to take and may be more appropriate for schoolchildren (as medication is not taken at schooltime), so is preferred.[BAP]
- **Lisdexamfetamine** is a pro-drug, which is metabolised to the active dexamfetamine, but it may be less liable to abuse than dexamfetamine.[BAP]
- **Guanfacine** may safely be given in combination with stimulants and atomoxetine.
- Stimulants and atomoxetine are cautioned in the presence of established or suspected cardiac disease.[BAP]

Drug	Time to efficacy	Abuse potential	Other notes	Drug interactions
Methylphenidate IR	Immediate	High		MAOIs – may cause hypertensive crisis (avoid concomitant use and for 14 days after stopping MAOI)
Methylphenidate MR	Immediate	Medium	Some products licensed in adults. Can be abruptly stopped if necessary	Fluoxetine/paroxetine/CYP2D6 inhibitors – may increase levels of dexamfetamine and lisdexamfetamine
Lisdexamfetamine	Immediate	?Low	Licensed in adults	Serotonin syndrome (theoretical) – caution with serotonergics
Dexamfetamine	Immediate	High	Avoid abrupt withdrawal	Antipsychotics antagonise stimulants
Atomoxetine	4 weeks at an effective dose	None	Second line. Probably less effective than stimulants	Avoid MAOIs, as per stimulants. Fluoxetine/paroxetine increase atomoxetine levels – slower titration. Strong caution with noradrenergic agents (venlafaxine, mirtazapine, imipramine). May prolong QT interval
Guanfacine	2-week titration; rapid at an effective dose	None	Second line. Can be given with stimulants. Requires retitration if two or more doses missed	CYP3A4/5: Inducers (phenytoin, CBZ, modafinil, rifampicin, St John's wort) may reduce efficacy. Inhibitors (clarithromycin, ciprofloxacin) may increase exposure and reduce tolerability

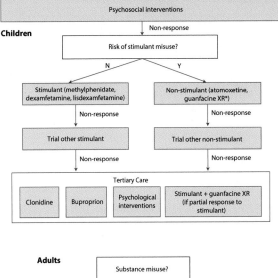

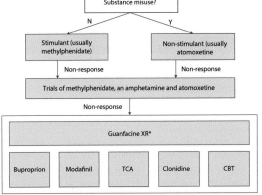

*As per Australian evidence-based guidelines and other recommendations, e.g. CADDRA

TREATMENT RESISTANCE

- Review diagnosis, patient motivation, co-morbidities and compliance. Ensure that medications have been given at effective doses.
- Other combinations of medications are commonly used, but there is no robust evidence for this strategy and there are limited data on adverse events (e.g. increased pulse and BP), which may be additive and are probably more common.[BAP]
- A combination of a stimulant and guanfacine is not a licensed treatment for ADHD; however, it may be useful if there is only a partial response to stimulant medication.
- Stimulants and α_2 agonists have complementary SEs making them an attractive choice, but the combination has not yet established sufficient evidence.[BAP]

NON-PHARMACOLOGICAL MEASURES

- Substance misuse is more common in people with ADHD and may complicate assessing efficacy of therapy. Liaise with drug and alcohol services.[BAP]
- All patients should be encouraged to implement personalised environmental modifications, e.g. alterations to seating arrangements, ↓noise, ↓distractions, headphones, frequent breaks and providing written instructions.[NICE]
- For children, provide parents and teachers with evidence-based information about ADHD.[BAP] Parental training: can be helpful in improving parenting and reducing oppositional behaviour,[BAP] but they do not help with ADHD.
- Educational interventions: teach child problem-solving or self-control strategies; assist teachers in adapting environment or teaching styles.
- Dietary interventions have shown some early promise, but the studies have numerous limitations.[BAP] Do not advise dietary elimination as part of standard care, but if there seems to be a link, recommend keeping diary tracking diet and Sx; if the diary shows a relationship, refer to a dietician.[NICE]

- CBT in adults can be helpful by encouraging memory aids, time scheduling and 'stop and think' techniques.[BAP]

STARTING

- Assess abuse or diversion potential for stimulants, including from relatives and carers.[BAP] Use of psychostimulants is popular for 'cognitive enhancement' in schools and universities.
- Conduct a structured dose titration, increasing doses according to effectiveness and tolerability.[BAP]
- ↑Dose until optimal Sx control. If SEs, limit titration up to an effective dose, consider medication switch.[BAP]
- Methylphenidate, dexamfetamine and lisdexamfetamine: titrate with weekly dose increases to optimal dose over 4–6 wks.[BAP]
- Atomoxetine: initial dose 0.5 mg/kg for 1 wk then increase to 1.2 mg/kg (max dose 100 mg) and monitor.
- Guanfacine: initially 1 mg od; increase by 1 mg every week (max dose 4–7 mg od depending on weight).
- Atomoxetine is metabolised by CYP2D6. In slow metabolisers, SEs are more pronounced, so slower titration is required. Suspect if intolerant to other drugs metabolised by CYP2D6 (see p. 382).[BAP]
- An adequate medication trial is 6 wks.[NICE]

SIDE EFFECTS

SE	Notes	Rx
HTN (stimulants, atomoxetine)	↑BP by average of 1–4 mm Hg, but in a few can be up to 10 mm Hg; monitor using age-specific charts	• ↓Dose • Drug holiday
↑HR (stimulants, atomoxetine)	Average just 1–2 bpm	• Monitor

(continued)

SE	Notes	Rx
Postural hypotension (clonidine, guanfacine)	Definition: ↓sys BP of 20 mm Hg or ↓dias BP of 10 mm Hg	• Standing up slowly • ↑Fluid and salt intake • Be careful with hot drinks and baths
↓Growth rate and weight loss (stimulants)	Cause small reduction Monitor weight: • Every 3 months for children 10 yr or younger • At 3, 6 months then 6 monthly for 11+ • Every 6 months for adults Monitor height every 6 months for all CAMHS	• Take first dose after breakfast • High-energy nutritious snacks • Drug holidays • Refer to paed endocrinology if extrapolating from growth charts gives a final ht below predicted • Consider switch if refractory to above management
Insomnia (stimulants)	Also common in unmedicated ADHD	• Sleep hygiene • Switch from stimulant to atomoxetine • Melatonin (see p. 271)
Abuse or drug diversion (stimulants)	To experience euphoria, must be snorted or injected*; prescription stimulants do not seem to result in higher rates of subsequent substance misuse	• Monitor at times of high risk, e.g. starting university[BAP] • Switch to atomoxetine or guanfacine • Involve substance misuse services
Suicidal thoughts (atomoxetine)	Rare	• Monitor carefully • Consider switch
Tics (stimulants)	Uncommon (evidence is mixed about role of stimulants in producing tics)	• Consider if drug induced • Assess if benefit of treatment outweighs impairment caused by tics

* Lisdexamfetamine does not not produce euphoria when snorted or injected.
Source: Graham et al., *Eur Child Adolesc Psychiatry* 2011; **20**(1): 17–37.[NICE]

Use the following formula to calculate predicted height:

$$\male \text{ predicted ht (cm)} = \frac{ht_{father} + ht_{mother} + 13}{2}$$

$$\female \text{ predicted ht (cm)} = \frac{ht_{father} + ht_{mother} - 13}{2}$$

MONITORING
- This is crucially important to outcomes and requires the use of structured tools, e.g. those used in the Dundee ADHD Clinical Care Pathway (Coghill & Seth, *Child Adolesc Psychiatry Ment Health* 2015; 9(52): 1–14). Ascertaining progress merely with vague or non-specific questions is not sufficient.
- Baseline assessment: ht, wt, pulse, BP, auscultation of heart and lungs, ECG (only required if cardiac disease, FHx of cardiac disease or abnormal cardiac exam), suicide/self-harm risk, stimulant abuse risk.[BAP]
- For atomoxetine, establish if there is any pre-existing liver disease, but in its absence, LFTs are not necessary.[BAP]
- Review efficacy at least annually[BAP] – use structured tools as previously noted.

STOPPING
- Continue medications as long as they are considered clinically useful, reviewing at least annually. Use the effects of any missed doses or drug holidays to aid this review.[BAP]
- Assess when transitioning from child to adult services to check whether medication still required.[BAP]
- Clonidine and guanfacine should be gradually tapered down to avoid rebound HTN. Atomoxetine may be stopped abruptly. The situation is less clear with stimulants, but drug holidays are possible with effective abrupt temporary discontinuation (Shier et al., *J Cent Nerv Syst Dis* 2013; 5: 1–17).

- If switching between medication classes, do not cross-titrate: start next Rx when previous has been stopped.

Drug holidays
- Purposes: (1) assess whether meds still required, (2) allow SE alleviation and catch-up growth (e.g. in school holidays) or (3) to accommodate a patient's preference to feel normal off meds.
- Duration varies between 2 days at the weekends to several months over a holiday.
- Less used in adults, as demands on concentration more constant.
- Limited, but favourable, evidence. (Graham et al., *Eur Child Adolesc Psychiatry* 2011; **20**(1): 17–37)

PRESCRIBING IN CHILDREN
- First-line Rx: Information and support, including advice on parenting and liaison with school.[NICE]
- Children <5 yr: Do not prescribe medications without specialist (ideally tertiary) input.[NICE]
- Children ≥5 yr: Offer medications if Sx are causing significant impairment in >1 domain after environmental modifications.[NICE]
- MR methylphenidate is often preferred in practice, as it is easy to take and is thought to be the better-tolerated stimulant.
- Whenever meds are used, it should be part of a package that includes behavioural, psychological and educational interventions.[BAP]
- For children who have benefited from medications but have impairment in >1 domain, consider course of CBT.[NICE]

PRESCRIBING IN SPECIAL GROUPS
Elderly
(Torgerson et al., *Neuropsychiatr Dis Treat* 2016; **8**(12): 79–87)

- ADHD less common with age, but Rx may still be helpful.

- Prior to prescribing meds, need thorough physical assessment to exclude co-morbidities.
- Titrate slowly.
- Be aware there is no safety data for older adults.

Pregnancy
Please refer to relevant section on perinatal psychiatry (page 321).

Physical health problems
- **Cardiac disease**: methylphenidate, amphetamines and atomoxetine are cautioned but may be used if slowly titrated and carefully monitored.[BAP]
  - Any concerns on baseline monitoring, or premature cardiac mortality in first-degree relatives, should warrant a cardiology opinion.
- **Epilepsy**: ADHD more common. Stimulants and atomoxetine are cautioned but can be used with careful monitoring. Avoid bupropion (Graham et al., *Eur Child Adolesc Psychiatry* 2011; **20**(1): 17–37).

Further information
Bolea-Alamañac et al., 'Evidence-based guidelines for the pharmacological management of attention deficit hyperactivity disorder: update on recommendations from the British Association for Psychopharmacology', *J Psychopharmacol* 2014; **28**(3): 1–25.

SUBSTANCE MISUSE

DIAGNOSIS
Substance misuse is a serious medical disorder. It is highly co-morbid with psychiatric disorders; for instance, up to 60% of people with schizophrenia smoke tobacco.

  According to ICD-11, a pattern of substance use can be categorised as dependence, harmful use or acute intoxication:

- **Dependence** requires ≥2/3 of impaired control over use, physiological features (e.g. tolerance, withdrawal) and substance use becoming a priority.
- **Harmful use** covers substance use that damages mental or physical health or causes harm to others.
- **Acute intoxication** can result in physical harm or even death.

TREATMENT

Treatment principles include:

- **Substitution:** giving medication with a similar mechanism of action but slower kinetics than drugs of abuse.
- **Detoxification:** medically assisted withdrawal from dependence on a substance in order to avoid symptoms, which are often very unpleasant.
- **Relapse prevention:** relapse rates after withdrawal may be high.

For drug overdose and withdrawal emergencies, see p. 400.

ALCOHOL

- Exercise caution in prescribing sedative drugs and gabapentinoids in patients who may be using alcohol, opioids or benzodiazepines.
- Drug metabolism is complex in chronic alcohol use, as CYP2E1 and CYP3A4 are induced, but liver failure delays metabolism of many drugs.

Drug	Mechanism	Use	Important SEs
Acamprosate	Anti-glutamatergic – reduces NMDA function	Relapse prevention	Nausea, diarrhoea, pruritic rash
Naltrexone	μ/δ/κ opioid antagonist	Relapse prevention	Nausea, sedation, headache, abdominal pain
Disulfiram	Inhibits aldehyde dehydrogenase	Relapse prevention	Only if alcohol ingested: N&V, flushing, headache, ↑HR, ↓BP

Nalmefene	μ/δ opioid antagonist; κ opioid partial agonist	Relapse prevention	Psychiatric effects, insomnia, dizziness, headache, nausea
Baclofen[1]	GABA_B agonist	Relapse prevention	Sedation, headache, nausea, polyuria, constipation
Benzodiazepines	Positive allosteric modulators of GABAA receptor	Detoxification	Sedation, confusion, paradoxical agitation, respiratory depression, gait instability

[1] Unlicensed in alcohol use disorder, but supportive evidence and used in clinical practice.

Units of alcohol
- 1 unit of alcohol = 10 mL pure ethanol (8 g).
- As a rough guide:
  - Beer: can (440 mL, 4% alcohol by volume (abv)) ~2 units; 1 pint (4–5%) ~2–3 units.*
  - Wine: small glass (125 mL, 10–14% abv) ~1–2 units, bottle (750 mL, 10–14% abv) ~7.5–10.5 units.
  - Spirits: 'shot' (25 mL, 40% abv) ~1 unit; bottle (700 mL, 40% abv) ~30 units.

*Some beers come in 'superstrengths' (e.g. 9% abv).

Alcohol dependence

Generally aim for complete abstinence, although reduced drinking may be a reasonable interim target for those who struggle to attain abstinence.[BAP]

Use motivational interviewing to help patients recognise problem and to encourage +ve change.[NICE]

Alcohol detoxification

Should be a planned part of a treatment programme.[BAP] Use medications if withdrawal Sx are present.[BAP]

Do not start medication if patient is currently intoxicated and withdrawal symptoms absent.[MPG]

Prescribe prophylactic B vitamins in those at risk of Wernicke's encephalopathy (see later section).[BAP]

Benzodiazepines (chlordiazepoxide or diazepam) are the usual choice and are effective for seizure prevention[BAP]:

- Consider lorazepam or oxazepam if ↓liver function.[MPG]
- Either fixed reducing-dose or symptom-triggered regimen may be used, but adequate monitoring is required if symptom-triggered regimen is used.[BAP]
- Chlordiazepoxide fixed-dose regimen[MPG]: consider total number of units of alcohol taken in a day, severity of alcohol withdrawal and if any previous complications.

Example fixed-dose chlordiazepoxide regimens[NICE]

Daily EtOH consumption					
Day	15–25 units		30–49 units		50–60 units
1	15 mg qds	25 mg qds	30 mg qds	40 mg qds	50 mg qds
2	10 mg qds	20 mg qds	25 mg qds	35 mg qds	45 mg qds
3	10 mg tds	15 mg qds	20 mg qds	30 mg qds	40 mg qds
4	5 mg tds	10 mg qds	15 mg qds	25 mg qds	35 mg qds
5	5 mg bd	10 mg tds	10 mg qds	20 mg qds	30 mg qds
6	5 mg nocte	5 mg tds	10 mg tds	15 mg qds	25 mg qds
7		5 mg bd	5 mg tds	10 mg qds	20 mg qds
8		5 mg nocte	5 mg bd	10 mg tds	10 mg qds
9			5 mg nocte	5 mg tds	10 mg qds
10				5 mg bd	10 mg tds
11				5 mg nocte	5 mg tds
12					5 mg bd
13					5 mg nocte

Chlordiazepoxide symptom-triggered regimen[MPG]:

- Administer the Clinical Institute Withdrawal of Alcohol (CIWA) Scale regularly.
- Prescribe chlordiazepoxide 20–30 mg up to hourly according to the CIWA score.

For delirium tremens, see p. 412.

Alcohol relapse prevention

- All pharmacological Rx should be accompanied by psychosocial support.[BAP]
- Offer pharmacological treatment for moderate-to-severe alcohol dependence.[NICE]
- First line: naltrexone or acamprosate.[NICE]
  - Start during or immediately after alcohol detoxification.[BAP]
- Disulfiram may also be used, but certain precautions required.[NICE, BAP]
  - Disulfiram inhibits aldehyde dehydrogenase, such that alcohol consumption causes a toxic build-up of acetaldehyde, causing nausea, flushing and palpitations.
  - An option for those aiming at abstinence without any CIs (decompensated HF, CAD, previous CVA, HTN, severe personality disorder, suicidal risk, psychosis).[BAP, SPC]
  - Supervised consumption improves outcome, e.g. friend or relative.[BAP]
  - Start disulfiram after ≥24 h of abstinence.[BAP]
- Baclofen probably helps people with alcohol use disorder at reducing the risk of relapse and increasing abstinent days. These effects may be more evident in those with concurrent anxiety symptoms. It does not currently have a licence.

Disulfiram: must warn patient of potentially severe reaction (flushing, sweating, tachycardia, hypotension, heart failure, arrhythmia, respiratory depression) if they drink alcohol, which can occur ≤7 days after stopping disulfiram.[BAP]

Alcohol present in food, perfumes and aerosols can cause a reaction. Disulfiram can also rarely cause hepatotoxicity, so patients should stop taking it if there is a sudden onset of jaundice.[MPG]

Monitoring

- Acamprosate, naltrexone: assess U&Es and LFTs at baseline and follow up any abnormalities as appropriate.[NICE]
- Disulfiram: baseline U&Es and LFTs (including GGT).[NICE] Clinical review every 2 wks for first 2 months, then every month for the next 4 months, then every 6 months thereafter.[BNF]

Stopping

- Acamprosate, naltrexone: consider stopping after 6 months or if drinking persists beyond 4–6 wks.[NICE]
- Disulfiram: consider stopping if no improvement.[NICE]

Wernicke's Encephalopathy (WE)

Occurs due to thiamine deficiency. Textbook triad of confusion, ataxia and ophthalmoplegia is rarely seen. A high index of suspicion is needed for subclinical presentations and patients at risk should be identified. Untreated, a proportion of patients progress to Korsakoff's syndrome, a form of irreversible alcohol-related brain disorder that is characterised by anterograde and retrograde amnesia, often accompanied by confabulation.

Prevention of WE is important during alcohol detoxification but can occur whenever there is a metabolic load on the brain, e.g. infection.[BAP] Rx of WE is a **medical emergency**; refer to general hospital.

Prophylaxis:

- If at risk (e.g. malnourished or unwell) or other suggestive signs (e.g. peripheral neuropathy), give Pabrinex 1 pair im/iv od for 3–5 days.

- If healthy and uncomplicated, give thiamine po 100 mg tds.

Treatment:

- Pabrinex 2 pairs im/iv tds for 3–5 days, then 1 pair od for 3–5 days, depending on response.[BAP]

OPIOIDS

Drug	Mechanism	Use	Important SEs
Naltrexone	μ/δ/κ opioid antagonist	Relapse prevention	Nausea, sedation, headache, abdominal pain
Methadone[1]	μ opioid agonist	Substitution and detoxification	Constipation, abdominal pain, sedation, QTc prolongation
Buprenorphine[2]	μ opioid partial agonist; δ/κ opioid antagonist	Substitution and detoxification	Constipation, nausea, diarrhoea, headache
Buprenorphine/naloxone[2,3]	μ opioid partial agonist; δ/κ opioid antagonist + μ/δ/κ opioid antagonist	Substitution and detoxification	
Lofexidine[4]	α_{2A}-adrenergic receptor agonist	Detoxification	Dry mouth, hypotension, sedation
Naloxone	μ/δ/κ opioid antagonist	Acute intoxication	Acute opioid withdrawal effects

[1] Methadone should be prescribed as a 1 mg/mL oral solution, as the tablets are easily crushed for injection.[BAP, MPG]

[2] Numerous formulations and dosing regimens available. Consult product literature.

[3] Naloxone only acts if given parenterally, so buprenorphine/naloxone (Suboxone) causes opioid withdrawal if injected or used intranasally.

[4] Not currently available in the UK.

Opioid dependence

Opioid substitution therapy (OST) can use methadone or buprenorphine, but consider patient choice and safety[BAP, NICE]:

- Offer alongside a psychosocial intervention.[BAP]
- Consider buprenorphine/naloxone (Suboxone) if significant concerns regarding injecting.[BAP]
- Should generally be supervised until titration complete and compliant with treatment programme.[NICE]
- Methadone and buprenorphine are controlled drugs, so there are certain additional requirements for prescriptions (see p. 336).
- When stopping, withdraw gradually.[NICE]

Considering OST	
Advantages	**Disadvantages**
• ↑Retention in treatment • ↓Drug-related behaviours that risk BBV transmission • ↓Heroin use	• OST diversion • Risk of overdose • Injection or snorting of OST • Accidental ingestion by children • Occupational difficulties • Most evidence relies on supervised consumption • Can use heroin in addition

Methadone versus buprenorphine	
Methadone	**Buprenorphine**
• Higher retention in treatment • Dose-related QTc prolongation • Cheaper	• Safer in overdose • Lower mortality around initiation • Less prone to CYP interactions • Less sedating

Monitoring

Methadone	ECG at baseline and annually if dose >100 mg/day or patient at ↑risk of QTc prolongation, e.g. cardiac disease, electrolyte abnormality, other medications[MPG]; monitor baseline LFTs then regularly at 6–9-month intervals.[NICE]
Buprenorphine	Monitor baseline LFTs then at regular intervals.[NICE]

Swapping

Swapping between methadone and buprenorphine is usually straightforward, but methadone to buprenorphine can precipitate opioid withdrawal.

Methadone daily dose	Action[MPG]
<40 mg	Stop methadone abruptly and commence buprenorphine after ≥24 h.
40–60 mg	↓Methadone dose as much as possible without patient becoming unstable, then stop abruptly. Delay buprenorphine until patient in opioid withdrawal (usually 48–96 h).
>60 mg	Aim to ↓methadone dose to ≤30 mg, but if not possible, admit to specialist inpatient unit.

Opioid detoxification

Can last up to 4 wks as an inpatient or up to 12 wks in the community[NICE]:

- Taper OST (methadone or buprenorphine).[BAP]
- Accompany pharmacological withdrawal with psychosocial interventions.[BAP]

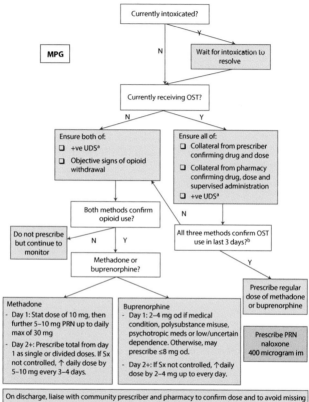

MPG

Currently intoxicated?

N → Y

Wait for intoxication to resolve

Currently receiving OST?

N — Y

Ensure both of:
- ❏ +ve UDS[a]
- ❏ Objective signs of opioid withdrawal

Ensure all of:
- ❏ Collateral from prescriber confirming drug and dose
- ❏ Collateral from pharmacy confirming drug, dose and supervised administration
- ❏ +ve UDS[a]

Both methods confirm opioid use?

N — Y

Do not prescribe but continue to monitor

All three methods confirm OST use in last 3 days?[b]

N — Y

Methadone or buprenorphine?

Prescribe regular dose of methadone or buprenorphine

Prescribe PRN naloxone 400 microgram im

Methadone
- Day 1: Stat dose of 10 mg, then further 5–10 mg PRN up to daily max of 30 mg
- Day 2+: Prescribe total from day 1 as single or divided doses. If Sx not controlled, ↑ daily dose by 5–10 mg every 3–4 days.

Buprenorphine
- Day 1: 2–4 mg od if medical condition, polysubstance misuse, psychotropic meds or low/uncertain dependence. Otherwise, may prescribe ≤8 mg od.
- Day 2+: If Sx not controlled, ↑daily dose by 2–4 mg up to every day.

On discharge, liaise with community prescriber and pharmacy to confirm dose and to avoid missing or duplicating a dose. See p. 259.

[a] Methadone is detected by standard UDS, but buprenorphine requires special kit or laboratory test.

[b] If OST use has not been supervised within last 72 h, tolerance cannot be guaranteed, so OST must be re-titrated.

Opioid relapse prevention

Refer for psychological interventions or self-help groups (e.g. Narcotics Anonymous).[NICE]

Consider naltrexone po for previously opioid-dependent patients who are highly motivated to remain abstinent.[BAP]

Acute intoxication

Pre-filled syringes with naloxone (e.g. Prenoxad) should be provided to patients, carers or hostel staff.

Provide training for patients and carers: call an ambulance, give rescue breaths if appropriate, place patient in recovery position, administer im naloxone.

OTHER SUBSTANCES

Benzodiazepines

Desired effects (acute): euphoria, anxiolysis.

Side effects (acute): sedation, confusion, paradoxical agitation, respiratory depression, gait instability.

Complications of long-term use: significant withdrawal syndrome (inc. seizures, death).

Addiction potential: physical – moderate; psychological – moderate.

Benzodiazepine misuse and withdrawal are covered in depth on p. 277. For benzodiazepine overdose, see p. 414. Maintenance prescribing is not generally recommended, but consider prescribing as part of a detox in someone who is dependent on benzodiazepines.[BAP] Manage any co-morbid opioid dependence first.[BAP]

Medical uses: multiple, varied (e.g. agitation, anxiety)

Cannabis and synthetic cannabinoid receptor agonists (SCRAs)

THC in cannabis and SCRAs are agonists at the cannabinoid CB1 receptor, but SCRAs bind with higher affinity. Some SCRAs also have pro-serotonergic activity. See page 351 for more information.

Desired effects (acute): relaxation, mild euphoria, (increased appetite).

Side effects (acute): anxiety, paranoia, dry mouth, impaired short-term memory, (increased appetite).

Complications of long-term use: respiratory pathologies. Heavy use may contribute to psychosis. Evidence gaps for SCRAs.

Dependence potential: physical – some; psychological – moderate.

Cannabis may be detected by routine UDS, but SCRAs sometimes cannot: clinical judgment may be required.[NEPTUNE]

Psychosocial interventions in milder cases should consist of brief advice, with consideration of formal psychological therapy and residential treatment for more severe cases.[NEPTUNE]

In the context of chronic SCRA use: manage psychosis with antipsychotics (SGAs preferred). If there has been acute SCRA intoxication, perform an ECG due to risk of vomiting-induced hypokalaemia.[NEPTUNE]

Manage depression with antidepressants.[NEPTUNE]

Medical uses: some neurological and psychiatric disorders, see p. 353.

GHB/GBL

GHB (and its precursor drugs GBL and 1,4-bd) are $GABA_B$ agonists.

Associated with the chemsex scene, also rarely used by bodybuilders. Often taken with other recreational substances.

Intoxication causes relaxation, disinhibition, ataxia and hallucinations.

Desired effects (acute): sociability, euphoria, anxiolysis, increased libido.

Side effects (acute): nausea, dizziness, agitation.

Interactions: acute toxicity and overdose can be life-threatening (e.g. coma, respiratory depression, seizures), particularly in combination with other sedatives, e.g. alcohol.

Complications of long-term use: severe withdrawal effects including seizures and death.

Dependence potential: physical – some; psychological – some.

Withdrawal causes pyrexia, severe anxiety, insomnia, tremors, paranoia and hallucinations, and can progress quickly to severe delirium, seizures and rhabdomyolysis, so consider inpatient admission.[BAP, NEPTUNE]

Rx of GHB/GBL withdrawal[TOXBASE]:

1. Ensure clear airway; monitor vital signs, ECG, bloods.
2. Hydration po/iv.
3. Diazepam 10–20 mg 2–4 hourly (max 100 mg/24 h) according to Sx.
4. Baclofen, e.g. 10 mg tds.
5. Monitor for seizures and delirium.

*Medical uses: Na form of GHB, sodium oxybate (**Xyrem SPC**), used for narcolepsy + catalepsy in specialist sleep centres in the US and Europe.*

Cocaine

Typically insufflated, injected, or smoked (particularly base/'crack' form).

DA reuptake inhibitor.

Desired effects (acute): euphoria, increased libido, increased energy, sociability.

Side effects (acute): agitation, psychosis, insomnia, bruxism, cardiovascular emergencies, stroke, pyrexia, hypertension.

Interactions: toxicity risk with MAOIs, TCAs, methyldopa, reserpine.

Complications of long-term use: CVD.

Dependence potential: physical – some; psychological – very high.

No specific medications recommended – symptomatic relief only. Use psychosocial interventions.[BAP]

For cocaine-induced psychosis, promote abstinence and give antipsychotics until resolution of Sx. If >1 episode of cocaine-induced psychosis, consider regular low-dose antipsychotic.[NEPTUNE]

Medical uses: Rarely used as an analgesic in some forms of head and neck surgery.

Amphetamines (inc methamphetamine)

Classical stimulant drug. Typically insufflated, injected or smoked (particularly meth form). DA release and reuptake inhibitor.

   Desired effects (acute): euphoria, increased libido, increased energy, sociability, cognitive enhancement, (appetite suppression).

   Side effects (acute): agitation, psychosis, insomnia, bruxism, GI upset (appetite suppression), rhabdomyolysis.

   Interactions: serotonergic drugs (risk of serotonin syndrome). Toxicity risk with MAOIs, TCAs.

   Complications of long-term use: CVD, may increase risk of PD in chronic heavy users.

   Dependence potential: physical – some; psychological – moderate.

   For amphetamine-induced psychosis, promote abstinence and give antipsychotics until resolution of Sx.[NEPTUNE]

Medical uses: Stimulants are used in medicinal forms as Rx for ADHD and off-licence for apathy.

Cathinones

Can be taken via chewing of khat leaves or insufflated as mephedrone powder (synthetic cathinone). Effects milder with chewed khat.

   DA release, monoamine reuptake inhibitor.

   Desired effects (acute): euphoria, increased wakefulness, (appetite suppression).

   Side effects (acute): short-term memory impairment, insomnia, bruxism, paranoia, tachycardia, (appetite suppression), HTN.

   Complications of long-term use: HTN, hepatotoxicity, renal toxicity, keratotic lesions at chewing sites. Oesophageal and gastric carcinomas have been observed in khat chewers.

   Dependence potential: physical – none; psychological – some.

   Mephedrone intoxication may be treated with benzodiazepines. Antipsychotics should be used with caution due to risk of seizures.[NEPTUNE]

MDMA

Also known as ecstasy when in pill form. Usually ingested or insufflated in powder form.

5-HT and DA reuptake inhibitor.

Desired effects (acute): euphoria, increased sociability, increased empathy, mild psychedelic effects.

Side effects (acute): insomnia, bruxism, paranoia, tachycardia, pyrexia/hyperthermia, dilutional hyponatraemia and hyponatraemic encephalopathy, cardiovascular emergencies.

Interactions: serotonergic drugs (risk of serotonin syndrome), protease inhibitors (inc concentrations).

Complications of long-term use: CVD, inconsistent evidence of neurotoxicity.

Dependence potential: physical – some; psychological – some.

In acute anxiety, provide reassurance and use benzodiazepines if necessary. Monitor for hyperpyrexia and arrhythmias.[NEPTUNE]

Medical uses: Under investigation for the Rx of psychiatric disorders, particularly PTSD.

Psychedelics

Numerous forms exist, e.g. psilocybin (in 'magic mushrooms'), LSD, DMT-containing compounds (e.g. ayahuasca), synthetic psychedelics. Most are ingested, some (e.g. DMT) are smoked.

$5\text{-}HT_{2A}$ partial agonists (pharmacology varies by substance).

Desired effects (acute): perceptual alterations, visual hallucinations, increased empathy, euphoria.

Side effects (acute): anxiety, agitation, paranoia, insomnia, appetite suppression.

Interactions: serotonergic drugs (risk of serotonin syndrome).

Complications of long-term use: hallucinogen persisting perceptual disorder (HPPD).

Addiction potential: physical – none; psychological – some.

In acute anxiety, provide reassurance; benzodiazepines may be used with antipsychotics as second line. HPPD is rare and may have anxious or functional aetiology.

Medical uses: Under investigation for the Rx of numerous neuropsychiatric disorders.

Ketamine

Commonly insufflated when used recreationally.

NMDA receptor antagonist.

Desired effects (acute): altered perceptions, (dissociation), euphoria.

Side effects (acute): sedation, dysphoria, delirium.

Complications of long-term use: urinary tract damage. Can precipitate DKA in type 1 DM.

Addiction potential: physical – some; psychological – moderate.

Withdrawal may be assisted with low-dose benzodiazepines, but evidence is very limited.[NEPTUNE]

Commonly used anaesthetic.

Nasal esketamine licensed for depression but not recommended by NICE.

Medical uses: Commonly used anaesthetic. Nasal esketamine licensed for depression but not recommended by NICE.
IV ketamine used off-licence for depression. Under investigation for alcoholism.

Nitrous oxide

Known as laughing gas or 'nos'. Commonly inhaled (e.g. through balloons).

Pharmacology unknown, likely broad effects.

Desired effects (acute): euphoria, mild hallucinations.

Side effects (acute): dizziness, disorientation, loss of motor control, hypoxia.

Complications of long-term use: functional B_{12} deficiency (irreversibly oxidises the cobalt moiety leading to inactivation).

Addiction potential: physical – limited evidence; psychological – anecdotal evidence.

Heavy use may lead to variety of neurological symptoms (motor, sensory, and ataxic) related to peripheral nerve and spinal cord damage. RX: Stop exposure, check vitamin B_{12} levels and supplement with vitamin B_{12}.

Withdrawal Sx are not significant.[NEPTUNE]

Used medically as analgesia/anaesthetic/anxiolytic ('gas and air').

Medical uses: Used medically as analgesia/anaesthetic/anxiolytic ('gas and air'). Under investigation for the Rx of psychiatric disorders (e.g. depression).

ABUSE OF PRESCRIPTION MEDICATIONS

Relevant medications covered in other sections: opioids (p. 255), benzodiazepines(p. 259 & 277), Z-drugs (p. 272), stimulants (p. 242), gabapentinoids (p. 232).

May start with legal prescriptions, but medications may also be purchased online.

General Mx: patient education, collaborative planning (lack of patient involvement may result in illicit purchase of drugs), gradual detoxification, establishing a single prescriber and psychosocial support.

NON-PHARMACOLOGICAL MEASURES

- Psychosocial intervention is main treatment for patients with harmful substance use but without dependence. In dependence, it is an important adjunct to medication.[BAP]
- Change can be conceived as five stages: precontemplation → contemplation → preparation → action → maintenance: psychosocial interventions can be seen to move patients from one stage to the next.
- Motivational interviewing aims to enhance a patient's motivation to change and can be easily integrated into routine care. It has several core skills:
  - Express empathy.
  - Develop discrepancy with the patient's values and their current behaviour.
  - Reflect back the patient's thoughts, amplifying those that support change.
  - Avoid confrontation.
  - Support confidence that change is possible.

PRESCRIBING IN SPECIAL GROUPS

Children and young people

Limited evidence, but generally follow adult treatment guidance, adjusting doses accordingly.[BAP]

Lower threshold for inpatient admission should be used.[BAP]

There is no evidence for the effectiveness of nicotine replacement therapy in adolescents, but it can be considered on an individual basis.[BAP]

NRT is recommended in children aged >12 years; NICE and NRT product licenses permit this.

Elderly

Limited evidence, but generally follow adult treatment guidance, adjusting doses accordingly.[BAP]

Offer full physical health screening.[BAP]

Lower threshold for inpatient admission should be used.[BAP]

Pregnancy

Please refer to relevant section on perinatal psychiatry (page 321).

Renal impairment

- For maintaining alcohol abstinence, avoid acamprosate,[BAP,BNF] but naltrexone may be used unless there is severe renal impairment.[BNF]
- For OST, buprenorphine is preferred,[BAP] though lower doses should be used.[BNF]
- For smoking, NRT should be used with caution in severe renal impairment. ↓Dose of bupropion. ↓Dose of varenicline if eGFR <30.

Hepatic impairment

- For alcohol withdrawal, use a short-acting benzodiazepine.[MPG] Oxazepam is often preferred. Seek specialist advice.
- Acamprosate should be avoided in severe hepatic impairment.[BNF] Naltrexone should be avoided in acute hepatitis, hepatic failure or severe impairment.[BNF]
- Methadone and buprenorphine should be avoided or used at a ↓dose.[BNF]

Physical health problems

- HIV: substance misuse can be associated with ↓compliance with antiretrovirals. Some interactions with antiretrovirals can be serious and even fatal.[NEPTUNE]
- NRT and varenicline are safe in patients with stable cardiac disease.[BAP]

Co-morbid mental health problems

- BPAD: substance misuse or withdrawal may contribute to (hypo) mania. Lithium + valproate may ↓substance misuse. Naltrexone should be first line to ↓alcohol consumption.[BAP] Bupropion is contraindicated due to risk of precipitating mania.
- Schizophrenia: preliminary data suggest clozapine may ↓substance misuse.[BAP]
- Depression: antidepressants with dual serotonergic and noradrenergic profiles may be more effective for depression with substance misuse than SSRIs, but avoid TCAs, as interactions with substances of abuse can cause fatal arrhythmias.[BAP]
- Anxiety: alcohol detoxification should usually be performed before treatment of anxiety disorder, but if this is not possible, follow treatment algorithms for anxiety.[BAP]

Further information

Bowden-Jones O & Abdulrahim D. 'Neptune clinical guidance: guidance on the clinical management of acute and chronic harms of club drugs and novel psychoactive substances, 2015. Available from: http://www.neptune-clinical-guidance.co.uk.

Lingford-Hughes et al. 'BAP updated guidelines: evidence-based guidelines for the pharmacological management of substance abuse, harmful use, addiction and co-morbidity. Recommendations from BAP', *J Psychopharmacol* 2012; **26**(7): 899–952.

NICE, 'Clinical knowledge summaries: opioid dependence', 2017. Last revised in April 2022. Available from: https://cks.nice.org.uk/topics/opioid-dependence.

NICE, 'Alcohol-use disorders: diagnosis, assessment and management of harmful drinking and alcohol dependence', Clinical guideline [CG115]. 23 February 2011.

Lindsey WT, Stewart D, Childress D. 'Drug interactions between common illicit drugs and prescription therapies', *American Journal of Drug and Alcohol Abuse*, 2012; **38**(4): 334–343.

Nutt D, King LA, Saulsbury W, Blakemore C. 'Development of a rational scale to assess the harm of drugs of potential misuse', *Lancet* 2007; **369**(9556): 1047–1053.

SLEEP DISORDERS

DIAGNOSIS

Insomnia is impaired sleep (in terms of onset, maintenance or waking) despite adequate opportunity, resulting in an impairment of daytime functioning. It increases the risk of HTN, depression, anxiety and road traffic accidents.

In **circadian rhythm disorder** the individual's sleep–wake cycle is out of sync with what is required of them. This often occurs in shift work, but other forms are **jet lag disorder** (worse when traveling eastwards), **delayed sleep–wake phase disorder** (onset of sleep and waking are consistently later than normal) and **non-24-h sleep–wake rhythm disorder** (sleep and waking times become progressively later each day).

Parasomnias cover a wide range of sleep disturbances and can occur in REM (e.g. nightmare disorder, REM sleep behaviour disorder) or non-REM (sleep terrors, sleepwalking) sleep. **Sleep terrors** (pavor nocturnus) are distinguished from nightmares by autonomic arousal and a lack of recollection. **Somnambulism** (sleepwalking) can involve familiar activities such as washing or making tea; it can be precipitated by drugs such as alcohol, hypnotics and lithium. **REM behaviour disorder** (RBD) is characterised by vivid dreams and failure of the normal skeletal muscle paralysis during REM sleep, resulting in acting out of dreams; it is strongly associated with α synucleinopathies. **Restless legs syndrome** (RLS) is characterised by an irresistible urge to move one's legs, usually while trying to sleep; it is associated with renal impairment, iron deficiency anaemia, pregnancy and many psychotropic drugs (e.g. SSRIs, SNRIs, TCAs, mirtazapine and antipsychotics).

Causes of insomnia:

Differential diagnosis

~½ have associated psychiatric disorder

- **Acute stress** (occupational, relational)
- **Depression** (early morning wakening)[1]
- **Anxiety**
- **Stimulant use** (caffeine, cocaine, amphetamines)
- **Sedative withdrawal** (benzodiazepines, Z-drugs, alcohol)
- **Schizophrenia** (circadian rhythm disorder)
- **PTSD** (insomnia, nightmares, non-REM parasomnia)

- **Pain** (especially MSK)
- **Restless legs syndrome**
- **Orthopnoea** (↑pillows to sleep due to breathlessness lying flat)
- **Paroxysmal nocturnal dyspnoea** (waking up breathless in the middle of the night)
- **Parkinson's disease** (tremor, rigidity, bradykinesia)
- **Hyperthyroidism** (↑HR, tremor, proptosis, diarrhoea; Ix: TFTs)
- **Prescribed medications** (β-agonists, methylphenidate, arousing SSRIs)

---

[1] Insomnia is a risk factor for depression, not simply a symptom of it.

Screening for other sleep disorders[BAP]:

Disorder	Qs
Obstructive sleep apnoea (OSA)	• Are you a very heavy snorer? • Do you ever wake up choking? • Does your partner say that you sometimes stop breathing at night? • Do you feel very sleepy during the day? • Do you wake up with a headache?
Restless legs syndrome (RLS)	• Do you have a sense of discomfort in your legs, or elsewhere in your body, that is worse at night, worse at rest and temporarily relieved by movement?
Periodic limb movements in sleep (PMLS)	• Do your legs twitch repeatedly while in bed? • Do you wake from sleep with jerky leg movements?
Narcolepsy	• Do you feel very sleepy during the day and find yourself falling asleep in inappropriate situations? • Do you have collapses or extreme muscle weakness triggered by emotion, for instance when you're laughing? (cataplexy)
Circadian rhythm sleep disorder	• Do you tend to sleep well but just at the 'wrong times' and are these times regular?
Parasomnias	• Do you have unusual behaviours associated with your sleep that trouble you or are dangerous? • Do you have unpleasant experiences before, during or after sleep, such as nightmares, paralysis or feeling, seeing and hearing things that aren't there? (Nightmare disorder is the sleep disorder most consistently associated with suicide.)

Source: Adapted from Wilson et al., *J Psychopharmacology* 2010; **24**(11):1577–1600.

Investigations for sleep disorders may include a collateral history (e.g. from a bed partner), a sleep diary or polysomnography. The **Epworth Sleepiness Scale** is a useful way of screening for excessive daytime sleepiness (EDS): 0–5 is low-normal, 6–10 is high-normal, 11–12 is mild, 13–15 is moderate and 16–24 is severe EDS.

TYPES OF MEDICATIONS

Class	Drug	Action	Equivalent po dose[1]	$T_{1/2}$ (h)[1]
Benzodiazepines	Alprazolam[2]	GABA-A PAM	0.5 mg	6–12
	Chlordiazepoxide		25 mg	5–30
	Clonazepam		1 mg	18–50
	Diazepam		10 mg	20–100
	Flurazepam		15–30 mg	40–250[3]
	Loprazolam		1–2 mg	6–12
	Lorazepam		1 mg	10–20
	Lormetazepam		1–2 mg	10–12
	Nitrazepam		10 mg	15–38
	Oxazepam		30 mg	4–15
	Temazepam		20 mg	8–22
Z-drugs	Zaleplon	GABA-A PAM with α_1 subtype		2[4]
	Zolpidem	specificity		2
	Zopiclone			5–6
Antihistamines	Diphenhydramine	H_1 ant		2–9
	Hydroxyzine			14–20
	Promethazine			5–14
Antidepressants	Amitriptyline	NRI>SRI		16–40
	Doxepin	SRI+NRI		8–24
	Mirtazapine	$5\text{-}HT_2 + 5\text{-}HT_3 + \alpha_2$ ant		20–40
	Paroxetine	SRI		~24
	Trazodone	$5\text{-}HT_2 + \alpha_1$ ant > SRI		5–13
	Trimipramine	SRI+NRI		23
Antipsychotics	Olanzapine	$D_2 + 5\text{-}HT_2$ ant		30–50
	Quetiapine	$D_2 + 5\text{-}HT_2$ ant		7
Other	Melatonin	$MT_1 + MT_2$ ag		4[5]

[1] Derived from authorative sources, inc.[MPG] and Ashton, 'Benzodiazepines: how they work and how to withdraw' (aka 'The Ashton Manual'), 2002. Available from https://benzo.org.uk/manual.

[2] Cannot be prescribed on the NHS but is sometimes prescribed privately and used recreationally.

[3] Active metabolite.

[4] Half-life from T_{max} is one hour. T_{max} occurs 1hr after ingestion.

[5] MR formulation (Circadin) has $T_{1/2}$ of 4 h, but IR form is <1 h.

CHOOSING A MEDICATION

Insomnia

- Short-acting benzodiazepines and Z-drugs are effective.[BAP] Z-drugs, temazepam, loprazolam and lormetazepam are recommended options for short-term use.[NICE]
- Initial treatment with a benzodiazepine or Z-drug should not normally extend beyond 2[NICE]–4[BAP] wks.
- $T_{1/2}$ is very important:
  - Benzodiazepines with shorter half-lives have a better SE profile. If $T_{1/2} > 6$ h, hangover effects likely.[BAP]
  - For initial insomnia, drugs with short $T_{1/2}$ are good. For mid- or late-insomnia, longer $T_{1/2}$ is better.[BAP]
  - All hypnotics reach T_{max} very quickly, so should be taken in the bedroom to avoid patients falling asleep prematurely. The exception is nitrazepam, where T_{max} is variable.
  - Due to their short $T_{1/2}$, **zolpidem** and **zaleplon** are not useful for early morning wakening or for maintaining sleep throughout the night.[BAP]
  - Zaleplon can, however, be taken up to 5 h before time of desired waking.[BAP]
- Consider the presence of substance misuse, when deciding on whether to prescribe drugs that can cause dependence.[BAP]
- Melatonin MR is effective if age >55 yr. It ↓s sleep latency and ↑s sleep quality.[BAP]
- Suvorexant (OR1 and OR2 antagonist) shows promise and is licensed in US but not available in UK.

Antihistamines

- Sedating antihistamines have some limited evidence for short-term use in insomnia.[BAP]
- Can be a useful strategy in patients where risk of dependence is high[BAP] and for difficulties with sleep maintenance (as they have longer half-lives).

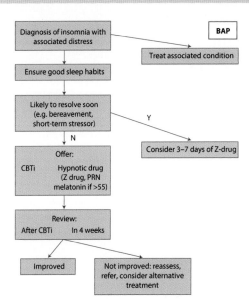

Antidepressants

- If depression is present, treat the depression appropriately with antidepressants at a therapeutic dose for depression.[BAP]
- Antidepressants used for insomnia are generally prescribed at lower doses than would be required for depression. Often the antihistamine action is the primary mechanism.
- There is some evidence for the antidepressants in the previous table, but they often have SEs ++ due to wide receptor actions.[BAP]
- TCAs are cautioned because of their toxicity in overdose even when low doses are prescribed.[BAP]

Antipsychotics

- Olanzapine and quetiapine seem to improve sleep but should not be used first-line due to high SE burden.[BAP]
- In patients taking antipsychotics for psychosis or BPAD, sleep tends to improve on switching from a typical to an atypical drug. Quetiapine tends to improve insomnia in SZ and BPAD.

Circadian rhythm disorders

- Melatonin is an effective treatment for jet lag disorder, delayed sleep phase syndrome and 24-h sleep–wake disorder, but timing is critical.[BAP]
- Melatonin is effective in blind people with 24-h sleep–wake disorder.[BAP]
- Light therapy is effective for delayed sleep phase syndrome,[BAP] but timing is critical and may be best done in specialist centres.

Parasomnias

- Weak evidence.
- ↓Triggers (e.g. frightening films, recreational drugs, late-night meals).[BAP]
- Ensure safety of patient and others, e.g. by separate sleeping arrangements, locking doors/windows, sleeping on ground floor.
- For NREM parasomnias, there is some evidence for clonazepam and antidepressants.
- For REM sleep behaviour disorder, use melatonin (3–12 mg) or clonazepam.
- Nightmares in the context of PTSD respond well to prazosin and may also be improved by trazodone (appears to have limited efficacy in non-PTSD nightmares).

NON-PHARMACOLOGICAL MEASURES

- Advise the person not to drive if they feel sleepy, but they do not need to inform the Driver and Vehicle Licensing Agency (DVLA) unless a primary sleep disorder is diagnosed or the sleepiness continues for 3 months or more.[NICE]

- Light therapy is a treatment for delayed sleep phase syndrome.
  - Requires exposure to bright light for 30–120 min depending on properties of the lamp.

Sleep hygiene techniques

- Exercise (but not near bedtime)
- Reduce caffeine, nicotine and other stimulants
- Reduce alcohol (helps with falling asleep but impairs sleep quality)
- Set a regular routine, getting up at the same time every day
- Take a warm bath before bed
- Avoid screens before bedtime
- If kept awake by worries, write down a plan for when you will deal with them

Source: nhs.uk

CBT for insomnia (CBTi)

- Individual or group. Also available in self-help books and online.
- Takes longer to work than medications, but the effects are more durable. With the exception of a single study, research shows that the effect of medication is lost once the medication is discontinued. However, the benefits of CBT endure long after the active therapy ends.
- Identifies a vicious cycle of racing thoughts → inability to sleep → further agitation in striving to sleep → further inability to sleep.
- Behavioural techniques: Rising at the same time every day, avoiding napping, going to bed later so that the time in bed closely matches the actual time asleep, changing the association with the bedroom by banning all activities from the bedroom aside from sleep and sex, and leaving the bedroom if one does not fall asleep to ensure there is almost no time spent awake in the bed.

STARTING

- Warn patients of risk of tolerance and dependence.
- Use lowest effective dose for the shortest period necessary.[NICE]
- Explain that this is a one-off prescription.[NICE]
- Do not issue further prescriptions without seeing the patient.[NICE]
- Intermittent doses may decrease the likelihood of tolerance and dependence. It is a good strategy if insomnia is intermittent and patients can predict when they are going to have insomnia.[BAP]

SIDE EFFECTS

- Benzos → ataxia, anterograde amnesia, dysarthria, confusion, dependence, falls (in elderly).
- SEs less severe for Z-drugs than benzos.
- Road traffic accidents are more common in people the day after taking benzos or zopiclone, although insomnia impairs driving performance as well.
  - The impairment in driving with benzos is similar to that when using alcohol.
  - If a patient is taking a medication that may impair driving performance, they should contact the DVLA.
- Benzos occasionally cause paradoxical excitement or disinhibition; this is more common in the elderly.
- Benzo dependence is more likely with drugs that have shorter half-lives.
- Benzo overdose can cause respiratory depression (see p. 403).
- Melatonin does not impair memory, and its SE burden is favourable.

MONITORING

- Review patient within 2 wks of starting a hypnotic.[NICE]
- If a patient is on long-term benzos, r/v every 3–6 months to consider weaning down.[BAP]

STOPPING

- In general, patients who have been on benzos for some time should be withdrawn gradually, unless there are significant risks.[BAP]
- Benzos should not be withdrawn rapidly due to a withdrawal syndrome, which can result in life-threatening seizures. Sx are agitation, insomnia, nausea, vomiting, muscle cramps, hyperhidrosis, depersonalisation and hyperaesthesia. This lasts longer following withdrawal from medications with a longer $T_{1/2}$, but usually persists for ~1 month.
- Risk factors for benzo continuation: substance misuse history, depression, dependent personality disorder, physical illness.
- One method to see if hypnotics are still providing any benefit is to periodically taper and assess Sx.[BAP]
- Benzo withdrawal may be monitored with the Clinical Institute Withdrawal Assessment Scale – Benzos (**CIWA-B**).
- Tips for tapering benzos:
  - Discuss with patient: lack of patient involvement may result in illicit purchasing.
  - Switch to a benzo with a longer $T_{1/2}$ (see following section on Swapping).[BAP]
  - Taper off over 2 wks (short-term use) or several months (long-term use).[BAP]
  - Consider offering prn benzos if Sx are intermittent.[BAP]
  - CBT alongside benzo withdrawal can help.[BAP]
- Suggested taper schedule[MPG]:

Current dose of diazepam	Recommended ↓in daily dose every 1–2 wks
>50 mg	10 mg
30–50 mg	5 mg
20–30 mg	2 mg
<20 mg	1 mg

SWAPPING

- Switching to a benzo with a long $T_{1/2}$ (e.g. diazepam or clonazepam) can be helpful when weaning a patient down, as this may ↓withdrawal Sx.
- Use the table on p. 271 to check dose equivalence, but err on the side of caution if giving high doses.

SPECIAL GROUPS

Children

- Behavioural treatment with sleep hygiene is usually effective.[BAP]
- Melatonin is a good first-line medication for initial insomnia or delayed sleep phase syndrome. It has an evidence base in autism, ADHD and learning disability.[BAP]
- Antihistamines only work in the context of behavioural treatments, but they may be useful adjuncts or short-term agents.[BAP] Some children may show paradoxical excitement due to the anticholinergic actions.[SPC]
- Clonidine is sometimes used, but it has a narrow therapeutic window.

Elderly

- CBTi is effective.[BAP]
- Melatonin MR has an evidence base for treatment up to 13 wks if age >55 yr (though frequently prescribed for longer), so it should be the first-line medication.[BAP]
- Benzos and Z-drugs have a complex relationship to risk of falls. The sedation and ataxia may ↑risk of falls, so use a medication with a short $T_{1/2}$.[BAP] However, insomnia may also be a RF for falls due to wandering; hypnotics may even ↓this risk.

Learning disability

- Insomnia is common and may be linked to some genetic syndromes (e.g. Smith–Magenis).
- Behavioural techniques and patient/carer education can be helpful.
- Melatonin is effective in this group for insomnia.[BAP]

Pregnancy

- If medications needed, diphenhydramine (ideally avoid in third trimester) is the best option. Discuss risks and benefits.[BAP]
- For RLS, DA agonists are contraindicated. Iron and folate supplementation are often effective, even if patient is not deficient. ↓ caffeine. Mild-to-moderate exercise in evening with stretching and massage helpful.[BAP]

Breastfeeding

- Z-drugs are preferred to benzos, as they tend to have shorter $T_{1/2}$ and only small amounts pass into breast milk. Use intermittent dosing for a short period of time. There is no particular preference for one Z-drug over another,[UKDILAS] but if all other factors are equal, general advice is to use a drug with a short $T_{1/2}$.
- Discourage co-sleeping when mother has taken a hypnotic.[UKDILAS]

Menopause

- ↑Rates of insomnia and OSA after menopause.
- General management of insomnia may be followed, but if perimenopausal, consider HRT.[BAP]

Renal impairment

- Benzos and Z-drugs are hepatically metabolised, so are relatively safe, although longer-acting benzos may show accumulation of active metabolites. Use short-acting drugs, start low and go slow. Risk of excessive sedation in renal impairment.

Hepatic impairment

- Rule out hepatic encephalopathy as a cause of sleep disruption.
- All benzos and Z-drugs are hepatically metabolised and precipitate coma, so they should be used with great caution. Best options are Z-drugs, lorazepam, oxazepam or temazepam.

Further information

Baldwin et al., 'Benzodiazepines: risks and benefits. A reconsideration', *J Psychopharmacol* 2013; **27**(11): 967–71.

Wilson et al., 'British Association for Psychopharmacology consensus statement on evidence-based treatment of insomnia, parasomnias and circadian rhythm disorders', *J Psychopharmacol* 2019; **33**(8): 923–947.

DEMENTIA

Dementia is a progressive brain disorder characterised by cognitive decline and ↓function (i.e. ↓ADLs) +/– behavioural/neuropsychiatric changes. Approximately 60% Alzheimer's disease (AD), 20% vascular dementia (VaD), 15% dementia with Lewy bodies (DLB) and 5% other (e.g. fronto-temporal dementia [FTD]).

There is mixed evidence regarding the utility of recognising pre-dementia syndromes, e.g. mild cognitive impairment (MCI).

Differential diagnosis: Important to consider +/– exclude other causes, especially if treatable (see box).

MILD COGNITIVE IMPAIRMENT

- 'Pre-dementia' stage (on cognitive decline 'continuum').
- Objective cognitive impairment, but help with ADLs not yet needed.
- Heterogeneous causes.
- Risk state for further cognitive and functional decline: 5%–15% develop dementia every year.
- However, ~50% remain stable at 5 years and minority have symptomatic resolution.
- A subset of those assessed for MCI will have functional cognitive disorder.

Other/treatable causes of dementia

Causes I AVOIDED

I	**I**nfection: ***Syphillis and HIV*** (rarely others[1])
A	**A**lcohol-related brain damage (including Korsakoff's)
V	**V**asculitis: Including sarcoid, systemic lupus erythematous
O	**O**ther autoimmune: Limbic encephalitis/channelopathies, e.g. anti-NMDAR Abs
I	**I**ntracranial: Tumour, NPH[2], subdural, injury (including repetitive minor = chronic traumatic encephalopathy)
D	**D**eficiencies: ***B12*** (also B1 and B6) and Excesses: Copper (Wilson's), toxins[3] (e.g. lead)
E	**E**ndocrine: ↓*T4* (also ↓/↑ cortisol, ↓/↑ PTH, ↑ Ca^{2+})
D	**D**epression, anxiety or functional cognitive disorder

[1] Viruses (especially HSV), Whipple's disease (*Tropheryma whipplei* ⟹ GI/rheum/neuro disease), Lyme disease (*Borellia* spp) TB and fungi, Creutzfeldt–Jakob disease (CJD).

[2] NPH = normal pressure hydrocephalus (suspect if gait +/– urinary dysfunction).

[3] Also includes drugs (especially anticholinergics) (see box on drugs that can commonly cause/worsen cognitive impairment).

Should be routinely excluded (Ix = HIV/syphilis serology, brain scan, B12, T4) – other causes normally only require investigation if suggestive features from history or neuro +/– psych exam. Rapid (<6 months) or young (<65 yr) onset should alert to previously discussed causes or rarer more rapid degenerative disorders (e.g. prion disease, CADASIL, etc.).

MCI definition (Langa & Levine, JAMA 2014)

- Concern of cognition changes from patient, knowledgeable informant or skilled clinician observing patient
- Objective evidence of impairment (from cognitive testing) in at least one cognitive domain including memory, executive function, attention, language, or visuospatial skills
- Preservation of independence with ADLs (but may show ↓efficiency/↑errors)
- No significant ↓in social or occupational functioning (i.e. not demented)

There are currently no evidence-based treatments. AChE-i and vit E do not ↓risk of AD[BAP].

However, the following is recommended:

1 Follow-up (e.g. 6 months)
2 Control/optimise vascular risk factors (stop smoking, control ↑BP/diabetes/dyslipidaemia/AF)
3 ↑Mental/physical activity
4 ↓Heavy alcohol/illicit drug use
5 Optimise vision, hearing and sleep-disordered breathing
6 ↓(Ideally stopping) any medications that can ↓cognition (see box)

Drugs that can commonly cause/worsen cognitive impairment
Anticholinergics (common action of many drug classes):

- Bronchodilators – e.g. atropine, ipratropium (also amino/theophylline)
- Antihistamines/antiemetics – e.g. cyclizine, cinnarizine, prochlorperazine
- Sleeping tablets – e.g. promethazine
- Allergies – e.g. cetirizine, loratadine, chlorphenamine
- Antispasmodics – e.g. hyoscine, procyclidine
- Bladder stabilizers – e.g. oxybutynin
- Tricyclic antidepressants – e.g. amitriptyline, lofepramine, dosulepin, trazadone

Other

- Opioids
- Benzodiazepines
- Antihypertensives – diuretics (e.g. furosemide), α-agonists
- Antiarrhythmic – e.g. digoxin
- Steroids – especially high dose and/or potency
- Chemotherapy – e.g. asparginase, cytosine, chlorambucil, ifosfamide, vinblastine/vincristine

ALZHEIMER'S DISEASE (AD)

Pathology: amyloid plaques and neurofibrillary tangles ⇒ neuronal loss and brain atrophy, especially medial temporal lobe (e.g. hippocampus) in early stages. Neocortical cholinergic neuronal loss predominates.

Diagnosis: largely clinical but excluding other causes important (see box on Other/treatable causes of dementia). Medial temporal lobe atrophy is highly suggestive. Biomarkers are of increasing diagnostic utility (especially CSF markers [$\downarrow A\beta_{1-42}$/$\uparrow$tau] and amyloid [PET] imaging) and may allow detection of prodromal/preclinical disease.

NIA diagnostic guidelines for AD (McKhann et al., Alzheimers Dement. *2011*)

Probable AD is diagnosed when the patient meets criteria for dementia and has the following characteristics:

A Insidious onset over months to years.

B Clear history of worsening cognition.

C Initial and most prominent deficits in one of the following:

    a   Amnesia, including impairment in learning and recall of recently learned information.

    b   Non-amnestic presentations: word-finding, visuospatial function, executive function.

D Do not apply the diagnosis in the presence of substantial cerebrovascular disease, non-dementia core features of dementia with Lewy bodies, prominent features of frontotemporal dementia or evidence for another disease or medications that could substantially affect cognition.

Treatment

Trials generally use the following:

- 1° outcome = MMSE or cognitive scale of AD Assessment Scale (ADAS-cog; total score = 70)
- Staging by MMSE: normal = 27–30, mild = 21–26, moderate = 10–20, severe = 0–9 (NICE 2011)
- NB: *MMSE is screening tool and not diagnostic.*

1 **Cognitive treatments**
   Currently two classes (see Table 2.1 for key comparisons):
   — **Cholinesterase inhibitors (AChE-i):** donepezil, rivastigmine
     and galantamine
     • All recommended for mild-mod AD (MMSE > 10)[NICE/BAP]
       although cognitive improvement over placebo small as are
       improvements in ADLs.
     • Switch to another drug if first not tolerated/effective.[BAP]
     • Benefits may persist in severe AD (e.g. Howard et al.,
       NEJM 2012).
   — **NMDA receptor antagonists:** memantine
     • Recommended for moderate-severe AD (MMSE <21)
       if cannot take/tolerate AChE-i[NICE/BAP]; benefits on
       cognition, ADLs and behaviour.

   NB: Benefits of giving both AChE-i and memantine unclear,[BAP]
   but a meta-analysis suggests improved cognition, behavioural
   disturbance, ADLs and global function for moderate-severe
   AD (Matsunaga et al., *Int J Neuropsychopharmacol* 2014; EFNS
   Guidelines, 2015). Consider adding memantine in moderate-
   severe disease.[NICE]

Table 2.1 Doses, SEs and cautions of cognitive treatments

	Donepezil	Rivastigmine	Galantamine	Memantine
Dose range	5–10 mg od	1.5–6 mg bd (or 4.6–9.5 mg/24 h patch[1])	4–12 mg bd (or 8–24 mg XL od)	5–20 mg od
Side effects	Commonly nausea, diarrhoea, vomiting, headache; also sleep disturbance, dizziness, ↓HR			Somnolence, dizziness
Cautions	Stop if: GI ulceration or ↓HR (e.g. heart block or other drugs that ↓HR)			Hepatic impairment, seizures/epilepsy

[1] Can ↑dose to 13.3 mg/24 h after 6 months in patient who have a meaningful cognitive deterioration and/or fn decline while on 9.5 mg/24 h.

All three licensed AChE-i have similar efficacy. Interrupting treatment course of AChE-i may ⇒ rapidly ↓and unrecoverable efficacy. Failure to respond and/or intolerance to one agent does not preclude a response/tolerability with another. Tolerability may be affected by dose or speed of titration.

2 **Other pharmacological treatment**

Optimise vascular risk factors and other factors. The following all currently lack evidence to justify use[BAP]: Latrepirdine, Ginkgo biloba, HRT, statins, folate+vitamin B12, vitamin E, multivitamins, omega-3 fatty acids, huperzine A, saffron and cerebrolysin. *NB: Some have significant side effects, and this should be factored into decisions to prescribe/recommend.*

NICE Guidance on AChE-i

- Donepezil, galantamine and rivastigmine for mild-to-moderate AD.
- Memantine for moderate AD if intolerant of AChE-i, or severe AD.
- Consider memantine in addition to an AChE inhibitor if they have moderate disease.
- Offer memantine in addition to an AChE inhibitor if they have severe disease.
- Treatment must only be initiated following specialist advice.
- Carer's view should be sought.
- Do not stop AChE inhibitors in people with Alzheimer's disease because of disease severity alone.
- Patients require regular review by a specialist team.
- Start with medication at lowest acquisition cost but take into account tolerance, adherence and the possibility of interactions and dosing profiles.

Clinicians should not rely solely on cognition scores in situations where any physical, sensory or learning disability or communication difficulty could influence the clinical picture. However, an alternative AChE inhibitor could be prescribed if it is considered appropriate when taking into account adverse event profile, expectations about adherence, medical co-morbidity, possibility of drug interactions and dosing profile.

3 **Non-pharmacological treatment**

Group cognitive stimulation and activities to promote well-being tailored to person's preferences are recommended. Ensure carer support.[NICE]

4 **Treatments in development**

There is a concerted effort to target disease progression. No drugs are currently licensed, but the following are the most promising agents.

Anti-amyloid

Immunotherapy: Active immunisation (Aβ 1-42 vaccination) research suspended as can ⇒ meningoencephalitis. Passive immunization (e.g. monoclonal Ab against amyloid, e.g. *bapineuzumab* and *solanezumab*) not supported by RCT evidence, which showed lack of efficacy and vasogenic oedema with bapineuzumab.

- *Secretase inhibitors (e.g. semagacestat):* targets buildup of Aβ fragments. Currently no evidence of efficacy.
- Aducanumab, lecanemab and donanemab (Aβ antibody treatments) have received FDA approval for use in US despite limited evidence for clinical efficacy and potentially severe side effects from ARIA (Amyloid Related Imaging Abnormalities) requiring MRI monitoring. None of these treatments currently approved in UK/Europe, although lecenemab is likely to be soon.

Anti-tau

- *Tau kinase inhibitors:* (↓tau hyperphosphorylation), tau aggregation inhibitors, microtubule stabilisation; under investigation, no current clear evidence of efficacy.

Neuroprotective/restorative

- Anti-inflammatory agents: e.g. NSAIDs, anti-oxidants and nerve growth factor; under investigation, no current clear evidence of efficacy.

VASCULAR DEMENTIA (VaD)

Pathology: Cerebrovascular disease, ranging from large infarcts and haemorrhages to deep white matter lesions and lacunes associated with ischaemia. Similar clinical picture to AD.

Treatment:

- No licensed treatments for VaD in the UK.
- Managing cardiovascular risk factors is primary intervention (especially BP, lipid profile, diabetes, smoking, diet, exercise, etc.).
- AChE-i and memantine not recommended, as although can improve cognition, global improvements not seen and adverse events common.[BAP]
- Clinically distinguishing VaD from AD can be challenging as the disorders can coexist, and it can be hard to distinguish age-related vascular MRI changes from VaD diagnosis. *Those with mixed VaD and AD may benefit from AChE-i or memantine.*[BAP]

'NINDS-AIREN' diagnostic criteria for VaD (Román et al., 1993 Neurology 43[2]:250–60)

1 Dementia: impairment in memory and two other cognitive domains
2 Evidence of cerebrovascular disease: on examination or brain imaging
3 A relationship between the two aforementioned conditions, or a relationship inferred by:
    a Symptoms within 3 months of a stroke
    b Abrupt ↓ in cognition
    c Fluctuating stepwise cognitive deterioration
4 Clinical features of VaD: gait disturbance, falls, urinary incontinence, pseudobulbar palsy, personality/mood changes

NB: VaD unlikely w/o focal neurological signs (e.g. gait disturbance) or cerebrovascular lesions on neuroimaging, and if early and progressive memory loss is the most prominent feature.

DEMENTIA WITH LEWY BODIES (DLB)

Pathology: Lewy bodies $\Rightarrow$ $\downarrow$dopaminergic and cholinergic neurons $\Rightarrow$ variable levels (and relative temporal onset) of cognitive, movement and neuropsychiatric disorders.

  Diagnosis: Dementia occurs before, or concurrently, with parkinsonism; if Parkinson's disease diagnosis ≥ 1 yr before dementia then called Parkinson's disease dementia (PDD).

Treatment:

- AChE-i: Can $\downarrow$cognitive and neuropsychiatric symptoms[BAP] and all agents equally effective.[BAP] There is high-quality evidence for rivastigmine and donepezil in Lewy body dementias.

Revised consensus criteria for probable and possible DLB
(McKeith et al., Neurology 2017; 89(1): 88–100)

Central feature – essential for any (possible or probable) diagnosis

- *Progressive cognitive decline* affecting social or occupational function.

NB: $\downarrow$Memory may not occur in early stages but usually evident with progression.
$\downarrow$Attention, executive function and visuo-spatial ability may be especially prominent.

Core features

- *Fluctuating cognition* – pronounced variations in attention and alertness
- *Recurrent visual hallucinations* – typically well formed and detailed
- *Parkinsonism* – triad of tremor, rigidity and bradykinesia
- *REM sleep behaviour disorder*

Supportive features (commonly present, but unproven diagnostic specificity)

- Repeated falls and syncope
- Transient, unexplained loss of consciousness

- Severe autonomic dysfunction e.g. orthostatic hypotension, urinary incontinence
- Hallucinations in other modalities
- Systematised delusions
- Depression
- Severe neuroleptic sensitivity
- Hyposmia
- Hypersomnolence

Indicative biomarkers:

- Reduced dopamine transporter uptake in basal ganglia demonstrated by SPECT or PET
- Abnormal (low uptake) [123]Iodine-MIBG myocardial scintigraphy
- Polysomnographic confirmation of REM sleep without atonia

Supportive biomarkers:

- Relative preservation of medial temporal lobe structures in CT/MRI scan
- Generalised low uptake on SPECT/PET perfusion/metabolism scan with reduced occipital activity +/- the cingulate island sign on FDG-PET imaging
- Prominent posterior slow-wave activity on EEG with periodic fluctuations in the pre-alpha/theta range

Diagnosis of DLB less likely if:

- Cerebrovascular disease evident from focal neurological signs or brain imaging
- Other physical illness present/brain disorder could account in part for symptoms
- Parkinsonism only appears for first time at stage of severe dementia

Probable DLB: ≥2 or more core clinical features with or without biomarkers
Probable DLB cannot be diagnosed on biomarkers alone
Possible DLB: 1 core clinical feature, no indicative biomarkers
OR ≥1 indicative biomarker with no clinical features

- Memantine: Can ↓cognitive symptoms and ⇒ global improvements.[BAP]
- Should be patient focused, depend on symptom severity and patient/carer wishes.[BAP]
- Start/↑ drugs cautiously: Treating one symptom can worsen others (e.g. antipsychotics can ↑parkinsonism, and antiparkinsonian drugs can ↑psychosis).

FRONTOTEMPORAL DEMENTIA (FTD)

Heterogeneous group of syndromes associated with degeneration/atrophy of prefrontal and anterior temporal lobes ⇒ behaviour changes and ↓executive function.

Pathology: Tau or TDP-43 protein (present in >90% of cases).

Diagnosis: Two main variants:

1 Frontal (fvFTD): Behavioural
2 Temporal (tvFTD): Language impairment

Includes Pick's disease, primary progressive aphasia and semantic dementia. Corticobasal degeneration (CBD) and progressive supranuclear palsy (PSP) are related 'tau-opathies' (aka 'Pick complex').

Treatment: No specific agents licensed. Treatment is symptomatic and prognosis poor.

- AChE-i and memantine not recommended[BAP] and may cause agitation.
- SSRIs have mixed evidence of improved behavioural (but not cognitive) symptoms.[BAP]
- Disease-modifying therapies (targetting Tau pathology) currently under investigation.

BEHAVIOURAL AND PSYCHOLOGICAL SYMPTOMS OF DEMENTIA (BPSDs)

BPSD = non-cognitive neuropsychiatric symptoms in dementia. Approximately 75% of dementia cases have ≥1 BPSD symptom; number/severity of symptoms variable.

> *Spectrum of BPSD symptoms*
> **Common**
>
> - Aggression
> - Agitation or restlessness
> - Anxiety
> - Depression
> - Sleep disturbance
> - Apathy
>
> **Other**
>
> - Psychosis: Delusions, hallucinations
> - Repetitive vocalisation, cursing and swearing
> - Shadowing (following others, e.g. carer, closely)
> - Sundowning (behaviour worsens after 5 p.m.)
> - Wandering
> - Non-specific behaviour disturbance, e.g. hoarding

Ensure other causes considered/treated (e.g. delirium, pain). Patients (and carers/families) should be involved in decision-making.

Treatment is divided into pharmacological and non-pharmacological therapies; non-pharmacological approaches should generally be considered first.

Non-pharmacological therapies

Behavioural analysis/intervention: 'ABC' (Antecedent-Behaviour-Consequence) charts to identify modifiable environmental, social or autobiographical factors.

Psychoeducation: For patients, carers and families (↓s anxiety/↑s empathetic care). Mild-moderate depression and/or anxiety in mild-moderate dementia may benefit from psychological therapy.[NICE]

Environment: Music and ↑calm/comfort/familiarity (= 'Snoezelen') Personalised activities to promote engagement, pleasure and interest (↓s distress/agitation/aggression)[NICE].

Complementary therapies: e.g. aromatherapy.

Pharmacological therapies

NB: start at low dose, ↑ slowly and review regularly with low threshold to ↓/stop.

Antipsychotics: NB: significant risks; ↑ all-cause mortality and cerebrovascular events. FGAs can ↑ arrhythmias, and SGAs can ↑ VTE and ⇒ aspiration pneumonia. Can ↓ aggression and psychosis. Currently only risperidone licensed; should be used cautiously in all dementias, especially in DLB (only under specialist supervision) when severe sensitivity reactions can occur; use in short courses (<6 weeks) for persistent aggression or psychosis. Can also ⇒ xs sedation, confusion, EPSEs and may accelerate cognitive decline. Antipsychotics should only be offered if patient is at risk of harming themselves/others, or they experience agitation/psychotic Sx that are causing them severe distress.

Cognitive treatments

- AChE-i recommended for non-cognitive, distressing or challenging symptoms when non-pharmacological approaches exhausted or antipsychotics inappropriate/ineffective.[NICE]
- Memantine may be useful in AD (and possibly also VaD) but evidence for efficacy limited.

Benzodiazepines

NB: avoid if possible or use with great caution as can ⇒ cognitive decline, falls & hip fractures in elderly. Can ↓ anxiety.

Antidepressants

Can counteract negative fx of depression on cognition, but overall limited evidence of efficacy and only recommended if treating pre-existing depression.[NICE] Sedating drugs (e.g. trazodone) may also ⇒ ↓irritability/agitation, and SSRIs may ↓agitation. TCAs should be avoided as ↑risk of falls/confusion due to anticholinergic fx – other drugs causing anticholinergic fx should also be avoided (or ↓dose) where appropriate.

Mood stabilisers

Currently insufficient evidence to support use, but may be justified if other treatments ineffective/not tolerated. Valproate is best avoided.

SUMMARY

Table 2.2 summarises the pharmacological management of each form of dementia.

Table 2.2 Antidementia drugs – summary of recommendations for cognitive treatments

Disorder		AChE-i	Memantine
MCI		–	–
AD	Mild	✔	–
	Moderate	✔	✔
	Severe	–	✔
VaD		✗	–
FTD		✗	–
LBD/PDD		✔	✔

Key: ✔ = recommended, – = not recommended, AD = Alzheimer's disease, FTD = fronto-temporal dementia, LBD = Lewy body dementia, MCI = mild cognitive impairment, PDD = Parkinson's disease dementia, VaD = vascular dementia.

Notes: MMSE staging; mild = 21–26, moderate = 10–20, severe = 0–9.

Further information

O'Brien et al., 'Clinical practice with anti-dementia drugs: a revised (third) consensus statement from the British Association for Psychopharmacology', *J Psychopharmacol* 2017; **31**(2): 1–22.

NEUROPSYCHIATRIC DISORDERS

EPILEPSY

Background

- Seizures can be categorised as (a) aware vs impaired awareness, (b) focal vs generalised or (c) motor or non-motor onset (tonic clonic/other motor onset).
  - Focal seizures can progress to generalised seizures.

- Usually requires two unprovoked seizures for diagnosis of epilepsy, which should be made by a a clinician with expertise in assessing first seizures and diagnosing epilepsy.
- International League Against Epilepsy definition: 'a disorder of the brain characterized by an enduring predisposition to generate epileptic seizures and by the neurobiologic, cognitive, psychological, and social consequences of this condition'.

Psychiatric effects of antiseizure medications (ASMs)

- Many ASMs have psychiatric side effects, too numerous to exhaustively list here. Important ones include levetiracetam (aggression, dysphoria) and topiramate (depression).
- Some ASMs, such as valproate, may have positive effects, e.g. mood regulation.
- Psychosis is a rare complication of several ASMs such as vigabatrin and topiramate.
- Pay special consideration to drug interactions: many ASMs and psychotropics have pharmacodynamic interactions via cytochrome P450.

Psychiatric drugs and seizure threshold

- It is generally safe to use most psychotropics in epilepsy and it is important to optimally treat psychiatric co-morbidity.
- Some psychotropics (serotonergics, TCAs, antipsychotics) can, at least theoretically, lower seizure threshold and can be part of review if epileptic seizures occur or are suspected.
- SSRIs are generally considered safe in epilepsy, and in fact may reduce seizures at a population level due to depression and anxiety having a pro-seizure effect.
- Clozapine may be particularly prone to inducing seizures during titration and after dose increases.
  - Nevertheless, clozapine has been successfully used in those on established epilepsy treatment: start low, go slow and monitor seizure frequency.
  - Consensus varies, but general expert opinion is not to start prophylactic ASMs in patients on higher doses of clozapine if they have not had a seizure.

Ictal psychoses

- Classified based on temporal relationship to seizure.
  - (Intra-)ictal psychosis: psychiatric phenomena within the seizure.
  - Post-ictal psychosis: seizure followed by psychotic symptoms (often with a 1–2-day 'lucid' period following seizure), typically resolves in a few days but can last up to a month.
  - Inter-ictal psychosis: usually in longstanding temporal lobe epilepsy, limited temporal relationship, may present very similarly to schizophrenia or schizophreniform disorder.
- There does not appear to be significant evidence that psychotropics are effective for ictal psychiatric phenomena.
- First principle in all ictal psychoses is to optimise seizure management: involve neurology.
- Guidance on treatment of post-ictal psychosis varies, mostly due to weak evidence base. Benzodiazepine +/− low-dose antipsychotic in the acute phase is recommended by expert opinion.
  - Some individuals who have recurrent post-ictal psychosis, particularly in the context of treatment-resistant epilepsy, may choose to remain on long-term anti-psychotic prophylaxis if consequences and risks of post-ictal psychotic symptoms are significant.
- Inter-ictal psychosis usually requires long-term antipsychotics; however, lower doses seem to be effective (no evidence on which to base choice).

Functional (or dissociative) seizures

- Patients can, and often do, have both epileptic and functional seizures, so identifying one type does not exclude the other. Ensure history taken from patient ± collateral of multiple seizure types (see page 420 for comparative semiology).
- Functional seizures have distinctive clinical features and will show absence of epileptic activity on ictal EEG.
- If functional seizures alone are diagnosed, it is the role of the (neuro)psychiatrist to support withdrawal of ASMs.
- Do not offer pharmacological treatment for functional seizures. Specialist MDT treatment, including CBT, may be helpful.

PARKINSON'S DISEASE (PD)

- Often referred to as the quintessential neuropsychiatric disorder: may be better viewed as a psychiatric disorder with associated motor characteristics.
- Presentations are a direct result of monoamine disruption (DA, ACh, NA, 5-HT).
  - Causes a predisposition to mood disorders, often precedes onset of motor Sx.
  - Differential rate of degeneration of the various dopaminergic pathways (see p. 376): some related to motor function (often first symptoms to appear), with others devoted to motivation, reward and salience following.
  - Medication used to treat movement disorders can result in a relative overdose in other pathways, with impulsive behaviours and psychosis resulting.
- There is additionally an organic personality change involving disinhibition (e.g. coarsening of humour, loss of empathy and reduced ability to understand the long-term consequences of actions) or 'pseudo-depressive' features (apathetic state that does not benefit from antidepressants).
- Often helpful to focus on the motoric function initially. Estimate the % of time the patient suffers with:
  - Excessive motor function – 'dyskinesias' (irregular jerking, wiggling, twitching): associated with psychosis and impulse control behaviours.
  - Poor motor function – where the patient is motorically 'off' (slow, stiff, shaky or low); associated with anxiety and depression.
  - Good motor function.

Treatment

Involve the patient's neurologist whenever possible. Treatment of the neurobehavioral features of PD depends on whether the Sx are due to excess or reduced dopamine.

Excess dopamine – this can be associated with excessive movements ('dyskinesias'). Can present as:

A. ICDs: gambling, compulsive shopping, hypersexuality and altered eating preference (increased eating of sweet foods).
B. Repetitive behaviours that can be either complex 'hobbyism' (excessive engagement in hobbies) or simple 'punding' (sorting, ordering or arranging items).
C. Psychosis: illusions, sense of presence, visual hallucinations (often of animals, people or children), delusions.
D. Compulsive medication use, where the patient takes more of their medication than prescribed.

Reduced dopamine – this can be associated with motor 'off' periods, including tremor, difficulty initiating movement and slower movement (bradykinesia).

- Psychiatric equivalent would be an apathy syndrome.
- Association also with depression and anxiety, especially around the time the medication wears off prior to the next dose.
- Anxiety is typically of a generalised pattern: impaired decision-making means that the day-to-day vicissitudes of life prove too burdensome a cognitive load.

Main oral treatments include

1. Dopamine agonists, typically used in the earlier stages. Have high affinity for D_2/D_3 receptors and are therefore more likely to cause the full spectrum of conditions listed in the 'Excess Dopamine' section.
2. L-dopa therapy, used in the more progressive phase of treatment.

Management

1. Excessive motor activity (i.e. dyskinesias), should prompt consideration of medication reduction. Often a delicate balancing act between motor function and symptom worsening.
   a. Cessation usually in the following order: (1) DA agonist, (2) amantadine or catechol-O-methyltransferase inhibitor and (3) L-dopa (not usually practical to stop, but the dose may conceivably be reduced/altered).

2. Poor motor activity should prompt consideration of increase in L-dopa/DA agonist.

Once clear that options 1 and 2 have been considered or determined not to be feasible, more specific treatment options should be considered:

- Antidepressants are often effective for depression or anxiety symptoms, not for apathy.
- (Low-dose) clozapine is effective for psychosis but SE limit use. Quetiapine sometimes tried (olanzapine or risperidone are CI). Only Rx such symptoms if distress present.
- Pimavanserin (5-HT$_{2A}$ inverse agonist) showing promise in psychosis in PD/DLB; currently available in US but not UK.
- CBT is effective for ICDs (and has secondary impact on depression and anxiety).
- Dopamine agonists may be beneficial for apathy but are often CI by the presence of disinhibitory symptoms or psychosis.

Neurocognitive disorders

Similar presentation to other cortical dementias, e.g. Alzheimer's. Symptoms comprise of the 4As: amnesia (problems with registration and recall), aphasia (difficulty with word production), apraxia and agnosia (e.g., increased tendency to get lost, or struggle to coordinate tasks such as putting on clothes in the right order).

- AChE-i (particularly rivastigmine) improve registration/recall in the context of cognitive impairment/dementia.
  - Also help reduce BPSDs, including psychosis, agitation and sometimes apathy.

HUNTINGTON'S DISEASE (HD)

Background

- Progressive autosomal-dominant neurodegenerative disorder featuring complex movement, cognitive and psychiatric symptoms.
- Caused by a CAG triplet repeat expansion in the *Huntingtin* gene (c4); number of repeats correlated with disease onset.

- Causes whole-brain neuronal loss; however, striatal D_2 neurons are particularly affected.
- Affects approximately 10–15/100,000. Onset most common aged 30–50 years but can occur at any age.

Clinical features

Neuropsychiatric and cognitive symptoms are often most debilitating, more so than motor symptoms.

- **Psychiatric symptoms:** depression, anxiety, apathy, irritability, personality change, OCD and, rarely, psychosis and mania. Apathy is the commonest and is tightly correlated with disease progression.
- **Cognitive symptoms:** rigidity, impaired set shifting, slowed cognitive processing, impaired executive function and impulse control and impaired emotion recognition. Cognitive Sx often interact with psychiatric Sx.
- **Motor symptoms:** chorea, dystonia, motor impersistence and a loss of postural stability. Parkinsonism (particularly bradykinesia and rigidity) and spasticity often develop later in the course of the disease.

Speech and swallowing problems commonly result from a combination of motor, cognitive and behavioural symptoms. Weight loss invariable. Patients eventually become bed-bound.

Management

Emphasise MDT approach. At present, there are no disease modifiers for HD; gene therapies are currently in clinical trial stage. Consider non-pharmacological approaches, esp at early stages before significant cognitive symptoms develop.

- **Psychiatric symptoms.** Specific evidence base is generally lacking. General principles include:
  1. Careful psychiatric assessment: treat common psychiatric disorders as described elsewhere in this book.
     a. Commonest prescribed psychiatric medications are SSRIs and SGAs.

      b. Use lowest effective dose; however, doses typically do
         not need to be adjusted from usual.

      c. May require second- or third-line treatments, inc ECT.

2. Where possible, rationalise medications and use those that
   may tackle multiple symptoms (e.g. SGAs for irritability,
   weight loss and chorea).

3. Avoid medications which may worsen dystonia, induce
   parkinsonism and/or cause high cognitive burden.

      a. Consider whether tetrabenazine is contributing to low
         mood/a psychiatric presentation.

4. There are no proven treatments for HD apathy – review
   for reversible causes (e.g. depression, sleep disorder, SEs).

5. Irritability may be treated with SSRIs and/or SGAs (e.g.
   olanzapine, risperidone, quetiapine), esp if concerns about
   violence.

      a. Mood stabilisers sometimes used for aggression.

- **Cognitive symptoms.** No current treatments.
- **Motor symptoms.** Chorea often more noticeable to onlookers
than to the patient; medications should only be used if chorea
distressing to the patient or comprises care.

   1. Tetrabenazine (vesicular monoamine transporter-2
   inhibitor) is licensed for chorea.

      a. Common SEs inc significant depression and anxiety.
         Not recommended for use in patients with HD and
         a significant psychiatric Hx. May also be associated
         with NMS and long QT syndrome.

   2. Although unlicensed, SGAs are commonly used to manage
   chorea.

      a. FGAs (like haloperidol) not recommended due to the
         high risk of EPSE.

   3. These medications do not work for motor signs beyond
   chorea (balance, gait, swallowing etc).

   4. Levodopa is used to reduce parkinsonian Sx but high
   doses are needed and the benefit is often limited.

5. Baclofen is used to reduce spasticity.
   a. For a small subset who have severe spasticity, targeted botulinum injections and/or intrathecal baclofen can be useful.

CATATONIA

Catatonia is a severe psychomotor disorder that can be caused by depression, psychosis, mania and a large range of other psychiatric and medical disorders, such as NMDA receptor encephalitis, benzodiazepine withdrawal, clozapine withdrawal and epilepsy.

Diagnose catatonia when ≥3 catatonic signs are present, as in the DSM-5 criteria: catalepsy, waxy flexibility, stupor, agitation, mutism, negativism, posturing, mannerisms, stereotypies, grimacing, echolalia and echopraxia.

Assessment

- Often challenging as Hx limited. Seek collateral Hx.[BAP]
- Catatonia examination: overall motor activity (stupor, agitation), spontaneous abnormal movements (posturing, mannerisms, stereotypies, grimacing), speech (mutism, echolalia), motor tone (catalepsy, waxy flexibility), compliance with instructions (negativism) and mimicry (echolalia, echopraxia).
- Score with Bush-Francis Catatonia Rating Scale (https://www.urmc.rochester.edu/psychiatry/divisions/collaborative-care-and-wellness/bush-francis-catatonia-rating-scale.aspx).
- Ix on basis of most likely diagnoses, e.g. TFTs, inflammatory markers, UDS, LP, EEG, MRI.
- If first episode or underlying Dx unclear, test for NMDA receptor antibodies (and others) in serum and CSF.[BAP]

Lorazepam challenge

Useful if presence of catatonia uncertain.[BAP]

1. Assess baseline catatonic features using Bush-Francis Catatonia Rating Scale

2. Give lorazepam 1–2 mg iv or im
3. Re-assess catatonic features after 5 min (iv) or 15 min (im).
   Positive response is 50% ↓ in catatonic features

Treatment

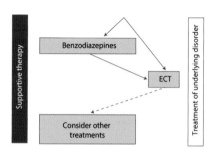

- Treat underlying disorder alongside catatonia, but antipsychotics
  are cautioned in catatonia, as risk worsening catatonia and
  triggering NMS.[BAP]
- First-line Rx: benzodiazepines and/or ECT. Consider SEs, ECT
  availability and presence of other disorder that might respond to
  ECT (e.g. depression).[BAP]
- Usual benzodiazepine Rx: start lorazepam 2–4 mg/day in
  divided doses. ↑ Dose daily to max 24 mg/day, catatonia treated
  or SEs develop. Monitor for sedation and respiratory depression.
- If catatonia due to benzodiazepine withdrawal, restart
  benzodiazepine.[BAP]
- If catatonia due to clozapine withdrawal, restart clozapine.[BAP]
- If catatonia due to antipsychotic use, consider stopping
  antipsychotic and caution with future antipsychotics.[BAP]
- If benzodiazepines and ECT not possible or ineffective, consider
  trial of amantadine or memantine.[BAP]
- In periodic catatonia, may prevent relapse with lithium.[BAP]

Preventing/managing complications

Complications	Prevention/management
Dehydration	Fluid monitoring, iv fluids
Poor food intake	Lorazepam 30–60 min before meals
Pressure sores	Pressure mattress, repositioning
Contractures	Mobilisation, physiotherapy
Venous thromboembolism (DVT, PE)	TEDS, low-molecular-weight heparin
NMS (catatonia is a strong risk factor)	Caution with antipsychotics

NEUROPSYCHIATRIC DISORDERS ASSOCIATED WITH HIV

Presentations
- The availability of effective ART has reduced CNS complications of uncontrolled HIV.
- Nevertheless, neuropsychiatric presentations can result in those with persistently high viral loads.
- Opportunistic infections (e.g. toxoplasmosis, PML, cryptococcal meningitis) may present with psychiatric features.
- HIV-associated neurocognitive disorder (HAND) is due to direct toxic effects of HIV virus on neurons: can lead to presentation which includes cognitive impairment, behavioural changes and motor impairments in late stages.

Treatment
- Treatment principles for HAND rest on effective ART: involve specialist as considering resistance is vital (may develop in those with incomplete treatment adherence).
- NICE and British HIV Association now recommend im depot formulation of cabotegravir + rilpivirine 2-monthly as an alternative to po medication in a select population of adults with viral suppression.

- This may help to improve adherence but comes with a ~2% risk of virological failure despite timely administration of injections.
- Some ARTs have recognised neuropsychiatric SEs, including sleep disturbance (particularly efavirenz and dolutegravir): discuss with HIV team who have prescribing responsibility.
- Numerous pharmacokinetic interactions between psychotropic drugs and ART, particularly non- nucleoside reverse transcriptase inhibitors (NNRTIs; vulnerable to subtherapeutic drug levels when co- administered with CYP450 inducers such as carbamazepine) and protease inhibitors (which are potent CYP450 inhibitors and can cause increased levels of drugs metabolised by P450 pathway, including benzodiazepines and phenobarbitone).
- Always use the Liverpool HIV drug interactions website to check for drug–drug interactions prior to prescription of new drugs with ART (https://www.hiv-druginteractions.org/checker).
- At standard doses, newer ART drugs do not generally cause prolonged QTc, but QTc is worth monitoring in the event of overdose of NNRTIs (e.g. efavirenz and rilpivirine).

AUTOIMMUNE ENCEPHALITIS

- AIE may present with florid psychotic symptoms, NMDAR encephalitis particularly commonly. It is a differential for severe acute psychiatric illness, however incidence is low.
- Very few quality trials evaluating treatments in AIE.
- Treatment principles largely borrowed from other related conditions.
- Good meta-analytical evidence that early initiation and, where necessary, escalation of immunotherapy leads to better long-term functional and neurocognitive outcomes.

Immunotherapeutic treatment

- First-line immunotherapy usually includes high-dose IV methylpred plus either plasma exchange or IVIG.

- Depending on the subtype of AIE, many patients may not require escalation immunotherapy (e.g. many pts with LGI1 encephalitis show a remarkable initial response to steroids).
- Second-line immunotherapy includes immunosuppressants e.g. cyclophosphamide or rituximab.
- Long-term oral steroid treatment is not advised as maintenance treatment. Use of steroid-sparing agents e.g. (mycophenolate mofetil and azathioprine) should be considered. Rituximab can be used to maintain remission.

Symptomatic treatment (acute)
- Pts can be treated for agitation with benzos or other sedating agents including promethazine.
- May be a role for treating catatonia with high-dose benzos although typically (e.g. in NMDAR encephalitis) catatonia most reliably resolves with successful immunotherapy.
- Antipsychotic medication should be considered second line, given limited evidence that in some cases of NMDAR encephalitis it can precipitate an NMS-type presentation (debate as to how much of this is treatment effect and how much is natural progression, given considerable clinical overlap between NMS and AIE).
- In general, the principle should be one of 'start low, go slow' and preference should be given for sedating 2GAs such as olanzapine.

Recovery
- Neuropsychiatric recovery from AIE can be protracted, sometimes taking many months.
- All newly introduced psychiatric medication should be cautiously weaned when there are no indications of an ongoing active encephalitis.
- Combination of oral steroids and antipsychotic medication significantly increases the risk of metabolic adverse effects.
- Re-emergence of psychotic symptoms on weaning antipsychotics in the early post-acute stage should raise suspicion of a partially

remitted or partially treated encephalitis rather than a de novo post-encephalitic psychotic disorder (although pts remain at risk for a variety of new-onset mental disorders for some years).

• Many patients with AIE require antiepileptic drugs in both acute and post-acute stages and these may interact with psychiatric medication.

Other prescribing considerations

PERINATAL PSYCHIATRY

GENERAL PRESCRIBING PRINCIPLES

- Potential adverse effects of any drug given in the perinatal period include the following: major congenital malformations, pregnancy complications, neonatal toxic or withdrawal symptoms and neurodevelopmental disorders.
- Exposure in the first two weeks results either in no adverse effect or in the demise of the conceptus.
- Sensitive period for a congenital malformation depends on the organ and may end in week 4 gestation (heart) or last as long as 16 weeks (CNS).
- Methodology in research of reproductive safety of psychotropic drugs has recently markedly improved:
  - Whilst RCTs cannot be conducted on ethical grounds, so quasi-experimental study designs are increasingly used with larger sample sizes and greater consideration of confounders.
  - Results of these show absence of many previously reported adverse outcomes or decrease in effect size to small or moderate (Wieck and Jones, 2020), with two main exceptions:
- **Evidence that valproate is highly toxic to the developing child in utero has continued to increase (see below).**
- Previously reported teratogenic properties of carbamazepine has also been confirmed (Wieck and Jones, 2020).

Making a decision about medication

- Decisions about prescribing psychotropics in the perinatal period involve balancing risks and benefits in the context of an individual patient, rather than blanket rules (McAllister-Williams et al, 2017).
- Carefully (re-) assess: accuracy of diagnosis, illness characteristics (course, severity, risk), psychiatric and physical co-morbidities, relapse frequency/triggers, (F)Hx of perinatal illness episodes, treatment Hx and social functioning.[BAP]
- Discuss treatment and prevention options with the patient and significant other, including potential benefits of medication,

harms associated with medication and what might happen if medication is stopped or changed.[NICE]

- Untreated mental illness can have a negative impact on pregnancy outcomes, due to higher rates of substance, misuse, poor self-care, suboptimal use of antenatal care and other fators.[BAP]
- Untreated maternal anxiety and depression in pregnancy are both reported to be associated with long-term behavioural and mental health problems in the offspring. Little is known on other disorders.[BAP]
- Note, that poor mental health in pregnancy predicts mental illness after childbirth.[BAP]

Choosing a medication

- According to current evidence, differences in the reproductive safety of psychotropic agents within the same drug class are small (some exceptions); therefore, a person's previous treatment response is an important consideration in selecting a psychotropic agent.
- Using a drug to which a patient has previously responded well may be preferable to one of unknown efficacy with a possible lower pregnancy risk.[BAP]
- Note the specific concerns regarding valproate and carbamazepine (see section above).
- Minimise number and dose of medications but avoid subtherapeutic doses.[BAP]

Pre-pregnancy period

- Since about 50% of pregnancies are unplanned, all persons of childbearing potential taking medication for mental illness should receive reproductive counselling: cover plans for childbearing, current contraception, adverse effects of medication on fertility, the effects of illness on childbearing (and childbearing on illness), the reproductive safety of the prescribed medication and an analysis of treatment risks and benefits. Consider referral for family planning.

- A person who is planning a pregnancy should be referred, if available, to the local specialist perinatal mental health service for preconception counselling.[BAP]
- If a woman is unable to conceive due to antipsychotic-induced hyperprolactinaemia and ovarian dysfunction, consider switch to prolactin-sparing antipsychotic.
- Explore and address substance misuse (including smoking), lifestyle and other issues that may affect maternal and infant outcomes.

Periconceptual folic acid supplements

- Low-dose folic acid supplementation (400 mcg/day) 3 months before and after conception has been shown to reduce the risk of neural tube and other major congenital defects.
- High-dose folic acid (4–5 mg daily) recommended for women with preconception BMI >/= 30, pre-existing diabetes,[NICE] and women whose diet is lacking folic acid.[BAP]
- Since low folate plasma levels are common in schizophrenia sufferers, it is reasonable to recommend a folate-rich diet and prescribe high-dose supplement in the periconceptual period.

During pregnancy

- Pregnancy does not protect against mental illness.[BAP]
- Pregnancies complicated by severe mental illness should be managed as high risk.
- Discuss risks/benefits of psychotropic medications as soon as possible on confirmation of pregnancy.[BAP]
- If medication is associated with significant risk of malformation, an urgent referral to the local maternity service/fetal medicine unit should be made for an assessment.
- Generally, avoid suddenly stopping medications on confirmation of pregnancy, as this can precipitate relapse.[BAP]
- Generally, avoid switching medications in pregnancy, unless benefits outweigh risks.[BAP]
- Ensure input from midwives, obstetricians, neonatologists/paediatricians, mental health team, social services, and any

other appropriate services. MDT antenatal-postnatal care plan to be ready by latest 32 weeks.

- In late pregnancy inform neonatologist/paediatrician of any potential drug-induced health problems in the neonate.

Delivery and immediate postnatal period

- Women with severe mental illnesses should deliver in hospital.[BAP]
- Particular care should be taken that the medication plan is followed throughout maternity care and post-discharge. No changes should be made without discussion with senior medical staff in the psychiatric team.[BAP]
- Women should bring medication into maternity service to avoid omitting doses at the most critical time for relapse.
- Neonatal toxic or withdrawal effects usually commence within 72 h of birth. Additional stay in hospital for monitoring and additional care may be necessary.

Breastfeeding

- Breastfeeding confers significant health advantages to parent and child.
- WHO recommends exclusive breastfeeding for first 6 months.
- The relative infant dose (RID, see box) is used in clinical practice to estimate infants' exposure to maternal drugs.
- Most psychotropic drugs have RID's <10% but there are exceptions.
- Sedative medications are cautioned due to impaired care for baby and feeding.[BAP]
- Since there are few known differences in safety within drug classes, it is usually best not to switch.[BAP]
- Do not recommend specific timing of feeding or discarding breast milk.[BAP]
- Exercise additional caution for premature/sick infants or during polypharmacy.[BAP]
- Monitor infant for potential adverse effects.[BAP]
- If mother is significantly sedated, advise to breastfeed with supervision.

> **Relative Infant Dose (RID)**
>
> $$RID = \frac{\text{Infant dose/kg/day}}{\text{Maternal dose/kg/day}}$$
>
> <10% of maternal dose is generally considered acceptable

Useful resources

The UK Teratology Information Service offers useful information on medicines in pregnancy for professionals (https://uktis.org/monographs) and similar information writen for patients (https://www.medicinesinpregnancy.org/Medicine–pregnancy). The Drugs and Lactation Database gives up-to-date evidence and clinical summaries for prescribers.

Psychosis in the perinatal period

- Be aware of the high morbidity in the perinatal period and the need for careful planning of treatment and monitoring.
- It is important that a pregnant woman with serious mental illness is as well as possible in pregnancy and after childbirth.
- Women with schizophrenia are at a high risk of inpatient admission in the perinatal period with a peak in the early postpartum.
- Around 60% of women with BD-I and II experience a recurrence in the perinatal period with depression more common than mania/hypomania in both.
- In women with BD-I, mania/psychosis during pregnancy is associated with a 7-fold increased risk of postpartum mania/psychosis (RR 7.0, p<0.001) (Perry et al. *J Affect Disord.* 2021; **294**:714–722).
- Irrespective of medication about 1/3 women with hx of bipolar disorder and postpartum psychosis have a postnatal recurrence.
- Discontinuing mood stabilizing medication at the beginning of pregnancy is associated with increased risks of bipolar recurrences in pregnancy.

- Some evidence that continuing medication in pregnancy prevents recurrences of bipolar disorder and postpartum affective psychosis (Wesseloo et al, 2016, **211**(1):31–36).
- Postpartum psychosis is closely related to bipolar disorder and requires similar management.
- Episodes of postpartum affective psychosis usually commence rapidly after childbirth, are often not identified in early stages, fluctuate markedly, escalate quickly, and are associated with high risks for mother and infant. They should be considered a psychiatric emergency. Suspected cases to be seen asap by experienced psychiatrists.

Use of antipsychotics in the perinatal period

- Recent evidence suggests that antenatal exposure of children to second-generation antipsychotics is not associated with major congenital malformations or neurodevelopmental disorders (Huybrechts et al, *JAMA Psych* 2023, 1;**80**(2):156–166).
- There is less research on first-generation antipsychotics but no evidence for differences to second-generation antipsychotics.
- Antipsychotic therapy is considered a modest risk factor for gestational diabetes (most likely with olanzapine, quetiapine and clozapine; OR < 2)
  - Pregnant women taking these drugs should be offered an OGTT at 24–28 weeks' gestation.[NICE]
- There is less evidence on the safety of newer drugs (e.g. Paliperidone, llurasidone, cariprazine). Additional caution is warranted.
- The plasma levels of quetiapine and aripiprazole but not olanzapine may decrease significantly in pregnancy (Westin et al, 2018 *Clin Pharmacol Ther.* 2018;**103**(3):477–484). Plasma levels should be monitored, ideally preconception, in each trimester and in the early postpartum. Little is known about other drugs.
- The choice of antipsychotic should be guided by past treatment response.

- For a patient stabilised on an antipsychotic, consider that switching poses a risk of destabilising illness without any benefit for fetus.[BAP]
- Depots can be used.
- If established on clozapine, benefits of continuation likely to outweigh risks.
- Late pregnancy exposure can occasionally cause neonatal EPSEs.[BAP]

Breastfeeding

- Consider infant's maturity at birth and health when starting or continuing antipsychotics.[BAP]
- Very low transfer into breast milk except for amisulpiride, supiride, haloperidol and risperidone.
- Few side effects reported (case literature): sedation, slowing of development, and irritability, especially when other antipsychotic or sedative medication co-prescribed.
- Monitor infant for sedation and EPSE.[BAP]
- Avoid clozapine (risk of agranulocytosis and seizures).[BAP]
- Several cases of impaired lactation during aripiprazole therapy described, incidence unknown.

Use of mood stabilizers in pregnancy

- Valproate is highly fetotoxic causing major congenital malformations (often several organs and severe) in 10% and neurodevelopmental disorders in 30%–40% of exposed children.[MHRA] For role of periconceptual folic acid supplementation see earlier section on page 310.
- Regulatory restrictions from Jan 2024: *valproate must not be started in new patients* (male or female) younger than 55 years, unless two specialists independently consider and document that there is no other effective or tolerated treatment, or unless there are compelling reasons that the reproductive risks do not apply.[MHRA]
- Any woman of childbearing potential should only be prescribed valproate if a pregnancy prevention programme is in place:

counselling, pregnancy tests, highly effective contraception (e.g. IUD or implant), annual reviews, signed informed consent.[MHRA]

- Women should not be prescribed valproate or carbamazepine in the postnatal period.[NICE]
- Women who have conceived during valproate therapy: see urgently and advise tocontinue valproate until then.[BAP]
- Restrictions in men result from concerns about fertility and potential transgenerational effects on neurodevelopment in humans seen in preclinical studies.[MHRA]
- Carbamazepine increases risk of major congenital malformation about 2-fold (4–6% of newborns) with no effects on neurodevelopment.[MHRA] It should not be prescribed to women with mental disorders who are pregnant, planning a pregnancy or are breastfeeding.[NICE]
- Lamotrigine can be prescribed in pregnancy as it does not seem to increase the risk of major congenital malformations or neurodevelopmental disorders (from data in epilepsy).
- Plasma levels can drop substantially (>50%) in pregnancy, but large interindividual variation. Recommend measuring levels, ideally before conception, in stable mental state, at least in each trimester, and twice within 2 weeks postpartum.
- Lithium: previously reported risk of extremely rare Ebstein's anomaly not confirmed in subsequent studies. There may be a small risk of other cardiac malformations (2.41% exposed vs 1.15% controls (adj RR: 1.65; CI 1.02–2.68) (Patorno et al. *N Engl J Med.* 2017;**376**(23):2245–2254).
- Lithium levels gradually decrease in first half of pregnancy and then increase again.
- Measure levels once a month in pregnancy and once weekly in 4 weeks before delivery and immediately following birth.[NICE] Adjust dose accordingly.
- Do not decrease or stop lithium pre-delivery or intrapartum – risks of bipolar recurrence are highest at this time. If plasma levels and kidney function are appropriately monitored there is little risk of maternal intoxication / worse outcome for the child (Wesseloo et al *Am J Psychiatry.* 2017;**173**(2):117–27).

Breastfeeding

- Caution with lamotrigine: infant plasma can be high; monitor infant for breathing difficulty, skin rash, excessive drowsiness and poor sucking.
- Case reports indicate that lithium plasma levels of breastfed infants can sometimes reach 50% of the maternal value. Several instances of infant health problems were described (suspected lithium intoxication, abnormal thyroid function tests, slow weight gain and delay in motor development.
- There are also numerous reports of infants without any signs of lithium toxicity or developmental problems. However, in the UK, clinicians generally advise against breastfeeding during lithium therapy.

Prescribing in clinical practice – bipolar disorder and postpartum psychosis

- Balance the risks of medications against the benefits of relapse prevention.
- Do not prescribe valproate or carbamazepine. Low-risk options for acute treatment or prophylaxis include antipsychotics, lithium and lamotrigine.
- Lithium is recommended as the initial long-term therapy for the prevention of bipolar episodes.[BAP]
- In a woman taking lithium who is planning a pregnancy or is in the first trimester, staying on lithium is an option if she needs continued medication and has responded to it, and that the risk of relapse would be high if it was discontinued or switched to an antipsychotic.
- If the woman is already taking an antipsychotic and requires a second mood stabilizer for the prevention of manic episodes, this should be lithium and not valproate or carbamazepine.
- If fetus exposed to lithium in first 4 weeks after conception refer for specialist fetal ultrasound to assess cardiac structures.
- An alternative to breastfeeding during lithium therapy is limited breastfeeding or the use of donor milk if available.

- If patient is planning to fully breastfeed, antipsychotic therapy is an alternative.
- ECT is an option for severe mania and depression in pregnancy and lactation, and for postpartum psychosis.
- No conclusive evidence yet for the best time and drug choice for medication prophylaxis in women with a hx of pure postpartum psychosis.
- If the patient requires an antidepressant during pregnancy, be mindful of manic switch if the mood stabiliser is withdrawn.

DEPRESSION

- On confirming pregnancy, avoid abrupt discontinuation of antidepressant.[BAP]
- Weigh risks and benefits. If depression is mild, consider tapering down antidepressant and discontinuing. If moderate/severe, consider continuing or switching to an antidepressant with beter safety evidence.[BAP]
- Also consider severity of past episodes and any prior postpartum episodes.

Pregnancy

- No current classes of antidepressants are absolutely contraindicated.
- Most safety evidence exists for SSRIs. Evidence base for less commonly used agents (individual tricyclics, venlafaxine, mirtazapine) is still small.
  - Not associated with changes in miscarriage rates.
  - Small effects (less than 2×) reported for pre-eclampsia (SSRIs), pre-term delivery (all antidepressants), postpartum haemorrhage (all antidepressants).
- Increased risk of persistent pulmonary hypertension of the newborn for offspring of patients on SSRIs during pregnancy (absolute risk, 3:1000 versus 2:1000 in general population).
- Antidepressant treatment (all classes) increase rate of poor neonatal adaptation from 1/10 to 3/10.[BAP] Symptoms are usually

mild and transient, sometimes infant requires monitoring in maternity service.
- There is a lack of evidence whether discontinuation close to delivery will alter risk of neonatal symptoms, but it places mother at increased risk of relapse at a critical time.[BAP]

Breastfeeding
- Antenatal depression predicts postnatal depression. If antidepressant effective in pregnancy, best to continue same agent rather than switch.[BAP]
- If antidepressant is restarted postnatally, prescribe drug to which patient has previously responded.
- If antidepressant therapy is initiated for a first depressive episode, select agents with low RIDs (sertraline, paroxetine).

ANXIETY DISORDERS
- If medication is selected as treatment option, antidepressants are usually used first line (for their reproductive safety see section on depression).

Pregnancy
- Discontinuation of antidepressants close to delivery is controversial (see Depression section).
- Early studies associated benzodiazepines with congenital malformations but recent evidence from research with improved methodology does not support this.
- If possible, avoid benzodiazepines near term due to risk of neonatal withdrawal and/or 'floppy infant syndrome'.[UKTIS]
- Recent reports of pregabalin being associated with very small increase in incidence of major congenital malformations and ADHD (Dudukina et al, 2023, 46(7):661–675) but evidence base is still small and residual confounding not excluded.
- MHRA advises counselling patient, avoiding use in pregnancy, and use of contraception during treatment.

- Although studies show no major safety concerns for gabapentin[UKTIS] evidence base is too small to draw conclusions. Avoid in pregnancy, if possible.

Breastfeeding

- Avoid regular use of diazepam which may accumulate in breastfed infants.
- Lorazepam has low RID and nursed infants show little adverse effects.
- RIDs for gabapentinoids low but limited data.
- Monitor infant for sedation.

INSOMNIA

Pregnancy

- Insomnia common in pregnancy due to nausea, back pain, urinary frequency, fetal movements, gastro-oesophageal reflux, pruritus and cramping. RLS also very common.[2]
- In mild cases of insomnia or RLS, reassurance that some sleep disruption in pregnancy is normal and may well resolve in postpartum period is often sufficient; however, more severe insomnia should be monitored closely and addressed.
- Minimise discomfort by treating pain and using pillow supports.[BAP]
- CBTi is effective, but little specific evidence for pregnancy.[BAP]
- If medications needed, zolpidem and zopiclone are best options.[BAP]
- Effective alternatives include olanzapine, quetiapine, risperidone and promethazine[BAP] which have low risks in pregnancy.
- For RLS, DA agonists are contraindicated. Iron and folate supplementation are often effective, even if patient is not deficient. ↓Caffeine.
- Mild-to-moderate exercise in evening with stretching and massage helpful.[BAP]

Breastfeeding

- Z-drugs are preferred to benzodiazepines as they tend to have shorter $T_{1/2}$ and only small amounts pass into breastmilk. No major issues reported, but limited data.
- Use intermittent dosing for a short period of time. There is no particular preference for one Z-drug over another,[UKDILAS] but if possible prefer drug with short $T_{1/2}$.
- When mother has taken hypnotic advise not to breastfeed at night without supervision and that co-sleeping is even more dangerous.

ADHD

Pregnancy

- Adolescents and young women with ADHD may engage in more risky sexual behaviour, so are at risk of unplanned pregnancies.
- No evidence that ADHD gets better or worse during pregnancy.
- Medications used in ADHD have been associated with some harm in animals, but there is no robust evidence in humans, though numbers of infants exposed are very small.[BAP]
- Methylphenidate does not appear to be linked to congenital malformations, although it is possible that it is associated with ↑risk of miscarriage (although this may be due to confounders).[BAP]
- If stimulants taken near to birth, neonatal withdrawal is likely.[BAP]
- Low birth weight has been reported with dexamfetamine; therefore, this is also likely with lisdexamfetamine.
- Benefits of continuing medications (↓maternal impulsive behaviour) should be weighed against risks to fetus.[BAP]

Breastfeeding

- Methylphenidate: limited safety evidence with differing advice (likely safe,[BAP] monitor,[SPS] avoid[BNF]). Likely to be safe, but sensible to seek expert advice on a case-by-case basis.
- Atomoxetine and amphetamines are cautioned.[BAP]
- Modafinil and bupropion should be avoided.[BAP]

SUBSTANCE USE DISORDERS

Pregnancy

- The UK Chief Medical Officers recommend not drinking alcohol at all during pregnancy.
- Alcohol detoxification should use chlordiazepoxide or diazepam, preferably as an inpatient.[BAP]
- Avoid medications for preventing alcohol relapse.[BAP]
- NRT may pose a risk to the fetus, but likely less harmful than smoking. First line: psychosocial interventions. Second line: NRT after risk–benefit analysis. Avoid varenicline and bupropion.[BAP]
  - For opioid dependence, offer methadone or buprenorphine substitution (but not buprenorphine/naloxone)[BAP]: buprenorphine may result in milder neonatal abstinence syndrome compared to methadone.[BAP]
  - Detoxification should be avoided in the first trimester and is cautioned in the third trimester – the best time is second trimester.[BAP]

Breastfeeding

- Women on methadone or buprenorphine should still breastfeed, but breastfeeding should not be abruptly withdrawn, as this can precipitate a withdrawal syndrome in the infant.[MPG]
- Seek specialist advice for women using crack cocaine or high-dose benzodiazepines.
- Varenicline and bupropion should not be prescribed.[BAP]

DELIRIUM

Diagnosis: **4AT** is first line[NICE]
(Maclullich et al., 2011)

1. Alertness:
   - Fully alert but not agitated – 0
   - Mild sleepiness for <10 sec after waking – 0
   - Clearly abnormal – 4
2. AMT4 (age, DoB, location, year):
   - No mistakes – 0

- Mistake – 1
- 2+ mistakes – 2

3. Attention (months of the year backwards):
   - 7+ months correctly – 0
   - Starts but scores <7 months or refuses to start – 1
   - Untestable (as too unwell, drowsy or inattentive) – 2
4. Acute change or fluctuating course in alertness, cognition or other mental function:
   - No – 0
   - Yes – 4

4+ Possible delirium ± cognitive impairment
1–3 Possible cognitive impairment
0 Delirium or severe cognitive impairment unlikely

Causes of delirium: **DDELIRIUMM** – **D**rugs (especially opioids, benzodiazepines, anticholinergics), **D**iscomfort (i.e. pain, sleep deprivation), **E**lectrolytes (especially $\downarrow Na^+$, $\uparrow/\downarrow Ca^{2+}$, $\uparrow urea$), **L**ungs ($\downarrow O_2$, $\uparrow CO_2$), **I**nfection, **R**espiratory failure (hypoxia, hypercapnia), **I**mpaction (of stools), **U**rinary retention, **M**etabolic ($\downarrow/\uparrow glucose$, $\downarrow/\uparrow thyroid$), **M**yocardial infarction.

Management[NICE]:
- If difficulty distinguishing from dementia, Rx delirium first. Consider hypoactive delirium which is easily missed.[NICE]
- Identify underlying cause(s) and Rx.[NICE]
- Reorientation (e.g. frequent explanations, clocks, photos).[NICE]
- Involve family and friends.[NICE]
- Consistency of staff.[NICE]
- Minimise moving room or ward.[NICE]
- Pharmacological treatments:
  - If delirium is in the context of alcohol or benzodiazepine withdrawal, give a benzodiazepine (see p. 412).
  - For other forms of delirium, there are no licensed drugs. If agitated, try non-pharmacological de-escalation first. If unsuccessful, may give haloperidol 0.5–2 mg po/im. Minimise length of treatment and use lowest effective

dose. Antipsychotics should only be used for symptom
management if the person is distressed or a risk to themselves
and/or others. Use with caution in older people.[NICE] Avoid
antipsychotics in Parkinson's or Lewy body dementia.[NICE]

- Benzodiazepines should generally be avoided as they
  may worsen confusion, so only use as last resort or if
  antipsychotics contraindicated.
- De-prescribing (e.g. of anticholinergics, opioids,
  anticonvulsants) is often more important than prescribing.

PRESCRIBING IN AUTISM

No medications have sufficient evidence to justify their routine use
for the core Sx of autism, but there are some possible treatments
directed at co-morbidities.

Disorder	Adult Rx[BAP]	Child Rx[BAP]
Core Sx of autism	–	–
Depression	Standard guidelines[a]	SSRIs
Anxiety disorders	Standard guidelines[a]	
Sleep problems	Standard guidelines[a] with early consideration of melatonin	Melatonin
Irritability	Consider trial of risperidone, aripiprazole or an SSRI, but behavioural/educational interventions should be tried first and continued	Consider trial of risperidone or aripiprazole, but behavioural/educational interventions should be tried first and continued
ADHD	Standard guidelines[a]	1. Methylphenidate 2. Atomoxetine 3. Clonidine/lofexidine
Tic disorders	Consider clonidine or guanfacine on a case-by-case basis	

[a] For these patients, cautiously follow the relevant guidelines for these conditions in the general
population, starting with low-dose treatment wherever possible.

PRESCRIBING IN EATING DISORDERS

- If using medication for psychiatric co-morbidities, be mindful of the effects of low or high body weight on pharmacokinetics.
- Consider methods of purging (vomiting, laxatives) which may affect drug absorption.
- Cardiac and metabolic consequences (e.g. low electrolytes) may place those with eating disorders at higher risk of side effects (e.g. arrhythmias). Be mindful of effects of medications (e.g. prolonged QTc).
- Insulin-dependent diabetes is an association and a complicating factor. Insulin may not be taken as prescribed to avoid weight gain. Specialist input may be sought on managing antidiabetic medications if food intake erratic or restricted.
- Refeeding syndrome refers to depletion of extracellular electrolytes, especially hypophosphatemia, due to too rapid reintroduction of food after a period of prolonged restricted intake. Refeeding syndrome may include serious neurological and cardiac consequences such as confusion, coma, cardiac arrhythmias and cardiac failure. Cautiously monitor patients' electrolytes in these cases. Multivitamin and mineral preparations are strongly recommended during refeeding.
- Patients can be detained under the MHA if their physical health is at serious risk directly related to their eating disorder.

Anorexia nervosa

- Generally, psychological therapies (specialised CBT or other disorder-specific psychological therapies), dietetic advice and physical monitoring are mainstays of treatment.
- Medication not recommended as the sole treatment.
- Antipsychotics which stimulate weight gain (e.g. olanzapine) are sometimes used in severe cases, although this is off-label. If antipsychotics are used, strictly avoid any which affect prolactin.

Bulimia nervosa

- Psychological treatment (guided self-help, CBT) first line.
- Medication not recommended;[NICE] however, fluoxetine (60 mg) is licensed for treatment.

Binge eating disorder

- Psychological treatment (guided self-help, CBT) first line.
- Medication not recommended.[NICE]
- Lisdexamfetamine is approved in some countries (e.g. US).
- There is also evidence for off-licence use of topiramate; pregnancy is a contraindication.

No pharmacological treatments advised for avoidant/restrictive food intake disorder, pica and rumination disorder.

PRESCRIBING IN PERSONALITY DISORDERS

The *International Classification of Diseases 11th Revision* (*ICD-11*) no longer codes specific personality disorders, opting instead for a dimensional model with mild, moderate and severe personality disorder as coded diagnoses.

Five domains act as diagnostic qualifiers: negative affectivity, anankastia, disinhibition, dissociality and detachment.

A borderline pattern descriptor has been added but this is not a diagnosis.

In the current NICE guidelines, no specific drug treatments are recommended for personality disorder even though they are widely used, often in complex polypharmacy.

MILD PERSONALITY DISORDER

Medications should not generally be used for the disorder or its symptoms but may influence choice and duration of medications for co-morbidities.

MODERATE PERSONALITY DISORDER

In moderate personality disorder, there are almost always additional mental state disorders present. As there is evidence that dependence on prescribed drugs is more likely to develop in the presence of personality disorder, this should be a factor in both initiating and determining the duration of drug treatment.

SEVERE PERSONALITY DISORDER

There is increasing evidence, not yet backed up by controlled trials, that clozapine may be effective in treating the symptoms and behaviour of severe personality disorder, but great care is needed in selecting patients for this treatment, particularly as it is likely to be long term.

APATHY

- Diminished motivation not attributable to decreased consciousness, cognitive impairment or emotional distress.
- Can be secondary to a large range of pathologies, inc depression, Alzheimer's, Huntington's, schizophrenia, stroke, PD, traumatic brain injury (TBI). Can also occur after lesions to the frontostriatal circuit.
- Treatment can be extremely difficult and no firm evidence for any pharmacological agent. Clinical significance of small changes shown in RCTs is unclear, and few studies use apathy as a primary endpoint. If secondary to other disease processes, these should be optimised.
- Post-TBI: Cochrane review inconclusive. Some experts suggest that dopaminergic drugs may be helpful, based on pathophysiology (mesolimbic dopamine reward system).
- Depression: weak evidence that SSRIs may worsen apathy; MAOIs may be better.
- PD: RCTs demonstrating benefit for rivastigmine, methylphenidate, apomorphine pumps, levodopa-carbidopa intestinal gel, rotigotine and pramipexole, but overall data are

poor. Optimise the dopaminergic therapy and then add (off-licence) cholinesterase inhibitors.

- Alzheimer's disease: Cochrane review suggests methylphenidate may be useful and have slight benefit for cognition and functional performance. Cholinesterase inhibitors may also help.
- Post-stroke: weak evidence for methylphenidate (case reports), bupropion (case reports) and donepezil (small open-label study).

BEHAVIOURAL ADDICTIONS AND IMPULSE CONTROL DISORDERS

Behavioural addictions

- Behavioural addictions share clinical features with substance use disorders (SUDs). There may also be some overlap with obsessive-compulsive disorders.
- **Gambling disorder** (GD) is included in DSM-5.
  - Epidemiological studies have indicated association between GD and prescription of aripiprazole (RR 5.2) and the DA agonists pramipexole and ropinirole (RR 7.6).
  - No licensed treatments.
  - Meta-analytic evidence indicates efficacy for antidepressants, opioid antagonists and mood stabilizers.
  - Some evidence to suggest placebo/expectancy may be contributing factor in treatment response.
  - Significant co-morbidities with SUDs.

Impulse control disorders

- Complications of Parkinson's disease include a range of ICDs, including eating, buying, compulsive gambling and sexual behaviours.
  - Epidemiological studies have confirmed association of ICDs with aripiprazole (RR 7.7) and pramipexole and ropinirole (RR 3.3).
  - Mx includes titrating down DA agonists.

- The DSM-5 also lists pyromania and kleptomania as impulse control disorders.
  - Disorders are rare and treatment evidence only from case reports/series.
  - Psychological therapy is mainstay.
  - Some indications of efficacy from SSRIs and opioid antagonists.

CONTRACEPTION

Background
- Contraceptive counselling has a key place in psychiatry:
  - Unintended pregnancy may be a risk associated with some disorders, e.g. mania in BPAD.
  - Unintended pregnancies are risk for poorer mental health in those of childbearing potential.
  - Several psychotropic drugs are teratogenic, particularly valproate.
- Hormonal contraception can interrupt menstruation, which may be useful in those whose Sx are worse at particular times in their cycle (e.g. in mood disorders, psychosis)
- Contraceptive and pregnancy advice should be given to all patients of childbearing potential with a mental health disorder.[NICE]

Interactions
- CYP3A4 inducers reduce effectiveness of COCP/ POP; COCP may also ↑clozapine levels (useful resource: fsrh.org/standards-and- guidance/documents/ ceu-clinical-guidance-drug-interactions-with-hormonal).
- If on enzyme-inducing medication, should be on IUD or depot or, if short-term user (<2 months), can use condoms + usual contraception during drug use and for 28 days after.
- Relationship between lamotrigine and hormonal contraception is complex. Briefly:
  - Lamotrigine dose may need to be adjusted with hormonal contraception.

- Be alert for signs of lamotrigine toxicity (dizziness, ataxia, diplopia) when using progesterone-only contraception.
- Additional use of condoms/alternative contraception are suggested if using CHC, SDI or POP; depot and LNG-IUD will not be affected.

Choosing contraception
- UKMEC (fsrh.org/documents/ukmec-2016) is a useful tool to help decide on safe contraception.
- No contraceptive method is perfect, but some are very effective.
  - Methods can be roughly grouped into those not dependent on user, those which depend on being remembered prior to intercourse and those used in emergency (i.e. post-intercourse):

Method	Action	Pregnancy rate, users per year (typical use)	Notes
Contraceptive methods not dependent on user			
Subdermal implants (SDI)	Secretes progesterone	<1/1000	Lasts for up to 3 years
Injectables/depot	Progesterone	6/100	Injection frequency, ~13/52
Intrauterine systems (LNG-IUD)	Secretes progesterone	<1/100	Lasts for 3–5 years
Copper IUD (Cu-IUD)	Prevents fertilisation and implantation	<1/100	Can also be used for emergency contraception (most effective means, <1/1000)
Sterilisation (male or female)	Stops fertilisation	1/2000 (male), 1/200 (female)	

(continued)

Method	Action	Pregnancy rate, users per year (typical use)	Notes
User-dependent methods			
Combined hormonal contraception (CHC; pill, patch or vaginal ring)	Inhibits ovulation, thins endometrium, thickens cervical mucus	9/100	Associated with mood changes (particularly adolescents)
Progesterone-only pill (POP)	Thickens cervical mucus	9/100	
Condoms (male or female)	Stops sperm entering vagina	18/100 (male), 21/100 (female)	Also reduces risk of STIs
Diaphragm/cap	Stops sperm entering uterus	12/100	Used with spermicide
Fertility awareness methods	Avoids sex out of fertile periods	24/100	
Emergency contraception (also see copper IUD, above)			
Ulipristal acetate	Inhibits ovulation (use within 120 h of intercourse)	1–2/100	
Levonorgestrel	Inhibits ovulation (use within 72 h of intercourse)	3/100	

Valproate
- MHRA currently advises that valproate must no longer be used in those of childbearing potential unless a Pregnancy Prevention Programme is in place:
  - ≥1 'highly effective' method of contraception, or 2 complementary forms of contraception (inc barrier method).
  - Examples of highly effective contraception:
    - Copper-IUD
    - Intrauterine systems – IUD
    - Subdermal implants
  - User-dependent methods must be used together with a barrier method.
  - Frequent pregnancy testing should be carried out.
- In future, prescribing valproate in those of childbearing potential may be further restricted.

PRESCRIBING FOR COMMON CO-MORBIDITIES IN SERIOUS MENTAL ILLNESS (SMI)

Many physical health conditions may be appropriately managed by psychiatrists with input and advice from primary and secondary care.

It may be appropriate (and appreciated by GPs) to initiate treatment for commonly encountered chronic conditions, particularly those seen more commonly in SMI or that arise as SEs from our Rx. (The below guidance is for adults.)

Hypertension
- Aim for BP <140/90 if using clinic measurements (150/90 in >80 years).
- Offer lifestyle interventions prior to commencing medication.
- Consider the following adapted flow chart when prescribing:

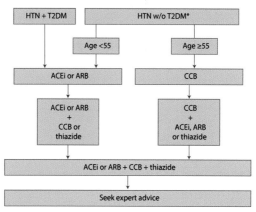

* NICE suggest offering CCBs to all patients of Black ethnicity at step 1, but this recommendation is not supported by all international guidelines.

- Consider interactions between psychotropic drugs and antihypertensives, e.g. ↑risk of postural hypotension with antipsychotics.

Type II diabetes
- Common in those on antipsychotics given common metabolic side effects, often seen alongside weight gain.
- Diagnosis based on:
  - HbA1c of ≥48 mmol/mol (6.5%).
  - Fasting plasma glucose level of ≥7.0 mmol/L.
  - Random plasma glucose of ≥11.1 mmol/L in the presence of Sx/signs.
- Repeat testing is sensible to confirm the diagnosis (required if asymptomatic).
- Always start with lifestyle modification advice.
- Treatment guidance:[NICE]

- Assess CV risk with QRISK2 and medical Hx (congestive heart disease, peripheral arterial disease, CVD, ACS/MI, angina, previous revascularisation).
- If low CVD risk, offer metformin (MR if GI disturbance); DPP-4 inhibitors, pioglitazone, sulfonylurea or an SGLT2 inhibitor can be alternative if metformin CI.
- Start metformin slowly, i.e. 500 micrograms od, then after a few days or a week increase to bd etc to reduce risk of GI SEs.
- If QRISK2 >10%, offer metformin (/MR), then consider SGLT2 inhibitor (monotherapy if metformin CI).
- If CHF, offer metformin (/MR), then SGLT2 inhibitor (monotherapy if metformin CI).
- If HbA1c not controlled, seek professional advice.

Thyroid disease

- Thyroid disease can be associated with many psychiatric disorders, particularly mood disorders and anxiety.
  - Psychiatric medication may cause thyroid disease, particularly lithium (either hypo/hyper).
- For hypothyroidism, NICE recommend:
  - Consider starting levothyroxine 1.6 micrograms/kg/day (rounded to the nearest 25 micrograms) for those <65 years of age with no Hx of CVD.
  - Consider starting levothyroxine at 25–50 micrograms per day with titration for adults aged ≥65 years and adults with a Hx of CVD.
- For new-onset hyperthyroidism, NICE recommends discussion with an endocrinologist.
  - Consider starting a beta-blocker (propanolol) if symptomatic (e.g. palpitations, tremor, anxiety) and no CI. Has the additional advantage that it partially blocks the conversion of T4 to T3.

SMOKING CESSATION

- Smoking is three times more common in SMI.
- Tobacco induces CYP1A2, leading to reduction in plasma levels of some important medications (see monographs), including clozapine, TCAs and some antipsychotics.[MPG]
- ↓Smoking has uncertain benefit, so aim for cessation.[BAP]
- Medication may be effective alone, but outcomes may be superior if combined with behavioural support (less so for bupropion or single form of nicotine replacement therapy [NRT]).[BAP, NICE]
- Three main options for pharmacological Rx[BAP, NICE]: NRT, bupropion, varenicline (latter not currently available).

Drug	Mechanism	Use	Important SEs
NRT	Nicotinic ACh agonist	Relapse prevention, temporary abstinence, smoking reduction (with or without cessation)	Skin irritation (patches), watery eyes (nasal spray), insomnia, headache
Bupropion	Noradrenaline–dopamine reuptake inhibitor + nicotinic ACh antagonist	Relapse prevention	Insomnia, headache, dry mouth, nausea, HTN, seizure risk
Varenecline	Nicotinic ACh partial agonist	Relapse prevention	Nausea, insomnia, vivid dreams, headache

NRT

Useful to reduce withdrawal symptoms in those addicted to nicotine who abruptly stop (e.g. psychiatric inpatients).

NRT is pure nicotine without the other components of tobacco smoke. There is no risk of cancer, and it is safe in stable coronary heart disease.[BAP]

NRT comes in numerous forms (e.g. patch, spray, inhalator, gum); recommended to give patients preference on form.[MPG]

Prescribe a combination of NRT: a transdermal patch + another form of NRT.[BAP] Continue for ≤8 wks and as long as necessary; no difference in outcome between tapering down versus abrupt discontinuation.[BAP]

- E-cigarettes advised on inpatient wards in place of tobacco smoking (latter not permitted in NHS hospital grounds).

Formulation		Dose	
		<20 cigarettes/day	≥20 cigarettes/day or smoking within 30 min of waking
Transdermal patch	16-h formulation	10 mg or 15 mg	25 mg
	24-h formulation	7 mg or 14 mg	21 mg
Nasal spray (0.5 mg/T)		T-TT to each nostril prn; max 2 sprays/h and 64 sprays/day	
Oral spray (1 mg/T)		T-TT prn; max 4 sprays/h and 64 sprays/day	
Lozenge (1 mg, 2 mg, 4 mg)		1 mg hourly	2–4 mg hourly; max 60 mg or 15 lozenges/day
Gum (2 mg, 4 mg, 6 mg)		2 mg hourly	4–6 mg hourly; max 60 mg/day
Inhalator (15 mg)		Max 6 cartridges of 15 mg/day	
Sublingual tablet (2 mg)		T-TT hourly	TT hourly; max 40 tablets/day
Mouth strips (2.5 mg)		One strip hourly; max 15 strips/day	

The NRT nasal spray can cause nose and throat irritation as well as watering eyes, so it should not be used while driving.[BAP]

Bupropion and varenicline

- Bupropion: nicotinic receptor agonist with dopaminergic and adrenergic action. Slight effect on seizure threshold which becomes relevant when co-prescribed with others with same (e.g. TCAs, antipsychotics).
  - Monitor BP during prescribing.
  - Discontinuation reaction not expected, but tapering may be considered.[SPC]
- Varenicline: nicotinic receptor partial agonist, first-line Rx, odds ratio for cessation at 1 year vs placebo, 3.2. Nil interactions with psychotropic medications. Increasing dose regimen: refer to monograph. **Not currently available in UK (withdrawn due to impurities found in medicine).**
  - No difference in neuropsychiatric SEs between people with and without mental illness, but it is good practice to monitor for any mood changes in anyone making an attempt to quit.
  - Advise patients that if they develop these Sx, they should stop varenicline and seek prompt medical advice.[BNF]

E-cigarettes

E-cigarettes can also be an effective aid for smoking cessation. Consensus view is harms from e-cigarettes far less than tobacco, though long-term harms are not yet established. Cannot be prescribed at present in UK but patients can be directed to their use.

CONTROLLED DRUGS (CDS)

In the United Kingdom, special 'prescription requirements' apply to 'schedule' 2 or 3 drugs. *NB: Special Home Office license is needed to prescribe Schedule 1 CDs.* The Department of Health recommends that quantity prescribed should not exceed 30 days. There must be a handwritten signature (if electronic prescribing used may accept advanced electronic signature). The following must be written 'so as to be indelible, e.g. written by hand, typed or computer generated':

> **Selected CDs**
>
> - Ketamine
> - Midazolam
> - Some opioids (morphine, diamorphine, fentanyl, methadone, buprenorphine, oxycodone)
> - Stimulants (methylphenidate, dexamfetamine, lisdexamfetamine)
> - Gabapentin and pregabalin (as of April 2019)

- Date signed (CD prescriptions valid for 28 days from the date signed).
- Patient's full name, address and age (if under 12 years).
- Drug name + form* + strength (when >1 strength available). If multiple strengths, then prescribe each one separately.
- Dosing regimen. 'As directed' is not acceptable, but '10 mg up to one hourly as required' is acceptable. 'Twice daily' is not acceptable, but '20 mg twice daily' is.
- Total amount of drug to be dispensed *in words and figures*.**
- Prescriber's address must be specified (should already be on the prescription form, e.g. hospital address) and should be within the United Kingdom.

*   Omitting the form (e.g. tablet/liquid/patch) is a common reason for an invalid prescription. It is often assumed to be obvious from the prescription (e.g. fentanyl as a patch or Oramorph as a liquid), but it still has to be written even if only one form exists.

** For tabs and other discrete formulations, state total number (in words and figures) of dose units to be supplied, e.g. '8 (eight) tablets of 10 mg'. For liquids, state total volume (in words and figures), e.g. '80 (eighty) mL'.

If prescribing prn, must be very specific, e.g. take ONE or TWO tablets prn.

These requirements *do not* apply to schedule 4 drugs (e.g. most benzodiazepines) and schedule 5 drugs (e.g. codeine, dihydro-codeine). For full details on controlled drug guidance in the United

Pharmacy Stamp	Age	Title, Forename, Surname & Address
	50	Miss Example
	D.o.B	
	01.06.1975	10 The Street New Town
Please don't stamp over age box		AB1 2CDE

Number of days' treatment
N.B. Ensure dose is stated

Endorsements

Morphine sulphate 10mg MR tablets
10mg 12 hourly
Supply 28 (twenty eight) x 10mg tablets
[No more items on this prescription]

X
X
X
X
X
X
X
X
X
X
X
X

D Foster

Date
01.06.2025

For dispenser No. of Prescns. on form

Dr Foster
The Village Clinic
44 The Avenue
New Town
AB1 3EFG
Tel: 01234 567891

NHS   FP10NC

Kingdom, see https://www.gov.uk/government/publications/information-about-controlled-drugs-regulations.

OFF-LICENSE PRESCRIBING

All medications have a market authorisation that specifies indications and doses that a medication may be used for, as described in a summary of product characteristics (SPC) (at https://www.medicines.org.uk/emc). The BNF takes account of the market authorisation as well as expert guidance. In the United Kingdom, the Medicines Act 1968 permits doctors to prescribe off-license, and guidelines sometimes recommend this (e.g. sertraline for anxiety). There are five reasons that prescribing may fall outside a product license: **D**emographic (e.g. age range, pregnancy), **D**isorder, **D**osage, **D**uration, **D**omain (different country).

Recommendations:

- Check that there is not a suitable licensed alternative.
- Be familiar with the evidence base for the off-license medication, including effectiveness, acceptability, side effects (SEs) and interactions.
- Obtain advice from another prescriber with expertise in this area (± specialist pharmacist) if you lack the expertise yourself, there is not an extensive evidence base or you have particular concerns.
- Consider and document potential risks and benefits, including considering children, elderly, childbearing potential, medical co-morbidity, impaired capacity.

(Royal College of Psychiatrists & British Association for Psychopharmacology, 'Use of licensed medicines for unlicensed applications in psychiatric practice, 2e', 2017)

- Discuss with patient and carers. Explain risks and benefits. If use is supported by authoritative guidance, explain in general terms why medicine is unlicensed. Otherwise, give a more detailed explanation. Obtain consent or consider lack of capacity. Document discussion.
- Start at a low dose and monitor carefully, involving other health professionals.
- If lack of benefit or risks outweigh benefits, withdraw the medication.

MENTAL HEALTH ACT (MHA) IN ENGLAND AND WALES

The MHA in England and Wales was passed in 1983 and is regularly revised. The MHA allows (1) detention of people suffering from mental disorder and then (2) their treatment, potentially against their will. For brevity, we do not include mental health legislation in Scotland and Northern Ireland. At the time of writing (2023), revisions of the MHA are before parliament, which broadly follow the recommendations of the Wessely Review (https://www.gov.uk/government/groups/independent-review-of-the-mentalhealth-act). It will be some years before the planned changes will been acted but the main aim of the reforms is to ensure that the views of patients about their treatment are central to care planning.

COMMONLY USED SECTIONS

Sections 2 (s2) and 3 (s3)

Patient must have mental disorder of a 'nature' (type of disorder) and/or 'degree' (severity) that makes it necessary for the patient to be detained in hospital for their health, their safety or the protection of others for the purposes of:

- s2: assessment or assessment followed by treatment.
- s3: treatment, and appropriate medical treatment is available.

Table 5.1 Summary of most frequently used MHA sections

Section	Aim	Maximum duration[a]	Authorised by	May apply to
2	Assessment and/or treatment	28 days	AMHP + 2 doctors (one must be s12 approved; in practice often both are s12 approved)	Inpatients or outpatients
3	Treatment	6 months[b]		
4	Emergency assessment	72 h	AMHP + doctor	
5(2)	Doctor's holding power	72 h	Doctor	Inpatients
5(4)	Nurse's holding power	6 h	Nurse	
17	Leave		RC	Patients detained under MHA
17A	CTO	6 months[b]	RC	Patients detained under s3 or S37
135	Conveyance to a place of safety by police	24 h (can be extended by up to 12 h)	Magistrate	Patients in a place authorised by a magistrate (which may include private residences)
136		24 h (can be extended by up to 12 h)	Police	Patients anywhere other than in a private residence

Note: AMHP, Approved Mental Health Practitioner, usually a social worker; CTO, Community Treatment Order, which allows the RC to place certain conditions on a patient's discharge from an s3 or 37; the patient may be recalled to hospital if they breach these conditions and there is significant risk or relapse; RC, Responsible Clinician, the professional with overall responsibility for the patient's care, usually a consultant psychiatrist.

[a] Sections should always be used for the miminum necessary time.

[b] s3 and a CTO last for 6 months in the first instance, but the RC may renew the Section with the agreement of another member of the team (s3) or an AMHP (CTO).

Pts detained under s3 may be considered for a CTO, and the patient may be recalled to hospital if they do not abide by the terms of the CTO and there is significant risk or relapse.

Section 5(2)

This is the most relevant section for junior doctors to allow emergency detention long enough for assessment for s2/3 if appropriate. The 72 h limit is to cover bank holiday weekends, but s2/3 assessments should be organised as soon as is practicable and the section reviewed regularly by the ward team.

Important points re s5(2):

- Patients must already be admitted: it only applies to inpatients (*not* A&E or outpatient departments, although 'clinical decisions units' may count as inpatient setting).
- For use in emergencies only; when not possible or safe to wait for completion of an assessment for s2 or 3.
- Appropriate least restrictive measures must have been considered and tried/failed.
- Give full address (including postcode) for hospital in which patient is to be detained. Incorrect/incomplete info can invalidate form.
- Appropriate sentence must be deleted regarding whether: (1) the clinician in charge of the treatment of the patient is filling in the form, or (2) a 'nominee' (a junior member of the team or the on-call clinician covering this team) is filling in the form.
- Give full reasons why informal treatment is no longer appropriate; include mental state abnormalities and potential risks to the patient and/or others.
- Form must be filed in the patient's notes and hospital MHA office informed. Generally, the MHA office holds the originals of detention papers. (Figure 5.1 presents example of completed form.)
- Reasons for using s5(2) should be documented clearly in patient's notes.

FORM H1 *Regulation 4(1)(g)*   **Mental Health Act 1983**
Section 5(2) – report on hospital in-patient

PART 1
(To be completed by a medical practitioner or an approved clinician qualified to do so under section 5(2) of the Act)

To the managers of *(name and address of hospital)*

> *St Elsewhere Hospital, London, S18 9GE*

I am *(PRINT full name)*

> *Dr Anthony Mally*

and I am *(Delete (a) or (b) as appropriate)*

(a) ~~the registered medical practitioner/the approved clinician (who is not a registered medical practitioner)~~ *(delete the phrase which does not apply)*

(b) a registered medical practitioner/~~an approved clinician (who is not a registered medical practitioner)~~* who is the nominee of the registered medical practitioner ~~or approved clinician (who is not a registered medical practitioner)~~ (*delete the phrase which does not apply)

in charge of the treatment of *(PRINT full name of patient)*

> *John Smith*

who is an in-patient in this hospital and not at present liable to be detained under the Mental Health Act 1983.

it appears to me that an application ought to be made under Part 2 of the Act for this patient's admission to hospital for the following reasons-
(The full reasons why informal treatment is no longer appropriate must be given)

> *This patient with a history of paranoid schizophrenia and with current active psychosis (auditory hallucinations and persecutory delusions) is trying to leave hospital despite having severe physical health problems (femoral and pelvic fractures, pneumonia). He lacks insight into his mental and physical health problems and is suspicious/untrusting of staff advice and intentions.*

(if you need to continue on a separate sheet please indicate here ( ) and attach that sheet to this form)

continue overleaf

Figure 5.1 Example of completed s5(2) form. (Reproduced from *BMJ*, Humphreys et al., 348, 2043, 2014, with permission from BMJ Publishing Group Ltd.)

Section 5(4)

Like s5(2), s5(4) applies only to patients admitted to hospital. A nurse who is suitably qualified, experienced and competent may detain a patient if a doctor cannot attend immediately and the patient is suffering from a mental disorder to such a degree that it is necessary for the patient to be detained. An s5(4) can detain a patient for up to 6 h or until a doctor can attend.

CONSENT TO TREATMENT

For patients who are not detained under the MHA, the Mental Capacity Act applies regarding consent to treatment. This also applies to patients detained under s5(2) or s5(4).

Treatment of informal patients is like that for a physical health problem – authority to treat flows either from the patient's capacitous consent or using the MCA. Authority to treat mental disorder for *detained patients* may be given under Part 4 of the MHA (Part 4A for CTO patients), but Part 4 does **not** apply to s5(2), s135(1) and s136 patients. *Treatment* includes nursing, psychological intervention, specialist mental health habilitation, rehabilitation and care; its purpose must be to alleviate, or prevent a worsening of, the disorders or its symptoms or manifestations.

If electroconvulsive therapy (ECT) is administered at any point or medication is given beyond the first **3 months** of detention, special certification requirements apply.

After 3 months, s58 of the MHA stipulates that treatment can only be given if there is either:

a. A completed **Form T2** certifying that the patient has **consented** to the treatment and is capable of understanding its nature, purpose and likely effects; or

b. A completed **Form T3** certifying that a **second opinion appointed doctor (SOAD)** agrees that the treatment is appropriate, and either the patient lacks capacity (according to MCA criteria) to consent to the treatment or the patient has capacity to consent to the treatment and is refusing it. The SOAD agrees a treatment plan and may amend the treatment plan of the Responsible Clinician (or Approved Clinician in charge of treatment); the SOAD then issues the T3.

Regardless of the time period, s58A of the MHA stipulates that adult patients may only be given ECT if there is either:

a. A completed **Form T4** certifying that the patient has **consented** to the treatment and is capable of understanding its nature, purpose and likely effects; or
b. A completed **Form T6** certifying that a **SOAD** agrees that (i) the treatment is appropriate, (ii) the patient has capacity to consent to the treatment and (iii) there is no prohibition on ECT by any advance decision or lasting power of attorney.

ECT at any point or other treatment beyond 3 months of detention may be given in **emergency** situations under **s62** MHA if the treatment is:

a. Immediately necessary to save the patient's life, or
b. Reversible and immediately necessary to prevent a serious deterioration, or
c. Reversible, not hazardous and immediately necessary to alleviate the patient's serious suffering, or
d. Reversible, not hazardous, immediately necessary and represents the minimum interference necessary to prevent the patient being a danger to himself or others.

s62 criteria: a) or b) must be met for urgent ECT – a), b), c) or d) must be met for medication.

MENTAL CAPACITY ACT (MCA) IN ENGLAND AND WALES

For the sake of concision, we do not include mental capacity legislation in Scotland and Northern Ireland. There is an enormous volume of case-law relating to the MCA and this legislation is in the process of being updated, with the replacement of Deprivation of Liberty Safeguards with Liberty Protection Safeguards. The act can be found at https://www.legislation.gov.uk/ukpga/2005/9/contents, and the official Code of Practice is at https://www.gov.uk/government/publications/mental-capacity-act-code-of-practice.

The MCA in England and Wales was passed in 2005. It provides a legal framework and a code of practice for assessing capacity and making decisions on behalf of those who lack capacity. It only applies to patients aged 16 and over.

Principles of the MCA:

- *Assumption of capacity*: A person must be assumed to have capacity unless it is established to be lacking.
- *Optimise decision-making*: A person is not to be treated as unable to make a decision unless all practicable steps to help him or her to do so have been taken without success.
- *Unwise decisions*: An unwise decision does not mean a lack of capacity.
- *Best interests*: Acts done, or decisions made, for incapacitous individuals must be in their best interests.
- *Use least restrictive options*: The least restrictive action or decision should always be employed.

Lack of capacity requires demonstrating both:

1 Impairment of, or disturbance in, functioning of the mind or brain
2 Because of (1), the person is unable to make a decision for himself or herself because he or she is unable to:
   - Understand the information relevant to the decision
   - Retain that information
   - Use or weigh that information as part of the process of making the decision
   - Communicate his or her decision (whether by talking, using sign language or any other means)

If a patient lacks capacity, a decision should be made to treat them in their best interests. This should take account of the patient's preferences, views of those close to the patient and the possibility of the patient regaining capacity. See the decision-making algorithm in Figure 5.2.

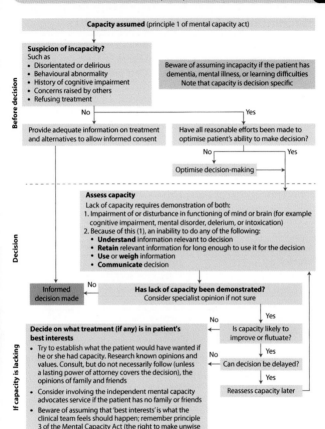

Figure 5.2 Assessment of Capacity. (Adapted by permission from Nicholson et al., *BMJ* 2008; **336**: 322–5.)

PSYCHIATRIC SIDE EFFECTS OF MEDICATIONS

Many non-psychotropic drugs can have neurobehavioural SEs. We highlight some of the most important here.

For a larger list of medications and their possible psychiatric SEs, see Turjanski et al. *BJPsych Adv* 2005; **11**(1):58–70.

Some possible SEs may simply be associations which arise by chance. Use causality assessment tools such as the Bradford Hill criteria to better establish causation or correlation.

Drug/Class	Psychotropic SEs
ACEIs	↑Arousal, psychomotor agitation
Anabolic steroids	Paranoia, aggression, mania, delirium
β-blockers	Sleep disorders, delirium, hallucinations, sedation
Corticosteroids	Depression, mania, psychosis, dependence
Efavirenz	Depression, mania, suicidal ideation
H₂ receptor antagonists	Depression, irritable withdrawal syndrome
Interferon	Depression
Isotretinoin	Depression, suicidal behaviour
Isoniazid	Mania, psychosis, serotonin syndrome
Levetiracetam	Depression, psychosis
Oestrogens and prostagens	Variable effects on mood
Valproate	Confusion, agitation

MEDICATION ADHERENCE

Medication non-adherence is a major risk factor for relapse. To optimise adherence, consider the following[BAP]:

- Devise a collaborative treatment plan
- Offer choices of medications, where possible
- Keep regimen simple: ↓frequency of dosing and ↓number of tablets

- Proactively monitor for and treat SEs
- Regularly check adherence by asking patient
- If there is a Hx of non-adherence, consider checking adherence with pill counting or drug plasma levels
- Consider long-acting injections, where available

Dossette boxes may also help if forgetting medications is a problem, but they do not help if lack of insight or motivation is the problem. Some medications (e.g. valproate, orodispersible formulations) are unsuitable for dossette boxes.

TAPERING MEDICATIONS

- Some psychotropic drugs may require tapering to decrease risk of relapse and/or withdrawal effects: relevant medications include benzodiazepines, antidepressants and antipsychotics.
- Of these, only benzodiazepines are addictive in the true sense of the word.
- It is imperative to counsel any patients starting on these medications that there is a risk of relapse and/or withdrawal effects on cessation. Always advise patients not to abruptly stop their medications.
- Tapering should always be undertaken in collaboration with the patient, who should look out for any Sx changes.
- Nevertheless, excessive focus on Sx checking by the patient or clinician may prove counterproductive.
- Both in terms of receptor occupancy and capacity to cause withdrawal effects, the final stages of tapering may prove the most challenging. It makes sense to use stepwise relative decreases (e.g. 50% reduction/wk).[MPG]
- If smaller doses required, tablets can be split or liquid formulations can be used.[MPG]

Relative risk of withdrawal effects from antidepressants

Highest risk	Moderate risk	Low risk
Amitriptyline	Citalopram	Bupropion
Clomipramine	Escitalopram	Fluoxetine
Paroxetine	Fluvoxamine	Agomelatine (lowest risk)
Venlafaxine	Lofepramine	
Duloxetine	Nortriptyline	
Imipramine	Mirtazapine*	
	Reboxetine	
	Sertraline	
	Trazodone	
	Vortioxetine	

* Rebound insomnia most common.

THERAPEUTIC DRUG MONITORING

General principles

- Also known as plasma 'level' monitoring. Can be used to help guide clinical decisions; however, is overused in some situations and can overcomplicate care.
  - As with all investigations, there is a risk of acting inappropriately on results with dubious clinical significance unless clear rationale (e.g. toxicity, suspected pharmacokinetic interactions, difficulty in confirming clinical response, narrow therapeutic index).MPG
  - Treat the patient, not the number (e.g. do not increase drug in a clinically stable patient even if level is 'low').
- Ensure samples are taken at correct times and the drug is at a steady state (usually five half-lives), except in overdose/suspected toxicity where this is irrelevant.MPG
- Routine plasma monitoring of most antipsychotics is not recommended (many do not have robustly established target ranges).MPG

Target ranges

- Exercise caution with target ranges; there are inherent difficulties in establishing clean signals in both research and clinical settings, but, of course, they can have some guidance value. Therapeutic ranges commonly available include[MPG]:
  - Clozapine: 350–600 micrograms/L.
  - Lithium: 0.6–1.0 mmol/L (>1.0 mmol/L may be required for mania).
  - Valproate: 50–100 mg/L.

Sample times

- Clozapine: trough (i.e. right before dose, often AM).
- Lithium: 12 hours post-dose (usually early AM if taking evening dose).
- Valproate: trough.

ONES TO WATCH

CANNABIS PRODUCTS

- Most cannabis products are not licensed in the UK, though were downgraded from Schedule 1 to Schedule 2 in 2018. Doctors on the GMC Specialist Register are permitted to prescribe off-licence within their own area of expertise.
- Important constituents of cannabis are THC, which is noticeably psychoactive (i.e. produces a high), and CBD, which is not. The latter is sold widely in food supplements.
- Cannabis compounds (except CBD) are contraindicated in those with a personal or family Hx of psychosis, or a Hx of any other serious mental illness.[BNF]
- Sativex (THC + CBD spray) is licensed for spasticity in MS, but not recommended by NICE. It has a modest evidence base for chronic pain.
- Nabilone (oral THC) is licensed for chemotherapy-induced N&V.

- Herbal cannabis (e.g. Bedrocan) is prescribed off-licence in non-NHS services for a number of neuropsychiatric indications. It must be inhaled via a vaporiser and not smoked.
- Oral cannabinoids (such as Epidiolex and Dronabinol) are not licensed in the UK but can also be prescribed on named-patient basis.
- CBD is being researched as an adjunct in psychosis and agitation in dementia, among other indications.

OTHERS

- Brexanolone: approved in the US for postpartum depression. Positive allosteric modulator of $GABA_A$ receptors; administered iv. Not licensed in the UK.
- Brexpiprazole: D_2 and $5\text{-}HT_{1A}$ partial agonist (atypical antipsychotic) with similar pharmacology to aripiprazole. Approved in the USA and EU for schizophrenia, but not available in the UK.
- Lumateperone: butyrophenone antipsychotic which has shown evidence for treatment of depressive episodes in BPAD-I and II. Currently approved by the FDA for these indications as well as schizophrenia. Not currently available in the UK.
- Pimavanserin: inverse agonist and antagonist at $5\text{-}HT_{2A}$. Approved in the USA for PD psychosis and under Ix for several other psychiatric disorders. Not available in the UK.
- Psilocybin and MDMA: Showing promise in international trials for numerous psychiatric disorders including depression, alcoholism and PTSD. Often given in combination with psychological therapy or support. Not available unless through a clinical trial.
- (Es)ketamine: nasal esketamine currently licensed for TRD; however, not NICE-approved. iv ketamine used off-label for TRD in specialist centres.

	Cannabis-based				Synthetic	
	Bedrocan	Tilray	Sativex	Epidiolex	Dronabinol	Nabilone
Profile	THC ± CBD	THC ± CBD	THC:CBD ratio 1:1	CBD	THC	THC
Formulation	Herbal cannabis	Oil	Oromucosal spray	Oral solution	Capsule or liquid	Capsule
Licensed indications	None	None	MS	None	None	Chemotherapy-induced N&V
Can be prescribed in the UK?	Consultants; named-patient basis	Consultants; named-patient basis	MS experts	No restrictions (specialist prescribers)	No restrictions; named-patient basis	No restrictions. (preferably in hospital; GPs continue Rx)

Source: (Adapted from Freeman et al. 'Medicinal use of cannabis based products and cannabinoids', *BMJ* 2019; **365**: l1141).

Non-pharmacological treatments

Non-pharmacological treatments may be alternatives to medications or may complement them. They range from basic communication skills to advanced treatments requiring specialist training.

EMPATHETIC LISTENING

- Empathetic listening can be an important therapeutic tool which can be incorporated into any psychopharmacological context.
- It is an active process of acknowledging and legitimising what is said in a calm and nonjudgmental way.
- Expectancy and placebo effects can be positively leveraged through factors such as a strong therapeutic alliance, which arises, in part, from empathetic listening.
- Symptoms may improve as a result of satisfying clinician contact, even in the absence of a direct treatment intervention.

PSYCHOEDUCATION

Psychoeducation should be part of any treatment plan as it can ↓Sx, ↓relapse rates and ↑compliance. Aim it at the patient and (ideally) carers. Before giving information, it is important to ask the patient about their current understanding of their diagnosis, medication etc, and what they would like to know. It often takes place in routine consultations, but may be formalised in group sessions, courses, patient information leaflets and online resources. Try to **individualise** psychoeducation to the patient in terms of their personal experiences, communication needs and level of education.

Cover:

- Diagnosis
- Symptoms
- Functional impact
- Prognosis
- Treatment

- Self-management
- Medication adherence
- Crisis planning
- Further sources of reliable information

Provide opportunities for questions.

CRISIS PLANNING

Crisis plans may help reduce the need for medication and other interventions. Anticipate medication non-adherence, social stressors and symptom breakthrough. Devise a **collaborative** written plan. Templates, such as the following example, can help.

Crisis plan for Joe Bloggs

- My diagnosis is emotionally unstable personality disorder
- My care coordinator is Sally Perkins (☎ 07999 999999, sally.perkins@mhtrust.uk)
- My carer is Jenny Bloggs (my wife) ☎ 07999 999990
- My warning signs that a crisis is developing:
  Not sleeping well. Relationship difficulties. Thinking too much about my past.
- I can remember that I want to live because:
  I have to be there for my daughter. People think I am a fun person to be with.
- My coping strategies are:
  Using a relaxation exercise. Going out for a walk. Calling a friend.
- If I need help, I can contact:
  My care coordinator (Monday-Friday 09:00-17:00)
  My GP: Dr Jones, Grove Surgery
  Samaritans on 116 123
  NHS helpline on 111
- In an emergency, I can attend my nearest A&E department

LIFESTYLE INTERVENTIONS

DIET

Nutrition is important to mental health in several ways. Specific **deficiencies** of cobalamin (vitamin B12), folate (B9), thiamine (B1), niacin (B3), vitamin D and vitamin C can cause psychiatric symptoms. Obesity is common among psychiatric patients. There is a growing body of research about the role of diet in mental well-being. Antimuscarinic side effects (SEs) of psychotropic meds ⇒ thirst and can contribute to high calorie intake with alcohol and soft drinks.

Principles for improving diet:

- Balance carbohydrates, fat and protein (see box)
- Eat five portions of fruit/vegetables each day
- Eat ≥2 portions of fish each week
- Eating foods high in omega-3 fatty acids (oily fish, walnuts) may be beneficial in depression and psychosis
- Ensure good calcium intake if ↑PRL in order to ↓risks from osteoporosis
- For serious problems, r/f to dietician

Good options from different food groups	
Carbohydrate	Brown rice, wholemeal bread, fruit, vegetables
Fat	Nuts, vegetable oils, whole grains
Protein	Fish, lean meat, whole grains

Occasionally, unwell psychiatric patients may become seriously **malnourished**. For example, this can happen in a patient with severe depression receiving ECT or in a patient with dementia who is self-neglecting. Dieticians generally prefer using 'real' food high in calories, but occasionally supplements may be necessary. Good options are **Complan Shake** (powder to be mixed with full-fat milk) or **Fortisip Compact**. For Complan Shake, prescribe 1–2 sachets/

day. For Fortisip Compact, prescribe 1 bottle bd or tds. Give between meals, rather than as a replacement for meals. Prescribe a flavour that patient prefers.

EXERCISE

Exercise may be helpful in prevention and treatment of depression and anxiety. It can ↑ sleep, ↑ self-esteem, ↑ concentration and ↓ drug cravings.

Each week, adults should do:

- 150 min of moderate aerobic exercise (e.g. walking, cycling) or 75 min of vigorous exercise (e.g. running, football) +
- Strength exercises on ≥2 days (e.g. lifting weights, press-ups)

For improving mental health, exercise that makes you out of breath is best, but anything is helpful.

Principles for ↑ physical activity:

- Find a form of exercise you enjoy
- Do it in a way you find fun (e.g. with music, with a friend, in an interesting place)
- Build it into your daily routine (e.g. journey to work, sports club)
- Start gently and ↑ gradually
- Avoid exercise close to bedtime, as it can make it harder to wind down

SLEEP HYGIENE

See p. 275.

SOCIAL INTERVENTIONS

VOCATIONAL REHABILITATION

Most patients wish to work, but in severe mental illness, unemployment rates are very high. Support may include:

- Training in employable skills
- Voluntary work
- Part-time work
- Special adjustments in the workplace (e.g. time out if experiencing anxiety, a quiet place to rest)

OT is helpful. Sometimes a letter from a health professional can be very persuasive with employers, e.g. in a patient with functional seizures, a letter from a psychiatrist stating that the patient needs reassurance and not calling an ambulance might allow the patient to remain in work.

PATIENT SUPPORT GROUPS

Usually helpful in providing peer support. Some are for people with any mental health problem (e.g. Mind, Rethink), others are for a specific disorder (e.g. Bipolar UK) and a few are highly specific (e.g. Maternal OCD). Sometimes groups can be against medication or compulsory treatment. Patients sometimes need a prompt to engage.

CARER SUPPORT

Where possible, involve carers in decision-making and care planning. Provide them with information. They are often keen to know what they can do to help. The Carers Trust provides support for carers. In the United Kingdom, local authorities are obliged to offer a carer's assessment. Financial support is sometimes available.

PSYCHOLOGICAL THERAPIES

COMMON FACTORS

All psychological therapies tend to be based on a confidential therapeutic relationship with active listening and empathy. There is a theoretical rationale for understanding the problem that guides the therapeutic techniques. The therapist's stance can vary from passive (e.g. psychoanalysis) to active (e.g. CBT) depending on the therapy.

There is evidence to indicate that the strength of the therapeutic alliance is a better predictor of recovery in many cases than the specific modality.

Factors to be considered when referring: patient's goals (insight versus problem resolution), ability to form a therapeutic alliance, psychological mindedness, readiness to change and good cognitive function.

COGNITIVE BEHAVIOURAL THERAPY (CBT)

CBT is probably the mostly widely used type of formal psychotherapy and spans 5–20 sessions. Its theoretical model emphasises how a person's interpretations of events shape their emotional and behavioural reactions. Patients learn to recognise and evaluate unhelpful thoughts and identify biases in their perceptions of themselves or the world around them. The behavioural aspect encourages a patient to test their thoughts through behavioural experiments or alter their actions, e.g. with relaxation training, graded exposure or behavioural activation. CBT techniques can often be applied in a less formalised way during medical consultations.

COUNSELLING

Counselling tends to be **non-directive** and places an emphasis on **active listening** with **reflecting** back a person's thoughts in order to help a patient better understand their feelings. There may be an element of problem-solving. It is particularly used with relationship problems and bereavement. It is offered by many charities and sometimes in primary care, but its effectiveness is modest. Debriefing after a traumatic event is not recommended,[NICE] as it can prolong Sx.

SUPPORTIVE PSYCHOTHERAPY

Supportive psychotherapy also emphasises listening skills and is often employed by health professionals in the course of their everyday work. It is supplemented by giving advice and providing hope. It is helpful for patients with enduring illnesses.

PSYCHODYNAMIC THERAPIES

Psychodynamic therapies aim to increase a patient's awareness of the role of unconscious processes on their mind and actions. In practice, this occurs through a close but professional relationship with a therapist in which the patient is encouraged to make **free associations** (say whatever comes into their mind). The therapist offers **interpretations** by linking the patient's current experiences and reactions to the therapist (**transference**) to childhood experiences. There are several forms of psychodynamic therapies:

	Frequency	Position
Psychoanalysis	5× weekly	Patient on a couch; not facing therapist
Psychoanalytic psychotherapy	3× weekly	Patient in chair; facing therapist
Psychodynamic psychotherapy	1× weekly	

Brief psychodynamic psychotherapy can be used where there is a focal problem to be addressed.

INTERPERSONAL PSYCHOTHERAPY

Problems are formulated as grief, role transitions, interpersonal deficits or interpersonal disputes. Specific strategies are then used to address each of these areas, including acknowledging differing expectations, learning to express emotion in alternative ways and examining patterns in relationships.

COGNITIVE ANALYTIC THERAPY (CAT)

CAT takes principles from psychodynamic therapy and CBT. Maladaptive behaviours (or problem procedures) are considered as **traps** (a false assumption generates an act that confirms the assumption), **snags** (abandoning appropriate goals because of assumptions about them) or **dilemmas** (false dichotomies in which the only options seen are unhelpful extremes). Treatment involves a written and diagrammatic reformulation of problems, recognising how procedures play out inside and outside the session and

NICE indications for psychological therapies

Disorder	1st-line intervention	2nd-line intervention	Other
Depression[a]	CBT, IPT, BA, couple therapy,	Brief psychodynamic, counselling, MBCT (as relapse prevention for recurrent depression)	
GAD[a]	CBT, applied relaxation		
Social anxiety disorder	CBT	Brief psychodynamic	
Panic disorder ± agoraphobia	CBT	Brief psychodynamic	
PTSD	CBT, EMDR		
OCD	CBT (with ERP)		
BDD	CBT (with ERP)		
IBS	CBT, hypnotherapy		
ME/CFS	CBT, graded exercise therapy, activity management		
Schizophrenia	CBT, family intervention		
Bipolar depression	CBT, IPT		
Alcohol misuse	CBT, couple therapy, behavioural therapies, social network and environment-based therapies		

ADHD	Parental training (children)
Autism	Individual or group social learning programme
Dementia	Group cognitive stimulation therapy
Borderline PD	Involve Pt in choosing the best intervention for them
Antisocial PD	Group cognitive and behavioural interventions
Self-harm	Psychological intervention for self-harm (DBT usually used)
Anorexia	CBT, MANTRA, specialist supportive clinical management
Bulimia[a]	

Note: ADHD, attention deficit hyperactivity disorder; BA, behavioural activation; BDD, body dysmorphic disorder; CBT, cognitive behavioural therapy; DBT, dialectical behavioural therapy; EMDR, eye movement desensitisation and reprocessing; ERP, exposure response prevention; GAD, generalised anxiety disorder; IBS, irritable bowel syndrome; IPT, interpersonal therapy; MANTRA, Maudsley Model of Anorexia Nervosa Treatment for Adults; MBCT, mindfulness-based cognitive therapy; ME/CFS, myalgic encephalomyelitis/chronic fatigue syndrome; OCD, obsessive-compulsive disorder; PD, personality disorder; PTSD, post-traumatic stress disorder.

[a] These disorders may benefit from guided self-help for mild Sx.

homework involving attempting a different behavioural strategy. Treatment spans 16–24 sessions.

DIALECTIC BEHAVIOURAL THERAPY (DBT)

DBT uses principles from CBT and mindfulness and is specifically directed at recurrent self-harm, often in the context of emotionally unstable personality disorder. As well as individual therapy, there are often group sessions with the option for telephone contact in crises. Patients are taught how to manage emotions and use alternative ways out of distressing situations.

GROUP PSYCHOTHERAPY

Group therapy often uses some of the models employed for individual therapy, but there is an emphasis on group members helping each other. There is a psychotherapist and up to eight members of the group. Group therapy may be particularly helpful for those who have difficulties relating to others. Members must be able to commit to attending and participating fully in the group.

THERAPIES FOR PERSONALITY DISORDERS

A number of evidence-based therapies are now available specifically for personality disorders. These include Schema Therapy (developed from CBT), Transference-Focused Psychotherapy and Mentalisation-Based Therapy (derived from psychodynamic therapy).

NEUROSTIMULATION

ELECTROCONVULSIVE THERAPY (ECT)

ECT entails administering a transcranial electric current to induce a generalised tonic-clonic seizure. Various mechanisms have been proposed. It can be an extremely effective acute treatment, but other therapy must be commenced, as patients often relapse in the weeks following ECT.

 In modern practice, a muscle relaxant (e.g. succinylcholine) is administered to ↓ risk of fractures. General anaesthetic is also necessary. Propofol is often used, but has the disadvantage of ↑ seizure threshold. ECT is classically given bilaterally; unilateral ECT can be given to the non-dominant hemisphere with the aim of ↓ memory loss, but unilateral ECT requires a higher dose. Typically, 8–12 sessions are required, but this should be carefully titrated to Rx response and SEs.

- Indications: Life-threatening or treatment-resistant cases of catatonia, mania or depression[NICE]
- No absolute contraindications (CIs). Relative CIs: ↑ICP, recent myocardial infarction/cerebrovascular accident, unstable fracture, severe osteoporosis, cerebral aneurysm
- SEs: Headache (Rx: paracetamol, NSAIDs), ↓ memory (especially autobiographical), death from anaesthetic (~1 in 100,000), asystole (ECT ⇒ ↑vagal tone), prolonged seizure (Rx: give more propofol or administer benzodiazepine)
- Workup:
  - Hx, including prior response to ECT, dental problems, personal/family anaesthetic reactions
  - Full physical examination, including inspecting for loose teeth
  - Mini-Mental State Examination (MMSE)
  - Bloods: Full blood count, urea and electrolytes
  - Electrocardiogram

OTHER FORMS OF NEUROSTIMULATION

Neurostimulation has mainly been developed for use in depression, although its use is now expanding to other disorders. None of the various techniques have the robust evidence base of ECT, but they are starting to enter clinical practice.

Vagal nerve stimulation (VNS) involves implanting a subcutaneous battery-powered device in the chest wall and connecting it such that it stimulates the vagus nerve in the neck. It has an established role in treatment-resistant epilepsy and has some evidence in depression, presumably by altering the vagal afferent signalling to the brain.

Repetitive transcranial magnetic stimulation (rTMS) uses an electromagnet applied externally to the cranium to induce an electric current in the underlying brain, increasing regional perfusion. It is safer than ECT and very well tolerated, but is less effective. NICE have approved rTMS for the short-term management of depression, although in practice it is not routinely used in the NHS. Private healthcare avenues exist.

Deep brain stimulation (DBS) is an invasive form of neurostimulation that was developed for Parkinson's. Like VNS, there is a battery-powered device implanted in the chest wall, but the leads are tunnelled beneath the skull to stimulate the brain. There is emerging evidence of efficacy for Rx-resistant OCD & Tourette's. NICE guidance (2021) acknowledges the promise of DBS in treating adult OCD, though recommends it only be used in research settings at present.

Transcranial direct current stimulation (tDCS) simply consists of two electrodes applied externally to the cranium with a current passed between them. Its advantages are its low cost and portability, but it remains investigational.

PSYCHOSURGERY

Psychosurgery gained a bad reputation with historical widespread use of frontal lobotomy for psychiatric disorders. Today, psychosurgery is rare, with only a few centres offering it with specific criteria for very severe and treatment-resistant cases. A few procedures have a limited evidence base:

Procedure	Indications
Anterior capsulotomy	OCD
Anterior cingulotomy	Depression, BPAD, OCD
Subcaudate tractotomy	Depression, BPAD, anxiety, OCD
Limbic leucotomy	Depression, BPAD, OCD

Source: Patel et al., *World Neurosurgery* 2013; 80(3–4): S31.e9–S31.e16.

Basic
psychopharmacology

Pharmacokinetics is what the body does to a drug.
Pharmacodynamics is what a drug does to the body.

PHARMACOKINETICS

Pharmacokinetics has four stages: (**ADME**) absorption →
distribution → metabolism → excretion.

ABSORPTION

- Absorption is the process of drug entry into the circulation from the site of administration.
- Drugs given intravenously are directly administered into the circulation.
- Oral drugs are absorbed through the gut mucosa, mostly in the small intestine, but some acidic drugs are absorbed in the stomach.
- If basic drugs (e.g. diazepam, imipramine, methadone) are taken after a meal, absorption is reduced, whereas absorption of acidic drugs (e.g. aspirin, ibuprofen, lurasidone) is accelerated.
- Some very lipophilic drugs require bile to emulsify them.
- Formulations can be engineered so that the release of active compounds is prolonged, which can make a drug with a short $t_{1/2}$ into one that can be given od. These are known as **modified release (MR)**, **extended release (ER)** or **sustained release (SR)**.
- Intramuscular drugs are absorbed almost completely, and speed depends on the chemical properties of the injection.
- Many long-acting injections (LAIs) or 'depots' use oil-based vectors which take longer periods to reach circulation where the active drug is cleaved from the long-chain fatty acid. Shorter fatty acid chains (e.g. in zuclopenthixol acetate [Clopixol Acuphase]) serve to deliver the drug more quickly. Other LAIs use alternative technology (e.g. Risperdal Consta).

DISTRIBUTION

- Distribution is the process of drug partitioning into body tissues from circulation.
- In the bloodstream, drugs are often partially bound to proteins:
  - Acidic and neutral drugs bind to **albumin**. Basic drugs bind to α_1-**acid glycoprotein**.
  - Only the unbound drug is active.
  - If a drug binds to the same place on a protein as another drug, it can displace it → ↑unbound (active) drug.
- Distribution to organs depends on (1) the blood supply to that organ and (2) how lipophilic the drug is.
  - **Hydrophilic** molecules tend to stay in the blood. **Lipophilic** drugs tend to distribute in adipose tissue.
- To diffuse across the blood-brain barrier, drugs must be (1) small molecules and (2) lipophilic. Some drugs are transported across the blood-brain barrier by transporter proteins, e.g. amisulpride and gabapentin.
- In the elderly, relative to body mass, there are higher levels of fat but lower water and albumin. Therefore, there is an ↑ volume of distribution for lipophilic drugs (→ ↑$t_{1/2}$), a ↓ volume of distribution for hydrophilic drugs (→ ↑initial levels) and ↑ free levels of drugs that are highly bound to albumin.

METABOLISM

- Metabolism is the conversion of drugs to (usually) inactive, hydrophilic compounds which can then be excreted by the kidneys. Metabolism occurs in the liver.
- Hydrophilic drugs (e.g. lithium) can be eliminated unchanged by the kidneys. Others must undergo **hepatic metabolism**.
- Two phases of drug metabolism:
  - Phase 1: **Modification**: alteration by oxidation, reduction, etc. This may result in a compound that is pharmacologically active.

- Phase 2: **Conjugation**: addition of polar group to make drug hydrophilic, e.g. glucuronide or sulphate. Products are pharmacologically inactive.

- The **cytochrome P450 (CYP)** enzyme system is the most important in drug metabolism, the most significant being CYP1A2, CYP2C9, CYP2C19, CYP2D6, CYP2E1 and CYP3A4. Some drugs have significant metabolism via other routes though.
  - Meta-analytic evidence indicates significant intra- and inter-ethnic differences in variability in CYP2D6 and CYP2C19 metabolism status; therefore, broad ethnic categories in themselves unlikely to be useful in stratifying an individual's risk (Koopmans et al., *Transl Psych* 2021; **11**, 141).
  - At present, individual genotyping is not common practice.
  - See p. 382.

- Drugs are carried from the gastrointestinal (GI) tract to the liver via the hepatic portal vein before reaching systemic circulation. During this stage, they undergo **first pass metabolism**. Extensive first pass metabolism can make the oral route unsuitable.

- In **liver disease**, both first pass metabolism and elimination metabolism are often impaired, leading to higher plasma concentrations of some drugs.

- Metabolites are sometimes pharmacologically active. In a few cases, the administered medication is a **pro-drug** for the active metabolite. Lofepramine is an example of a pro-drug that is metabolised to desipramine.

- In children, side effects may be more marked and less predictable, so it is advisable to start at lower doses relative to weight than in adults. However, due to children's faster metabolism, their final dose may be higher in terms of mg drug/kg body weight.

EXCRETION

- Excretion is the loss of a drug or its metabolites from the body.
- Drugs and their metabolites may be excreted by the kidneys into urine, via the faeces (e.g. clozapine) or by the liver into bile, which can lead to some drugs being re-absorbed from the GI tract (e.g. oral contraceptives).
- Most psychotropic drugs undergo some hepatic metabolism prior to excretion, but **lithium, amisulpride, sulpiride** and **paliperidone** are prominent examples of psychotropic drugs that are renally excreted unchanged.
- Renal impairment → accumulation of renally excreted drugs.
- There are two patterns for drug elimination kinetics.
  - **Zero-order kinetics:** A fixed *amount* of drug is eliminated per unit of time, e.g. 10 mg in the first hour, then 10 mg in the second hour, etc., until it is fully eliminated. A few psychotropic drugs follow zero-order kinetics, notably **ethanol, fluoxetine, paroxetine** and **phenytoin**. Small increases in doses can lead to unpredictably large increases in plasma levels.
  - **First-order kinetics:** A fixed *proportion* of drug is eliminated per unit of time; e.g. for a starting concentration of 20 mg, 10 mg may be eliminated in the first hour, then 5 mg in the second hour, then 2.5 mg in the third hour, etc. The vast majority of drugs follow first-order kinetics.
  - However, enzymes that usually metabolise drugs with first-order kinetics can be **saturated** at high doses, resulting in zero-order kinetics.
- In first-order kinetics, **half-life** ($t_{1/2}$) is the time it takes for a drug to reach half its plasma concentration. The $t_{1/2}$ is constant, such that after $2 \times t_{1/2}$, a quarter of the original concentration will remain, etc.
- Drugs reach a steady state in plasma after $4{-}5 \times t_{1/2}$, and take the same period of time to effectively be eliminated when they are no longer taken.
- In the elderly, renal function tends to be reduced, resulting in slower excretion of many drugs.

PHARMACODYNAMICS

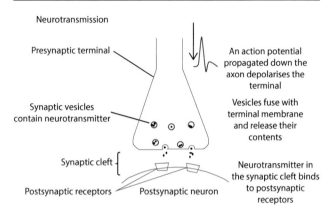

Adapted from *Fundamentals of Clinical Psychopharmacology*, Anderson & McAllister-Williams 2015.

THE SYNAPSE

Neurotransmission starts with an electrical impulse in an axon. This causes calcium influx in the presynaptic terminal, resulting in exocytosis of vesicles containing neurotransmitters. These neurotransmitters may cross the synapse and bind to postsynaptic or presynaptic receptors. The receptor may open an ion channel or activate a G-protein, resulting in an intracellular enzyme cascade. Neurotransmitter is removed from the synapse, either by breakdown by an enzyme or by re-uptake into the presynaptic terminal. Breakdown may also occur in the presynaptic neuron. Neurotransmitters in the presynaptic terminal can then be packaged into vesicles ready for exocytosis.

DRUG TARGETS

- Psychotropic drugs have four main mechanisms:
    1. Influencing receptor activation
    2. Enzyme inhibition
    3. Transporter interference
    4. Ion channel stabilisation

Receptor binding

Presynaptic receptors may increase or decrease the activity of the neuron on which they sit. When activated by the transmitter used by the neuron, they are usually **autoreceptors** that exert a negative feedback effect on release of the neurotransmitter. There are several possible actions on a receptor:

- An **agonist** binds the receptor in the same location, and stimulates the receptor to the same degree, as the neurotransmitter; e.g. methadone is an agonist at the μ opioid receptor.
- An **antagonist** binds the receptor in the same location as the neurotransmitter, but it does not stimulate it, blocking the neurotransmitter from acting; e.g. most antipsychotics are antagonists at the dopamine D_2 receptor.
- A **partial agonist** binds the receptor in the same location as the neurotransmitter, but it stimulates it to a lower degree than the neurotransmitter. If levels of the neurotransmitter are low, a partial agonist will increase the postsynaptic response by providing some receptor stimulation. If levels of the neurotransmitter are high, a partial agonist will reduce the postsynaptic response by blocking the neurotransmitter from binding the receptor. For example, aripiprazole is a partial agonist at the dopamine D_2 receptor, and buspirone is a partial agonist at the serotonin $5\text{-}HT_{1A}$ receptor.
- A **positive allosteric modulator** binds to a different site on the receptor from the one that the neurotransmitter binds to; it increases the response of the receptor to the neurotransmitter. For example, benzodiazepines bind to the $GABA_A$ receptor at a site different from the GABA binding site and facilitate the opening of the chloride channel by GABA.

- A **negative allosteric modulator** binds to a different site on the receptor from the one that the neurotransmitter binds to; it reduces the response of the receptor to the neurotransmitter. For example, ketamine binds to the ion channel of the glutamatergic NMDA receptor, reducing its activity.

Although drugs are often labelled as having activity at one particular receptor, in reality they often bind to multiple receptors. This can account for SEs of a medication. For example, olanzapine causes extrapyramidal symptoms (EPSEs) and ↑prolactin due to D_2 antagonism; however, it also has antihistaminergic and antimuscarinic SEs.

Once a receptor is stimulated, it activates a downstream signalling cascade by one of these mechanisms:

- **Ligand-gated ion channels:** Some receptors are coupled to an **ion channel**. When the receptor is activated, the ion channel opens, allowing influx or efflux of an ion. For example GABA acts on the $GABA_A$ receptor to open a Cl^- channel, resulting in Cl^- influx and consequent hyperpolarisation of the cell membrane.
- **G protein-coupled receptors:** Receptors are coupled to a '**G protein**'. When the receptor is activated, it causes a conformational change in the G protein, which then changes the activity of an enzyme or an ion channel. The effect depends on which G protein is coupled to the receptor.
  - G_s stimulates adenylyl cyclase → ↑cAMP synthesis → ↑transcription of specific genes
  - G_i inhibits adenylyl cyclase → ↓cAMP synthesis → ↓transcription of specific genes
  - G_q stimulates phospholipase C → IP_3 and DAG signalling → opening of Ca^{2+} channels
  - G proteins may also couple to ion channels, e.g. the 5-HT_{1A} receptor couples to potassium and calcium channels (as well as to G_i)

Enzyme inhibition

- Drugs may inhibit enzymes that **degrade** neurotransmitters. For example, monoamine oxidase inhibitors reduce the activity of the enzyme monoamine oxidase, which is responsible for the breakdown of 5-HT, DA and NA.

Transporter interference

- Drugs may block the **reuptake transporters** that remove neurotransmitters from the synapse, e.g. SSRIs block the serotonin reuptake transporter SERT/5-HTT.

Ion channel modulation

- Some ion channels in the cell membrane open in response to a **depolarisation**, allowing an influx of ions.
- Drugs can block these ion channels. For example lamotrigine and carbamazepine bind voltage-gated sodium channels and stabilise them in the inactive state; gabapentin and pregabalin bind to the presynaptic voltage-gated potassium channel, reducing release of neurotransmitters.

NEUROTRANSMITTER SYSTEMS

Many neurotransmitters involved in psychopharmacology are known as **monoamines** because they contain a single amine group. They include the **catecholamines** (DA, NA and adrenaline), **tryptamines** ([5-HT] and melatonin) and histamine. Glutamate, GABA and opioid systems are also important.

DOPAMINE (DA)

Synthesis and inactivation

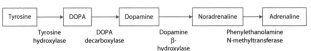

As well as being a neurotransmitter, DA is also a precursor to adrenaline and noradrenaline. DA is either inactivated in the extracellular space by **COMT** or taken up into the presynaptic terminal by the dopamine transporter (**DAT**). In the presynaptic terminal, it may be repackaged into vesicles or broken down by MAO A or B.

Pathways

Name	From	To	Function	Effect of blockade
Mesolimbic	Ventral tegmental area	Nucleus accumbens	Motivation, reward	Antipsychotic
Mesocortical	Ventral tegmental area	Prefrontal cortex	Cognition, emotion	Cognitive impairment, blunted affect
Nigrostriatal	Substantia nigra	Striatum	Movement initiation	EPSEs
Tuberoinfundibular	Hypothalamus	Anterior pituitary	Inhibits prolactin release	↑Prolactin

Receptors

The five dopamine receptors are categorised as the D_1 type (D_1 and D_5) and the D_2 type (D_2, D_3 and D_4).

Receptor	Group	Target	Synaptic location	Brain location
D_1	D_1 type	G_s	Postsynaptic	Limbic system
D_2	D_2 type	G_i	Pre- and postsynaptic	Limbic system, basal ganglia, pituitary
D_3	D_2 type	G_i	Pre- and postsynaptic	Limbic system, basal ganglia
D_4	D_2 type	G_i	Pre- and postsynaptic	Limbic system
D_5	D_1 type	G_s	Postsynaptic	Basal ganglia, hypothalamus

Example drugs

Most antipsychotics act by antagonism at the D_2 receptor, although aripiprazole is a D_2 receptor partial agonist. Some also bind to the D_3 receptor, such as amisulpride, a D_2/D_3 antagonist and cariprazine, a D_2/D_3 partial agonist. The antiemetics metoclopramide and domperidone are also D_2 receptor antagonists. Pramipexole is a selective D_2/D_3 agonist used in difficult-to-treat mood disorders.

SEROTONIN (5-HT)

Synthesis and inactivation

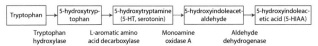

Tryptophan	→	5-hydroxytryp-tophan	→	5-hydroxytryptamine (5-HT, serotonin)	→	5-hydroxyindoleacet-aldehyde	→	5-hydroxyindoleac-etic acid (5-HIAA)
		Tryptophan hydroxylase		L-aromatic amino acid decarboxylase		Monoamine oxidase A		Aldehyde dehydrogenase

Serotonin action in the synapse is terminated by its reuptake into the presynaptic terminal via **SERT/5-HTT**. Here it can be packaged into vesicles or degraded by **MAO-A**.

Receptors

Receptor	Location	Target	Function
5-HT$_1$ (5-HT$_{1A}$, 5-HT$_{1B}$, 5-HT$_{1D}$)	Raphe nuclei, hippocampus, smooth muscle	G_i	Cortical postsynaptic receptors (5-HT$_{1A}$), autoreceptors on 5-HT neurons, vasoconstriction
5-HT$_2$	Central nervous system (CNS), platelets, smooth muscle	G_q	GI motility, platelet aggregation, CNS excitation/inhibition
5-HT$_3$	Area postrema, PNS	Na$^+$/K$^+$/Ca^{2+} ion channel	Vomiting, nociception
5-HT$_4$	GI tract, CNS	G_s	Cognition
5-HT$_5$	Olfactory bulb	G_s	Unknown
5-HT$_6$	Hippocampus	G_s	↑ ACh release
5-HT$_7$	CNS, GI tract, blood vessels	G_s	Circadian rhythms

Example drugs

SSRIs and some TCAs block SERT, causing ↑ levels of synaptic 5-HT. MAOIs cause ↓5-HT breakdown. Atypical antipsychotics usually have some antagonism at 5-HT_2 receptors. The anxiolytic drug buspirone is a partial agonist at the 5-HT_{1A} receptor. The antiemetic ondansetron is a 5-HT_3 receptor antagonist. For migraine, the 5-HT_2 antagonist pizotifen is used in prophylaxis, while the $5\text{-HT}_{1B/D}$ agonists are effective in acute treatment.

HISTAMINE

Synthesis and inactivation

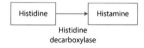

There is no presynaptic transporter for histamine, so its breakdown is dependent on one of two enzymes: histamine methyltransferase (**HMT**) and diamine oxidase (**DAO**).

Receptors

Receptor	Location	Target	Function
H_1	Mast cells, CNS	G_q	Inflammatory response (vasodilatation, ↑ vascular permeability); wakefulness
H_2	Stomach, neutrophils	G_q	↑ Gastric acid
H_3	Presynaptic terminals in CNS and PNS	G_i	↓ Release of other neurotransmitters
H_4	Mast cells, eosinophils, monocytes	G_i	Modulates allergic response

Example drugs

The first-generation 'antihistamines' (e.g. chlorphenamine, promethazine) are antagonists at the H_1 receptor, so can treat various allergic conditions; however, they cross the blood-brain barrier, so they also cause drowsiness. Second-generation H_1 antagonists (e.g. cetirizine, loratadine) are less prone to crossing the blood-brain barrier, so they cause less drowsiness. H_2 antagonists (e.g. cimetidine, ranitidine) are a second-line Rx for GORD.

MELATONIN

Synthesis

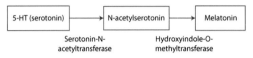

Synthesis only occurs in the pineal gland.

Receptors

Receptor	Function	Location	Target
MT_1	↓ SCN activity, promotes sleep	SCN, retina, cardiovascular system	G_i
MT_2	Shifts circadian rhythms		

Example drugs

Synthetic melatonin is an MT_1 and MT_2 agonist; it is used as a hypnotic. Agomelatine is an antidepressant that also has MT_1 and MT_2 agonism, so it tends to promote sleep.

GLUTAMATE

Glutamate is the brain's main excitatory neurotransmitter.

Synthesis and inactivation

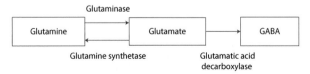

Receptors

Receptor	Location		Target	Function
AMPA	CNS	Postsynaptic	Cation	Fast excitatory
Kainate		Postsynaptic	channel	neurotransmission
NMDA		Postsynaptic		Slow excitatory neurotransmission, long-term potentiation
Metabotropic ($mGlu_{1-8}$)		Pre- and postsynaptic	G_q/G_i	Modify glutamate release and the response to other glutamate receptors

Example drugs

Memantine is a voltage-dependent NMDA antagonist used in Alzheimer's disease to block putative neuronal excitotoxicity. The recreational drugs ketamine and PCP are non-voltage-dependent NMDA.

GAMMA-AMINO-BUTYRIC ACID

GABA is the brain's major inhibitory neurotransmitter.

Synthesis and inactivation

GABA is synthesised from glutamate (see above). The **GABA transporter** (**GAT**) can remove it from the synapse, and **GABA transaminase** may then degrade it.

Receptors

Receptor	Location	Target	Function
$GABA_A$	CNS	Cl⁻ channel	Hyperpolarises cell membrane → sedative, myorelaxant and anxiolytic effects
$GABA_B$	CNS	G_i	Slow hyperpolarisation

Example drugs

Benzodiazepines and Z-drugs are positive allosteric modulators at the $GABA_A$ receptor, enhancing the action of endogenous GABA. The anticonvulsant and mood stabiliser sodium valproate inhibits GABA transaminase, reducing GABA breakdown.

OPIOID

Synthesis

Endogenous opioids (**endorphins**) are synthesised in the anterior pituitary gland from a precursor molecule **POMC**. They preferentially act on the μ-opioid receptors.

Receptors

Receptor	Location	Target	Function
μ	Brain, spinal cord, GI tract	G_i	Analgesia, respiratory depression, euphoria, ↓ GI motility, sedation
δ	Brain, GI tract	G_i	Analgesia, respiratory depression, ↓ GI motility
κ	Brain, spinal cord, GI tract	G_i	Dysphoria, sedation, analgesia

Example drugs

Classic opioids (such as morphine, diamorphine and methadone) are agonists at the μ-opioid receptor. Naloxone and naltrexone are antagonists at all three opioid receptors, with highest affinity for the μ-receptor. Buprenorphine is a μ partial agonist and a δ/κ antagonist. Nalmefene is a μ/δ antagonist and a κ partial agonist.

ACETYLCHOLINE (ACh)

Synthesis and inactivation

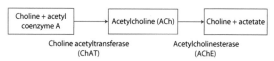

Choline + acetyl coenzyme A → Acetylcholine (ACh) → Choline + actetate

Choline acetyltransferase (ChAT)　　　　　Acetylcholinesterase (AChE)

Receptors

Receptor	Location	Target	Function
Nicotinic (nAChR)	CNS and neuromuscular junction	Na$^+$/K$^+$/Ca^{2+} ion channel	(*in CNS*) Cognition, memory, reward; (*at neuromuscular junction*) muscle contraction
Muscarinic (mAChR)	Smooth muscle, myocardium, CNS	G$_q$/G$_i$	Exocrine secretion, GI motility, urination, bradycardia, cognition

Example drugs

Nicotine in tobacco products is an agonist at the nAChR, while varenicline is a partial agonist. Many drugs for Alzheimer's disease (donepezil, rivastigmine and galantamine) inhibit acetylcholinesterase. Many psychotropic medications (e.g. TCAs, SGAs) have antimuscarinic SEs, causing dry mouth, urinary retention and constipation.

DRUG INTERACTIONS

ENZYME INTERACTIONS

- Drug interactions can be due to changes in the activity of an enzyme that metabolises one or both drugs. The CYP system is most commonly implicated.
- Drugs may be **substrates** of an enzyme (they are metabolised by it), **inhibitors** of an enzyme (they ↓ its activity) or **inducers** of an enzyme (they ↑ its activity).
- Enzyme inhibition tends to happen immediately and resolves promptly after stopping the inhibiting drug. The effects of induction can take days to weeks to appear, as induction involves production of new enzymes. When the drug is withdrawn, the enzymes need to be broken down for the effect to be reversed, which also takes days to weeks.
- CYP interactions can have serious consequences. They should be considered when **starting** and **stopping** a drug. For example:

- The OCP is metabolised by CYP3A4. Carbamazepine and St John's wort induce CYP3A4, so they can cause failure of the OCP.
- Tobacco smoking (not NRT) induces CYP1A2, which metabolises clozapine. Stopping smoking (e.g. on admission to hospital) can cause clozapine toxicity.
- Fluvoxamine inhibits several CYP enzymes that metabolise Warfarin, so it can result in a raised INR.
- Carbamazepine induces its own metabolism: after a few weeks from an initial dose, the serum level can be much lower. It therefore requires dose adjustments after initial dosing.

Class	Drug	CYP1A2	CYP2C9	CYP2C19	CYP2D6	CYP2E1	CYP3A4
Antidepressants and anxiolytics	Agomelatine	M					
	Amitriptyline		M	M	↓M		M
	Bupropion				↓		
	Buspirone						M
	Citalopram			M	M		M
	Clomipramine				M↓		
	Duloxetine	M			M↓		
	Escitalopram			M	↓		
	Fluoxetine				M↓		↓
	Fluvoxamine	M↓	↓	↓	M		↓
	Imipramine				M		M
	Mirtazapine						M
	Nortriptyline				M		
	Paroxetine				↓		↓
	Reboxetine						M
	St John's wort		↑	↑			↑
	Trazodone						M
	Venlafaxine				M		M
	Vortioxetine				M		
Antipsychotics	Aripiprazole				M		M
	Clozapine	M			↓		

(continued)

Class	Drug	CYP1A2	CYP2C9	CYP2C19	CYP2D6	CYP2E1	CYP3A4
	Haloperidol				M↓		M
	Lurasidone						M
	Olanzapine	M			M		
	Quetiapine						M
	Risperidone				M		
	Zuclopenthixol				M		
Anticonvulsants	Carbamazepine	↑	↑	↑			M↑
	Lamotrigine		M				
	Phenytoin	↑	M	M			M↑
	Valproate		M				
Sedatives	Alprazolam						M
	Clonazepam						M
	Diazepam			M			M
	Melatonin	M					
	Midazolam						M
	Nitrazepam						M
	Z-drugs						M
Substance misuse	Alcohol (acute)[1]					M↓	M↓
	Alcohol (chronic)[1]					M↑	↑
	Buprenorphine						M
	Caffeine	M					
	Codeine[2]				M		
	Disulfiram					↓	
	Methadone						M
	Tobacco (**not** NRT)	↑					
Cognitive enhancers / stimulants	Amphetamines				M		
	Atomoxetine				M		
	Donepezil						M
	Galantamine				M		M
	Modafinil		↓	↓			M
Cardiovascular	Amiodarone	↓	↓		↓		↓
	ARBs		M				
	Diltiazem/verapamil						M
	PDE inhibitors						M
	Statins						M
	Warfarin	M	M	M			M

(*continued*)

Class	Drug	CYP1A2	CYP2C9	CYP2C19	CYP2D6	CYP2E1	CYP3A4
GI	Cimetidine	↓		↓	↓		↓
	Omeprazole			M↓			
Antibiotics	Azole antifungals		↓	↓			↓
	Ciprofloxacin	↓					↓
	Clarithromycin/ erythromycin						M↓
	Cobicistat				M↓		M↓
	Efavirenz	↓	↓	↑			↑
	Metronidazole		↓				
	Protease inhibitors (not ritonavir)						M↓
	Rifampicin	↑	↑	↑			↑
	Ritonavir			↑	↓		M↓
Other	Calcineurin inhibitors						M
	Cyclophosphamide			M			
	Grapefruit juice	↓					↓
	NSAIDs		M				
	OCP						M
	Tamoxifen²				M		M
	Theophylline	M					

Source: **MPG**, Flockhart DA. 2007. *Drug Interactions: Cytochrome P450 Drug Interaction Table*. Indiana University School of Medicine. Available from https://drug-interactions.medicine.iu.edu. Accessed 15/10/2018.

Note: M, substrate of the enzyme (see 'metab by **P450**' in common drugs section entries); ↓, inhibitor of the enzyme; ↑, inducer of the enzyme. Interactions in **bold** are considered important by the sources that follow, but note that the potency of many interactions is not known.

[1] In occasional drinkers, the main enzyme responsible for metabolising *alcohol* is alcohol dehydrogenase, but in heavy drinkers, CYP2E1 is induced and has the greatest effect on alcohol metabolism.

[2] *Codeine* and *tamoxifen* are pro-drugs that *require* metabolism by CYP2D6 to become active. Pharmacological inhibition of CYP2D6 has been shown to ↓ the effectiveness of tamoxifen and ↑ risk of Ca recurrence.

Below are some of the most important interactions of psychotropic medications, along with a few important interactions of non-psychotropic medications. This table is **not** exhaustive.

Interactions with non-medicinal products

These are commonly used and easily forgotten about when taking a drug history or explaining how to take a medication.

- **St John's wort** induces CYP2C9, CYP2C19 and CYP3A4.
- Drinking **alcohol** as a one-off inhibits CYP2E1 and CYP3A4, but chronical alcohol use induces these enzymes. Patients who return from a one-off binge should have their medications reviewed before being administered (a) to avoid compounding respiratory depression and (b) to ensure there is no important pharmacokinetic interaction. In chronic alcoholism, dosing is complex because some cytochrome enzymes are induced, but active drug concentrations may be higher because of lower blood proteins.
- **Tobacco** induces CYP1A2, but NRT does not have this effect. Therefore, active smoking reduces clozapine levels, but smoking cessation causes an increase in clozapine levels.
- **Grapefruit juice** inhibits CYP1A2 and CYP3A4, so should generally be avoided by patients taking medications that are metabolised by these pathways.

OTHER IMPORTANT INTERACTIONS

- Many pharmacodynamic interactions are additive from multiple drugs with similar effects. Such interactions are often responsible for QTc prolongation, sedation and respiratory depression.
- **MAOIs** can cause a hypertensive crisis if taken in combination with foods high in tyramine or some nasal decongestants (see p. 223).
- Serotonin syndrome usually occurs in patients taking >1 medication or substance with **pro-serotonergic activity** (see p. 410).
- **Lithium** is renally excreted. **Diuretics, NSAIDs** and **ACEIs** can directly or indirectly impair lithium excretion, raising serum levels. Acetazolamide can increase lithium excretion.

- **Carbamazepine** has an active metabolite, carbamazepine-10,11-epoxide, which mediates many of the adverse effects of the drug. **Valproate** inhibits the enzyme that degrades it, increasing levels of carbamazepine-10,11-epoxide and worsening SEs.
- **Lamotrigine** is metabolised by UGT2B7, which is inhibited by valproate. If valproate is co-prescribed with lamotrigine, the dose of lamotrigine should be halved.

SIDE EFFECT PROFILES
Knowledge of these, together with a drug's mechanism(s), will simplify learning and allow anticipation of drug SEs.

Cholinoceptors
ACh stimulates nicotinic and muscarinic receptors. Anticholinesterases ⇒ ↑ ACh and ∴ stimulate both receptor types and have 'cholinergic fx'. Drugs that ↓ cholinoceptor action do so mostly via muscarinic receptors (antinicotinics used only in anaesthesia) and are ∴ more accurately called 'antimuscarinics' rather than 'anticholinergics'.

Cholinergic fx	Antimuscarinic fx
Generally ↑ secretions	*Generally ↓ secretions*
Diarrhoea	**Constipation**
Urination	**Urinary retention**
Miosis (constriction)	**Mydriasis ↓ accommodation**[2]
Bronchospasm/bradycardia[1]	**Bronchodilation/tachycardia**
Excitation of CNS (and muscle)	**Drowsiness, Dry eyes, Dry skin**
Lacrimation ↑	
Saliva/sweat ↑	
Commonly caused by	
Anticholinesterases:	Atropine, ipratropium
MG Rx, e.g. pyridostigmine	Antihistamines (including cyclizine)
Dementia Rx, e.g. rivastigmine, donepezil	Antidepressants (especially TCAs)
	Antipsychotics (especially 'typicals')
	Hyoscine, Ia antiarrhythmics

[1] Together with vasodilation ⇒ ↓BP.

[2] ↑blurred vision and ↑IOP.

Adrenoceptors

α generally excites sympathetic system (except*):

- $\alpha_1 \Rightarrow$ GI smooth-muscle relaxation*, otherwise contracts smooth muscle: vasoconstriction, GI/bladder sphincter constriction (uterus, seminal tract, iris). Also ↑ salivary secretion, ↓ glycogenolysis (in liver).
- $\alpha_2 \Rightarrow$ inhibition of neurotransmitters (especially NA and ACh for feedback control), Plt aggregation, contraction of vascular smooth muscle, inhibition of insulin release. Also prominent adrenoceptor of CNS (inhibits sympathetic outflow).

β generally inhibits sympathetic system (except*):

- $\beta_1 \Rightarrow$ ↑ HR*, ↑ contractility* (and ↑ salivary amylase secretion).
- $\beta_2 \Rightarrow$ vasodilation, bronchodilation, muscle tremor, glycogenolysis (in hepatic and skeletal muscle). Also ↑ renin secretion, relaxes ciliary muscle and visceral smooth muscles (GI sphincter, bladder detrusor, uterus if not pregnant).
- $\beta_3 \Rightarrow$ lipolysis, thermogenesis (of little pharmacological relevance).

Serotonin (5-HT)

Relative excess: 'Serotonin syndrome'; seen with antidepressants at ↑ doses or if swapped without adequate 'tapering' or 'washout period'. Initially causes restlessness, sweating and tremor, progressing to shivering, myoclonus and confusion, and, if severe enough, convulsions/death.

Relative deficit: 'Antidepressant withdrawal/discontinuation syndrome' occurs when antidepressants stopped too quickly; likelihood depends on $t_{1/2}$ of drug. Causes 'flu-like' symptoms (chills/sweating, myalgia, headache and nausea), shock-like sensations, dizziness, anxiety, irritability, insomnia, vivid dreams. Rarely ⇒ movement disorders and ↓ memory/concentration.

Dopamine (DA)

Relative excess: Causes behaviour changes, confusion and psychosis (especially if predisposed, e.g. schizophrenia). Seen with

L-dopa and DA agonists used in Parkinson's (and some endocrine disorders, e.g. bromocriptine).

Relative deficit: Causes extrapyramidal fx, ↑prolactin (sexual dysfunction, female infertility, gynaecomastia), NMS. Seen with DA antagonists, especially antipsychotics and certain antiemetics such as metoclopramide, prochlorperazine and levomepromazine.

Dopamine withdrawal syndrome can occur if a pro-dopaminergic drug, e.g. pramipexole, is suddenly stopped.

Extrapyramidal effects

Abnormalities of movement control arising from dysfunction of basal ganglia.

- *Parkinsonism:* Rigidity and bradykinesia ± tremor.
- *Dyskinesias* (= abnormal involuntary movements); commonly:
  - *Dystonia* (= abnormal posture): dynamic (e.g. oculogyric crisis) or static (e.g. torticollis).
  - *Tardive (delayed onset) dyskinesia:* Especially orofacial movements.
  - *Others:* Tremor, chorea, athetosis, hemiballismus, myoclonus, tics.
- *Akathisia* (= restlessness): Especially after large antipsychotic doses.

All are commonly caused by antipsychotics (especially older 'typical' drugs) and are a rare complication of antiemetics (e.g. metoclopramide, prochlorperazine – especially in young women). Dyskinesias and dystonias are common with antiparkinsonian drugs (especially peaks of L-dopa doses).

Most respond to stopping (or ↓dose of) the drug – if not possible, does not work or immediate Rx needed add antimuscarinic drug (e.g. procyclidine) but does not work for akathisia (try β-blocker) and can worsen tardive dyskinesia: seek neurology ± psychiatry opinion if in doubt. See p. 389.

Cerebellar effects

Especially antiseizure medications (e.g. phenytoin, valproate) and alcohol.

- **D**ysdiadochokinesis, dysmetria (= past-pointing) and rebound
- **A**taxia of gait (wide-based, irregular step length) ± trunk
- **N**ystagmus: Towards side of lesion; mostly coarse and horizontal
- **I**ntention tremor (also titubation = nodding-head tremor)
- **S**peech: Scanning dysarthria – slow, slurred or jerky
- **H**ypotonia (less commonly hyporeflexia or pendular reflexes)

PLACEBO/EXPECTANCY EFFECTS

- Placebo effects are due to the context surrounding medical treatment. They affect every treatment and every medical encounter to varying degrees.
- Placebo incorporates expectancy, suggestion and numerous other factors.
- Often seen as nuisance variables which complicate the interpretation of clinical trials, but modern research is beginning to take into account the potential positive effects.
- Research on open placebos (patient is told the treatment is a placebo) has indicated that even these have positive effects.
- Treatments which follow elaborate procedures in medical settings, e.g. sham rTMS, are more likely to show larger placebo effects.
- Placebo effects have robust neurobiological correlates, including activation of frontal cortices, ventral striatum and brainstem.
- The neurobiological correlates overlap with those of disorders such as depression, which show some of the larger placebo tendencies.
- Neurotransmitters implicated in placebo include endogenous opioids, dopamine, serotonin, cholecystokinin and oxytocin.
- Some have called for the leveraging of placebo effects in the treatment of neuropsychiatric disorders (Burke et al., *J Neuropsychiatry Clin Neurosci* 2020; 32:101–104).

FURTHER READING

Anderson & McAllister-Williams, *Fundamentals of Clinical Psychopharmacology*, 2016.

See also:
Ritter et al., *Rang & Dale's Pharmacology*, 8e, 2015.
Stahl, *Stahl's Essential Psychopharmacology: Neuroscientific Basis and Practical Applications*, 2013.
Davies & Nutt, *Psychiatry* 2004; 3(7): 268–72.

Emergencies

Most emergencies require transfer to a general hospital for definitive treatment, though some mild cases may occasionally be managed in a psychiatric setting. Emergency management may also be required prior to transfer. In all cases, include the following specific management as part of an **ABCDE** assessment.

In the following text, assume the emergency is taking place in a psychiatric inpatient environment with limited access to specialist medical care prior to transfer.

RAPID TRANQUILISATION (RT)

RT is parenteral pharmacological intervention with the goal to achieve a state of calmness without sedation, sleep or unconsciousness, but sedation may be considered an appropriate interim strategy.[BAP] There are several phases of the management of acute disturbance[BAP]:

- Pre-RT – de-escalation
- Pre-RT – by mouth (po)/inhaled (inh)/buccal treatment
- RT – intramuscular (im) treatment
- RT – im combinations
- RT – intravenous (iv) treatment

Some degree of physical restraint will often be required to administer RT safely.[BAP]

The skills and equipment for iv sedation are unlikely to be available in psychiatric settings, and thus routine use of iv medications in such settings cannot be recommended.[BAP]

Use of iv medications should be exceptional and restricted to appropriate settings, such as an emergency department.[BAP]

DE-ESCALATION

Should precede and accompany RT[NICE]

De-escalation techniques[BAP]:

- Continual risk assessment
- Self-control techniques (ensure own emotional regulation)
- Avoidance of provocation (be aware of known triggers)

- Respect patient space (↓ perceived threat)
- Management of environment (move other patients away or move patient to a more appropriate space)
- Passive intervention and watchful waiting (minimise cognitive load)
- Empathy (verbal and non-verbal)
- Reassurance
- Respect and avoidance of shame
- Appropriate use of humour
- Identification of patient needs (seeking to resolve them)
- Distraction
- Negotiation
- Reframing events (provide alternative interpretations)
- Non-confrontational limit setting (prevent a choice within certain boundaries)

MEDICATIONS

Adverse effects are frequently dose related, with higher doses and combinations having higher risks. Parenteral dosing is more likely to cause side effects compared with oral dosing. The following gives a list of drugs covered in this section; not all are recommended for RT.

Medication[BAP]	Route	Bioavailability	T_{max}	Side effects (SEs)
Promethazine	po	25%	2–3 h	Antimuscarinic fx, sedation, drowsiness, agitation, confusion, central nervous system (CNS) depression, hypotension, ↓seizure threshold, rarely extrapyramidal symptoms (EPS) and rarely neuroleptic malignant syndrome (NMS)
	im	100%	2–3 h	

(continued)

Medication[BAP]	Route	Bioavailability	T_{max}	Side effects (SEs)
Lorazepam	po	100%	2 h	↓ GCS, over-sedation, drowsiness, hypotension with risk of falls, **respiratory depression**, ataxia, cardiovascular collapse, amnesia, disinhibition (rare), dependence, tolerance (may ↓ efficacy)
	im	100%	1–1.5 h	
	iv	100%	sec–min	
Midazolam	Buccal	75%	30 min	
	im	>90%	30 min	
	iv	100%	sec–min	
Clonazepam	po	90%	1–4 h	
	im	93%	3 h	
Diazepam	po	76%	30–90 min	
	iv	100%	≤15 min	
Loxapine	inh	91%	2 min	Antimuscarinic fx, hypotension (particularly olanzapine and benzodiazepines combination), dystonia, akathisia, oculogyric crisis, parkinsonism, QTc prolongation (particularly haloperidol), NMS (see p. 409) Loxapine can ⇒ bronchospasm (consider prescribing prn salbutamol)
Aripiprazole	po	87%	3–5 h	
	im	100%	1 h	
Haloperidol	po	60–70%	2–6 h	
	im	100%	20–40 min	
	iv	100%	sec–min	
Olanzapine	po	Unknown	5–8 h	
	im	Unknown	15–45 min	
	iv	100%	sec–min	
Quetiapine	po	Unknown	1.5 h	
Risperidone	po	67%	1–2 h	
Droperidol	po	75%	1–2 h	
	im	100%	≤30 min	
	iv	100%	sec–min	
Zuclopenthixol acetate (Clopixol Acuphase)[SPC]	im	100%	36 h	

Source: Schwinghammer et al., *Biopharm Drug Dispos* 1984; **5**(2): 185–94; Beradis et al., *Int J Mol Sci* 2017; **18**(2): 349.

- When deciding between options, consider patient preference, health problems/pregnancy, intoxication, previous response, SEs, interactions and total dose prescribed.[NICE]
- For im RT, use lorazepam rather than an antipsychotic if no info about previous response, no ECG, pre-existing cardiac disease or antipsychotic-naïve.[NICE]

T_{max} is the time taken to reach maximum plasma concentration of a drug, although some effect (usually level of sedation) is usually observed earlier than this point.

Do not normally exceed BNF max doses (**including regular and PRN medication**) and only do so under direction of a senior doctor.[NICE]

Avoid prescribing multiple antipsychotics (including regular) where possible.

> **Akathisia** is a feeling of restlessness and an inability to stay still. It is a SE of antipsychotics and can resemble agitation. Avoid giving further RT as additional antipsychotics may worsen it.[BAP]

PO/INH/BUCCAL TREATMENT

- No difference in efficacy between typical and atypical antipsychotics.[BAP]
- Do not use oral **clonazepam** or **diazepam** acutely: no evidence for efficacy and they can accumulate.[BAP]
- Buccal midazolam may have a more rapid onset of action and be associated with greater sedation and respiratory depression than other benzodiazepines, but is shorter acting.
- Administration of buccal medication may be difficult in an acute disturbance setting.
- Orodispersible formulations act no more quickly than normal tablets, but it is easier to ensure compliance.[BAP]
- ECG advisable before giving haloperidol.[SPC]
- Inhaled **loxapine**[BAP]:
  - Requires some patient cooperation.

- Due to the risk of bronchospasm, it is contraindicated in respiratory distress or active airways disease (e.g. asthma, COPD).
- Assess respiratory function before administering.
- Have a salbutamol inhaler to hand in case of bronchospasm (often within 1 h).

IM TREATMENT

- **Haloperidol** can cause acute dystonia, so should not be used as monotherapy, but the addition of promethazine $\Rightarrow \downarrow$ EPSEs, so the combination is an option. Haloperidol + lorazepam is also an option.[BAP]
- Leave 1 h between im **olanzapine** and IM **benzodiazepine** due to risk of hypotension and respiratory depression.[BAP]
- High doses of antipsychotics do not cause more rapid or effective sedation, but they $\uparrow$ SEs.[BAP]
- **Lorazepam** may cause respiratory depression; increased risk in those with lung pathology or if administered in combination with other sedating medications, particularly opioids and/ or alcohol. Some guidelines recommend having iv flumazenil available, but there are numerous CIs and it should only be used by those experienced with its use or in rare cases of severe isolated benzodiazepine toxicity. In practice, the emphasis should be on an ABCDE approach and emergency transfer to medical care.
- **Haloperidol** or **droperidol** in any formulation should only be used with a pre-treatment ECG.[BAP]
- **Droperidol** is structurally similar to haloperidol, but is more sedative. It was withdrawn from use in the United Kingdom in 2001 due to QTc prolongation, although there is some recent evidence supporting its use.[BAP]
- **Promethazine** is useful in benzodiazepine-tolerant patients.[BAP]

IV TREATMENT

- Only use IV treatment in settings where resuscitation equipment and clinicians trained for medical emergencies are available.[BAP]

- If giving IV **diazepam**:
  - Flumazenil must be confirmed as immediately available.
  - Use emulsified formulation (Diazemuls), not the aqueous solution.[BAP]
  - It can accumulate.[BAP]
  - Give 1 mL/min (not bolus).[BAP]
  - Keep patient supine for ≥1 h after administration.[BAP]
- Only give IV **haloperidol** or droperidol with continuous cardiac monitoring to detect QTc prolongation and arrhythmias.[BAP]
- IV **olanzapine** is effective, but should be used with caution due to risk of respiratory depression and lack of reversal agent.[BAP]
- Others e.g. dexmedetomidine may be effective in general hospital settings (Castro & Butler et al., *Journal of the Academy of Consultation-Liaison Psychiatry*, 2024)

ZUCLOPENTHIXOL ACETATE
(CLOPIXOL ACUPHASE)

- IM injection form of the typical antipsychotic, often known by its brand name Clopixol Acuphase. It must be distinguished from the long-acting depot zuclopenthixol *decanoate*.
- Not a form of RT as the sedative effect can take several hours to develop and has a prolonged duration, but it is sometimes an option once RT options have been exhausted.[BAP]
- Main advantage is ↓ number of injections.[BAP]
- However, marked risks, including coma and fatal arrhythmia. Do not give if patient accepting oral treatment, antipsychotic naïve, sensitive to EPSEs, unconscious, pregnant or with hepatic/renal/cardiac disease. Do not give at the same time as other parenteral antipsychotics (wait at least 1 h for IM, 15 min for IV before giving Acuphase). It is often given at the same time as lorazepam and can be given safely as the T_{max} is different.
- Perform an ECG before use.[BAP]

BAP/NAPICU ALGORITHM

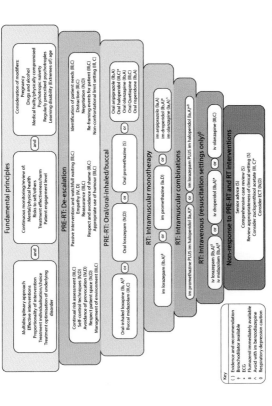

Reprinted from Patel & Sethi et al. *Journal of Psychopharmacology*, 32(6), 601–640, 2018, SAGE Publishing, https://doi.org/10.1177/0269881118776738.

PREGNANCY

- Complex area, so seek senior advice.
- Try to avoid medications, but weigh against risks of untreated illness and/or physical restraint.[BAP]
- Medications with short half-lives are recommended.
- No contraindications for promethazine, lorazepam or haloperidol.[BAP]
- Giving meds immediately before birth should be avoided. When given in late pregnancy, benzos ⇒ floppy baby syndrome, while antipsychotics ⇒ neonatal EPSEs.[BAP]
- If RT is required during labour, an iv benzodiazepine with an anaesthetist and paediatrician present should be considered.

MINIMUM MONITORING POST-INTERVENTIONS

Intervention		Physical monitoring[BAP]	Psychiatric observations[BAP]
Pre-RT		News hourly for ≥1 h	Hourly
im RT[a]	Most patients	News every 15 min for ≥1 h	Every 15 min
	Patient over-sedated, asleep or physically unwell	News every 15 min for ≥1 h + continuous pulse oximetry until ambulatory	Continuous (within eyesight)
iv RT		Continuous monitoring with availability of resuscitation facilities	Continuous (within arm's length)

[a] Buccal midazolam and loxapine may require monitoring according to im schedule due to risk of respiratory dysfunction.

DRUG TOXICITY SYNDROMES

Unless you are familiar with the up-to-date management of the specific overdose in question, the following sources should always be consulted:

- *Toxbase website (https://www.toxbase.org):* Authoritative and updated regularly by the NPIS. Should be used in the first instance to check clinical features and Mx of the poison(s) in question. If you use the website, you will need to sign in under your departmental account; if your department is not registered, contact your A&E department to obtain a username and password. An app exists and requires an nhs.net email address to register.
- *NPIS:* If in the United Kingdom, phone 0344 892 0111 (if in Republic of Ireland 01 809 2566) for advice if unsure of Toxbase instructions and for rarer/mixed ODs.

Check paracetamol concentration in all patients who have taken an overdose and are unable or unwilling to give an accurate history.

OPIOID OVERDOSE

(Thanacoody, *BMJ Best Practice* 2018, https://bestpractice.bmj.com/topics/en-gb/339)

Signs: Respiratory depression (e.g. RR <12 when awake) and failure, miosis, ↓ consciousness.

NB: Hypercapnia is commonly present; clinically significant hypoxia is a terminal event.

Give naloxone according to the regimen below:

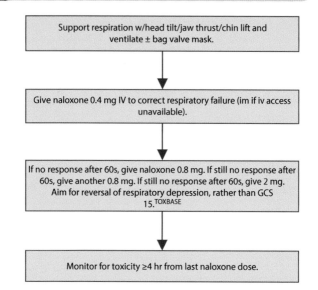

Support respiration w/head tilt/jaw thrust/chin lift and ventilate ± bag valve mask.

Give naloxone 0.4 mg IV to correct respiratory failure (im if iv access unavailable).

If no response after 60s, give naloxone 0.8 mg. If still no response after 60s, give another 0.8 mg. If still no response after 60s, give 2 mg. Aim for reversal of respiratory depression, rather than GCS 15.TOXBASE

Monitor for toxicity ≥4 hr from last naloxone dose.

- In the case of cardiac arrest, administer naloxone while giving CPR.
- Examine the patient for opioid patches, which may be causing the toxicity.
- Be aware naloxone may not be fully effective in reversing buprenorphine and tramadol overdosage due to their complex pharmacology.
- Naloxone is generally safe and has no contraindications. However, its action is much shorter than the duration of many opioids, so it is common for toxicity to return once naloxone has worn off.
- Naloxone will precipitate withdrawal in dependent individuals, but opioid withdrawal is not fatal. Consider transfer to general hospital.

BENZODIAZEPINE OVERDOSE

Signs: ↓Consciousness, mild respiratory depression, ataxia. Respiratory depression with oral benzodiazepines alone is rare and more commonly occurs when co-ingested with other substances (e.g. alcohol or opiates).[MPG]

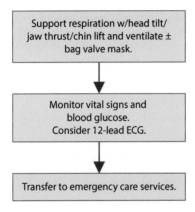

Support respiration w/head tilt/ jaw thrust/chin lift and ventilate ± bag valve mask.

↓

Monitor vital signs and blood glucose. Consider 12-lead ECG.

↓

Transfer to emergency care services.

- Main focus should be to resuscitate according to ABCDE approach and transfer care to emergency services.
- Flumazenil should generally only be given by those with previous experience of its use.[BNF, MPG]
- Use is hazardous and it risks causing seizures and ventricular arrhythmias.[MPG]
- Unlike naloxone, **flumazenil** can only be given IV and should not be given in those with epilepsy, benzodiazepine dependence, prolonged QT or who have co-ingested other drugs (contraindicated in mixed OD) due to risk of causing seizures.
- Flumazenil will induce withdrawal in benzodiazepine-dependent individuals.

- If there is no response after the patient has received a total dose of 2 mg within a few minutes it is unlikely that flumazenil will reverse the respiratory depression.
- Consider transfer to general hospital.

PARACETAMOL OVERDOSE

Significant OD is >75 mg/kg in any 24 h period (toxicity may occur if >150 mg/kg, toxicity uncommon if 75–150 mg/kg).

If paracetamol OD is suspected, urgent assessment is required, as treatment must be commenced within 8 h.

Initial management

This depends on time since ingestion. 0–8 h post-ingestion:

- *Activated charcoal:* If available and within 1 h of significant OD.
- *Acetylcysteine:* Wait until 4 h post-ingestion before taking urgent sample for paracetamol concentration (results are meaningless until this time). If patient presents at 4–8 h post-ingestion, take sample ASAP.

If concentration is above the treatment line (see Figure 6.1), use the following dosing regimen for acetylcysteine: First dose: 150 mg/kg body weight (maximum 16.5 g) in 200 mL 5% dextrose or 0.9% sodium chloride over 1 h; Second dose: 50 mg/kg body weight (maximum 5.5 g) in 500 mL 5% dextrose or 0.9% sodium chloride and infuse over 4 h; Third dose: 100 mg/kg (maximum 11 g) in 1 L 5% dextrose or 0.9% sodium chloride and infuse over the next 16 h

OR

First dose: acetylcysteine 100 mg/kg body weight (maximum 11 g) in 200 mL 5% glucose or 0.9% sodium chloride over 2 h; Second dose: 200 mg/kg body weight (maximum 22 g) in 1 L 5% glucose or 0.9% sodium chloride and infuse over the next 10 h.

Strongly consider transfer to general hospital.

> Do not delay acetylcysteine beyond 8 h post-ingestion if
> waiting for paracetamol concentration and if OD is >150 mg/
> kg (beyond 8 h, efficacy ↓s substantially) – ivi can be stopped
> if concentrations come back as below treatment line and
> international normalised ratio (INR), alanine (-amino)
> transferase (ALT) and creatinine normal.

In staggered ODs, patients who have taken >150 mg/kg in 24 h
should have acetylcysteine immediately.

8–24 h post-ingestion:

- *Acetylcysteine:* Give regimen as previously stated ASAP if
  >150 mg/kg OD taken. Do not wait for urgent paracetamol
  concentration.

>24 h post-ingestion:

- Acetylcysteine is controversial when presenting this late.
- Give acetylcysteine immediately to all patients if it is thought
  that ≥150 mg/kg paracetamol has been ingested as an acute
  overdose, or if patient is symptomatic with jaundice or hepatic
  tenderness.
- If the patient is asymptomatic and has ingested <150 mg/kg,
  wait for blood results before considering treatment with
  acetylcysteine.
- Consider transfer to general hospital.
- Check creatinine, LFTs, INR, glucose and paracetamol
  concentration, and consult Toxbase or NPIS for individual
  cases.

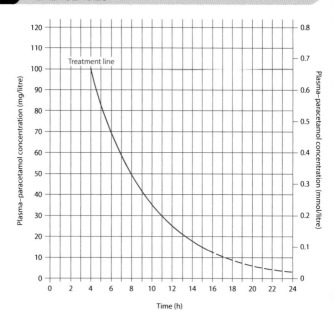

Figure 6.1 Treatment lines for acetylcysteine treatment of paracetamol overdose. (Reproduced with permission of the MHRA under the terms of the Open Government Licence (OGL) v3.0.)

Medical clearance

Patients may be *medically* fit for discharge once acetylcysteine ivi is completed, and INR, ALT, creatinine and HCO_3^- ($\pm$ pH) are normal (or recovering in two successive checks if additional acetylcysteine has been administered). In patients with laboratory abnormalities despite acetylcysteine, consult Toxbase $\pm$ NPIS for advice on further acetylcysteine and specialist referral.

ANTIPSYCHOTIC OVERDOSE^{TOXBASE}

Features: CNS depression, acute dystonia, blurred vision, fluctuating mental state. Less commonly, ↓/↑blood pressure (BP), ↓/↑heart rate (HR), seizures, renal failure, coma. NMS (see next section) can occur at any point in Rx, but it is **not** especially common in overdose.

Clozapine toxicity is increased in clozapine-naïve patients. Features can persist for several days.

Serotonin syndrome (p. 410) may occasionally occur in overdose of atypical antipsychotics.

Patients require a medical assessment (in addition to a psychiatric assessment) if dose > toxic dose (see table below), ≥2 drugs taken, symptomatic or phenothiazine taken by a patient who does not usually take phenothiazines.

Drug	Suggested toxic po dose
Haloperidol	0.5 mg/kg
Chlorpromazine	6 mg/kg
Sulpiride	25 mg/kg
Trifluoperazine	0.4 mg/kg
Flupentixol	0.13 mg/kg
Fluphenazine	0.2 mg/kg
Zuclopenthixol	0.6 mg/kg
Olanzapine	1.5 mg/kg
Risperidone	1 mg/kg
Paliperidone	0.4 mg/kg
Quetiapine	15 mg/kg
Amisulpride	25 mg/kg
Clozapine	10 mg/kg
Lurasidone	10 mg/kg
Aripiprazole	1 mg/kg

Mx includes: Consideration of activated charcoal (if presenting within 1 h), provided airway can be protected. 12-lead ECG, checking for QT prolongation. Magnesium sulphate for torsade de pointes, VF or VT preceded by prolonged QT. A single brief seizure does not need treatment; otherwise use benzodiazepines. Procyclidine or diazepam for acute dystonia. Fluids for hypotension.

Observe for ≥6 h post-ingestion (≥12 h for clozapine). Following clozapine overdose, full blood count (FBC) must be monitored weekly for ≥3 wks to check for agranulocytosis.

Acute dystonia may rarely occur some days after overdose in naïve patients. Patients should be warned of this possibility and advised to seek treatment if this occurs.

ANTIDEPRESSANT OVERDOSE^{TOXBASE}

Features: Tremor, agitation, tachycardia, QTc prolongation (more with citalopram), torsade de pointes, ↑/↓ BP, rhabdomyolysis, serotonin syndrome (see next section).

In addition, TCAs can cause antimuscarinic fx (sinus tachycardia, confusion, drowsiness, dry mouth and dilated pupils), convulsions, coma, ↑tone and hyperreflexia. Arrhythmias can occur shortly after ingestion.

Patients require a medical assessment (in addition to psychiatric assessment) if dose>toxic dose (see table below), ≥2 drugs taken or symptomatic.

Fatalities are rare when SSRIs or mirtazapine are taken alone. TCAs and MAOIs can be very dangerous.

Mx is mainly supportive, but can include: consideration of activated charcoal (if presenting within 1 h), provided airway can be protected. Magnesium sulphate for torsade de pointes, VF or VT preceded by prolonged QT. Monitoring of ABGs, U&Es, blood glucose and SpO_2. Treat seizures and agitation with benzodiazepines. For TCAs, consider iv sodium bicarbonate.

Observe for ≥6 h post-ingestion.

Drug	Suggested toxic dose	Drug	Suggested toxic dose
Citalopram	2 mg/kg	Doxepin	4 mg/kg
Escitalopram	1 mg/kg	Trimipramine	5 mg/kg
Sertraline	7 mg/kg	Mirtazapine	5 mg/kg
Fluoxetine	6 mg/kg	Mianserin	4 mg/kg
Fluvoxamine	15 mg/kg	Trazodone	15 mg/kg
Paroxetine	3 mg/kg	Phenelzine	2.5 mg/kg
Duloxetine	5 mg/kg	Tranylcypromine	0.4 mg/kg
Venlafaxine	7 mg/kg	Isocarboxazid	0.6 mg/kg
Clomipramine	4 mg/kg	Moclobemide	30 mg/kg
Amitriptyline	3 mg/kg	Vortioxetine	1 mg/kg
Dosulepin	3 mg/kg	Reboxetine	0.5 mg/kg
Imipramine	4 mg/kg	Bupropion	6 mg/kg
Nortriptyline	2.5 mg/kg	Agomelatine	3 mg/kg
Lofepramine	4.5 mg/kg		

NEUROLEPTIC MALIGNANT SYNDROME (NMS)

Wadoo et al. *BJPsych Advances.* 2021, 27(6).

- *Risk factors:* Parkinson's, alcohol-related brain damage, learning disability, agitation, dehydration, high-potency first-generation antipsychotics, rapid antipsychotic dose ↑, multiple antipsychotics, abrupt withdrawal of anticholinergics
- *Clinical features:* Muscle rigidity, hyperpyrexia, altered consciousness and autonomic instability, usually with an insidious onset
- *Blood markers:* ↑CK, ↑WCC, ↓iron and ↑LFTs
- Management in a psychiatric unit mostly consists of urgent transfer to general hospital. Cease dopamine antagonists and consider im benzodiazepines.[MPG]

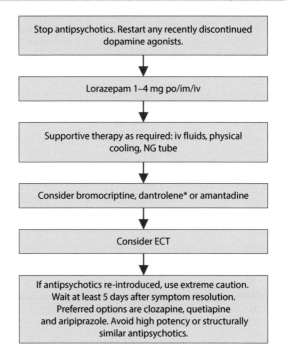

Stop antipsychotics. Restart any recently discontinued dopamine agonists.

↓

Lorazepam 1–4 mg po/im/iv

↓

Supportive therapy as required: iv fluids, physical cooling, NG tube

↓

Consider bromocriptine, dantrolene* or amantadine

↓

Consider ECT

↓

If antipsychotics re-introduced, use extreme caution. Wait at least 5 days after symptom resolution. Preferred options are clozapine, quetiapine and aripiprazole. Avoid high potency or structurally similar antipsychotics.

* Dantrolene not to be used as monotherapy due to increased mortality rates, but can be added as an adjunct to dopamine agonists.

SEROTONIN SYNDROME

(Boyer & Shannon, *NEJM* 2005; **352**(11): 1112–20; Ellahi, *BJPsych Adv* 2015; **21**(5): 324–32)

- Occurs in up to 1% of patients on SSRI monotherapy but 15% of those with antidepressant overdose.
- Serotonin toxicity is common following SSRI/SNRI overdose. Co-ingestion with olanzapine or risperidone ↓risk 2–6-fold and moclobemide ↑risk 5-fold.

- *Drugs responsible (often in combination or with CYP inhibition):* serotonergic antidepressants, lithium, St John's wort, some opioids (tramadol, pethidine, fentanyl, buprenorphine, dextromethorphan), certain Abx (linezolid, isoniazid), selegiline, some recreational drugs (cocaine, amphetamine, MDMA), carbamazepine, methylphenidate, certain antipsychotics (risperidone, olanzapine), triptans.
- *Features:* Agitation, (myo)clonus, autonomic instability, pyrexia, hyperreflexia*, tremor, diaphoresis, diarrhoea, midriasis*, rigors and rigidity, usually with a rapid onset. Death can occur within 24 h.

* Symptoms used to help differentiate serotonin syndrome from NMS.

Management:

- Stop serotonergic drugs. Look for and remove opioid patches.
- Avoid physical restraint, as can worsen lactic acidosis.
- Diazepam for agitation.
- General hospital: cyproheptadine (5-HT$_{2A}$ antagonist) po 12 mg stat, then 2 mg every 2 h for ongoing Sx.
- Physical cooling.

LITHIUM TOXICITY

(^{TOXBASE} Haussmann et al., *Int J Bipolar Disord* 2015; 3(1): 23)

If a patient on lithium has accidentally taken twice their daily dose, advise them to omit their next dose and then continue as normal. In all other cases of lithium overdose, a patient should have medical assessment, including an urgent lithium concentration measurement.

- *Risk factors:* Dehydration, hyponatraemia, renal impairment, certain drugs NSAIDs, ACE-i, thiazide diuretics)

- *Features:* Coarse tremor, nausea, drowsiness, confusion, diarrhoea, seizures, ECG changes (heart block, bradycardia, ST elevation)

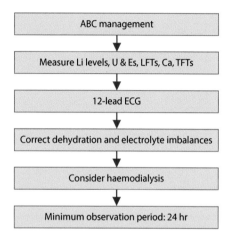

Activated charcoal is not helpful in lithium toxicity.

Symptoms may be delayed and repeat lithium concentrations are necessary (see TOXBASE). Lithium toxicity is often more profound in those already established on lithium, as lithium has saturated their tissues.

ALCOHOL AND DRUG WITHDRAWAL SYNDROMES

ALCOHOL WITHDRAWAL
(Shuckit, *NEJM* 2014; **371**(22): 2109–113); also see www.asam.org/quality-care/clinical-guidelines/alcohol-withdrawal-management-guideline)

This covers more severe alcohol withdrawal and delirium tremens. For milder Sx, see p. 252.

The diagnostic criteria for alcohol withdrawal are met when two or more of the following are present:

- Autonomic hyperactivity (e.g. sweating or pulse >100bpm)
- Increased hand tremor
- Insomnia
- Nausea or vomiting
- Transient visual, tactile or auditory hallucinations or illusions
- Psychomotor agitation
- Anxiety
- Grand mal seizures

Withdrawal begins 10–72 h after last drink.

The revised Clinical Institute Withdrawal Assessment for Alcohol (CIWA-Ar) scale should be used to determine both the severity of withdrawal and the need for treatment. Patients should be treated with regimens that are patient-specific and flexible to respond to changes in severity of withdrawal (symptom triggered). Fixed treatment schedules, where the patient is given a standard regimen irrespective of their symptoms, are inappropriate.

Treatment should be initiated when the CIWA-Ar score is >8; this will benefit the patient symptomatically. When the CIWA-Ar score is ≥15, the use of a symptom-triggered regimen reduces the risk of major complications developing.

- Consider transfer to intensive care unit.
- Bloods: U&E, FBC, LFTs.
- Monitor CIWA-Ar score and vital signs at least every 30 min.
- Pabrinex iv, one pair of ampoules daily for 3–5 days. Consider regular thiamine and vitamin B compound strong after.
- Rehydration po/iv.
- Benzodiazepines (preferably iv), e.g. diazepam 10–20 mg iv, repeated as required to control features. Initially, doses may be needed every few minutes if diagnosis has been delayed.

- If antipsychotic effect required, use haloperidol 0.5–5 mg po/im. Many other antipsychotics should be avoided due to proconvulsant effect.
- Provide reorientation (see Delirium p. 321).

OPIOID WITHDRAWAL

Features: Yawning, sweating, salivation, lacrimation, urination, defaecation, abdominal pain, muscle cramps

Opioid withdrawal can be extremely unpleasant, but it is not life-threatening. See p. 257.

BENZODIAZEPINE WITHDRAWAL

(Puening et al., *J Emerg Med* 2017)

- *Features:* Anxiety, panic, tremor, hallucinations, hyperventilation, generalised tonic-clonic seizures. Timing dependent on $t_{1/2}$ of the benzodiazepine.
- Normally managed in the community (see p. 277), but if there is abrupt discontinuation, delirium, seizures or psychosis can develop, requiring hospitalisation.
- Prolonged seizures in benzodiazepine withdrawal can be life-threatening.
- Treat symptomatically with po diazepam (iv if patient unable to swallow). Re-evaluate regularly.
- May use haloperidol (as in delirium tremens) if psychosis does not respond to benzodiazepines.

GHB/GBL WITHDRAWAL^{TOXBASE}

- *Features:* Agitation, insomnia, confusion, hallucinations, seizures, rigidity. $t_{1/2}$ <1 h, so withdrawal can be rapid and severe. Withdrawal resembles alcohol withdrawal with more prominent neuropsychiatric features, and may be more prolonged (up to 2 wks).

- *Management:*
  - Ensure clear airway, monitor vital signs, ECG and bloods
  - Hydration po/iv
  - Diazepam 10–20 mg 2–4 hourly (max 100 mg/24 h) according to Sx
  - Baclofen 10–20 mg qds
  - Monitor for seizures

ACUTE DYSTONIA

More common with typical antipsychotics (can occur with atypicals and antidepressants) and takes several forms: **laryngeal dystonia** (stridor, dyspnoea and respiratory distress), **torticollis** (twisted neck), **opisthotonus** (back arching), **trismus** (limited jaw opening), **blepharospasm** (eyelids forced shut) and **oculogyric crisis** (eyes fixed in upward gaze). Onset can be delayed by hours or a few days. May be more common in younger patients, and those antipsychotic-naïve.

Management:

- Secure airway (rarely needed)
- Consider procyclidine 5–10 mg im/iv stat
- Review antipsychotic prescription

HIV POST-EXPOSURE PROPHYLAXIS (PEP)

(Cresswell et al. 'UK guideline for the use of HIV post-exposure prophylaxis 2021', *HIV Medicine* 2022; **23**(5): 449–569)

- Risky sexual practices are common in mania and acute psychosis.
- Needle sharing may occur in IVDUs.

Exposure

- Involve infectious disease expert +/– occupational health (if staff affected).

- All those with potential exposures should have counselling and be offered support.

When to give PEP:

	Source HIV status		
	HIV+		**High-risk group with unknown HIV status**
	Viral load >200/mL or unknown	**On ART with sustained viral load <200/mL**	
Receptive anal sex	✓	✗	✓
Insertive anal sex	✓	✗	C
Receptive vaginal sex	✓	✗	✗
Insertive vaginal sex	C	✗	✗
Needle sharing	✓	✗	✗
Needlestick injury	✓	✗	✗*

Note: ✓, give PEP; C, consider PEP; ✗, do not give PEP.
* Unless exceptional circumstances, see full guideline.

High-risk groups in the UK are men who have sex with men, intravenous drug users (IVDUs) from high-risk countries (e.g. Eastern Europe and Central Asia) and immigrants from countries where HIV prevalence >1% (e.g. Sub-Saharan Africa).

PEP is not generally recommended following oral sex or human bites. Ideally, start PEP within 24 h of exposure, but it can be considered up to 72 h. Prescribe Truvada **(tenofovir disoproxil fumarate 245 mg and emtricitabine 200 mg) 1 tab od + raltegravir 1200 mg od for 28 days.** Always check for drug interactions (including with psychotropic drugs), so check at https://www.hiv-druginteractions.org/checker.

Baseline bloods should include HIV/hep B/hep C/syphilis serology, hep B sAg, U&E, LFT. Also perform baseline STIs screen, urinalysis and pregnancy test as appropriate. Pregnancy does not contraindicate PEP, but testing allows an informed discussion.

PEP may be initiated out-of-hours by a non-specialist, but there should be prompt discussion with an HIV specialist with arrangement for follow-up.

Attempt to gain history from source if confirmed HIV+: current treatment and resistance may, rarely, warrant deviation from standard PEP.

HANGING

1. **Call for help,** particularly if you are on your own, but minimise delays to step 2.
2. **Remove any ligature** from around neck. If patient still suspended, support the body while doing this. Support the C-spine as best you can.
3. Standard **ABC assessment** and management, considering the following:

> C-spine injuries are only common if patient has dropped from more than their body height. In practice, most attempted hangings have not generated forces likely to injure the bony spine. Though C-spine injury should always be considered, airway compromise and asphyxia, and reduced cerebral perfusion are the most likely causes of injury and death. Restoring the airway and circulation is therefore the highest priority of First Aid in attempted hanging, over C-spine control.

   a. *Airway:* Lie patient on floor and assess. Support airway if necessary, preferentially with a **jaw thrust,** to avoid destabilising the C-spine.

With the patient supine, this is achieved by approaching the patient from behind (cranially, with their body directed away from you). The heels of the hands grasp the sides of the patient's head as a solid base of support, and the index fingers are placed behind the mandible, to displace it anteriorly. Specifically try to avoid the 'Head tilt, chin lift' technique of opening a compromised airway – this technique tends to extend the neck, which may be unsafe in the setting of cervical spinal injury. However, if a jaw thrust is unsuccessful, other airway-opening techniques should be employed to prevent death from asphyxiation. More is to be lost by inadequately managing an airway than the unlikely event of destabilising an injury of the cervical spine.

b. *Breathing and circulation:* If not breathing, or pulseless, initiate Basic Life Support (BLS). The patient may be apnoeic but have a pulse, in which case rescue breaths are indicated. Continue to administer BLS until help arrives. If breathing and circulation are intact, place the patient in the recovery position. This is best achieved by two people, with one attempting to maintain the C-spine in an anatomically neutral position, neither flexed, nor extended. This position may be supported manually, until help arrives. Ensure that breathing and circulation are maintained.

Petechiae in the face and conjunctivae are common.

SELF-LACERATION

Often superficial with only simple dressing required. Occasionally, there is risk of significant haemorrhage. The principles of haemorrhage control in first aid are *pressure* and *elevation*. Most commonly, bleeding of the limbs can be controlled by these measures alone. Penetrating injuries to the torso, thighs (particularly groin), head or neck, require urgent specialist assessment.

- Ensure your own safety – do not proceed if there is a risk of injury to yourself.

- Apply gloves.
- Remove any clothing necessary to expose the wound.
- If there is an object in the wound, do not remove it, but apply pressure to either side of it. Apply direct pressure to wound, with gauze and a bandage. If not available, use any material to hand, particularly if bleeding is brisk.
- Raise the affected limb with the injury higher than the heart to reduce blood flow. Lie the patient flat.
- If bleeding is not controlled, ensure that pressure is being properly applied over the wound. Sometimes, in the urgency to control haemorrhage, pressure is ineffectively applied, and then masked by a bandage. A cool head, and recommencing an assessment from scratch, is often the most effective strategy. Thereafter, try to disturb the wound as little as possible.

Lacerations to specific areas
- *Limb:* If bleeding remains uncontrolled despite firm local pressure and elevation, a tourniquet may be applied, proximal to (above) the bleeding point. This is uncommonly required but may be lifesaving in acute, severe haemorrhage. A tourniquet may be a belt or any ligature, tied tightly enough that the bleeding is controlled, in combination with local pressure and elevation. Facilitate urgent transfer to A&E by ambulance. Ensure that all parties are aware that a tourniquet has been applied.
- *Torso/abdomen:* Apply pressure to control external haemorrhage. It will not be possible to control internal haemorrhage. Lie the patient flat and facilitate urgent transfer to A&E by ambulance.
- *Neck:* Sitting the patient up can decrease bleeding, particularly from veins, and often provides effective haemorrhage control, in combination with manually applied, local pressure. Sitting the patient up achieves elevation of the injury – be aware that lying the patient flat may increase bleeding. However, if the patient's level of consciousness drops, suggestive of cerebral hypoperfusion, the patient should be laid flat. Never apply a circumferential bandage to the neck, for obvious reasons.

- Complete ABCDE assessment – Part of E is ensuring that all penetrating injuries are accounted for. You may have perfectly managed their superficial wrist wounds, but is there an occult, penetrating wound to the abdomen?

SEIZURES (EPILEPTIC AND FUNCTIONAL)

(Adapted from Mellers J, *Postgrad Med J* 2005; **81**(958): 498–504)

	Functional seizure	Epileptic seizure
Distinguishing features		
Timing		
• Gradual onset	Common	Rare
• Waxing and waning	Common	Very rare
• Duration >5 min	Common	Rare (but serious)
Motor		
• Side-to-side head movement	Common	Rare
• Asynchronous thrashing movements	Common	Very rare
• Pelvic thrusting	Occasional	Rare
Eyes		
• Eyes closed	Common	Rare
• Unreactive pupils	Rare	Common
Post-ictal		
• Recall for unresponsive period	Common	Very rare
Acute management[a]	• Avoid benzodiazepines (worsen dissociation) and other anticonvulsants	(SIGN 143) *Initial management:* • Secure airway • High-flow O_2 • Vital signs • Obtain iv access • Time seizure

(*continued*)

	Functional seizure	Epileptic seizure
	• Ensure safe in surroundings, e.g. by removing hard or sharp objects if able to. • Adopt a calm, non-judgemental tone with patient; reassurance during seizure may be beneficial. • Avoid calling for emergency medical support or treatment if certain patient has an established Dx and is currently having a functional seizure.	*If seizure persists >5 min give one of:* • Midazolam 10 mg buccal/ intranasal (preferred option) • Lorazepam 4 mg iv (if midazolam not available) • Diazepam 10 mg pr/iv (if other options not available) *If no response within 10 min, may repeat dose of benzodiazepine and transfer to A&E for iv anticonvulsant (e.g. phenytoin, levetiracetam, valproate). Exclude or treat reversible metabolic causes, especially ↓O$_2$, ↓glucose (give thiamine as well as glucose in alcoholic or malnourished patient)*

a If type of seizure is uncertain, treat as an epileptic seizure and seek a specialist opinion.

NB:

• Patients can, and often do, have both epileptic and functional seizures, so identifying one type does not exclude other types occurring, too. Ensure history taken from patient ± collateral of multiple seizure types.
• Many psychotropics (serotonergics, antipsychotics) can lower seizure threshold and should be reviewed if epileptic seizures occur or are suspected.
• Clozapine is particularly prone to inducing seizures during titration and after dose increases.

ACUTE CORONARY SYNDROMES (ACS)

In the psychiatric setting, the onus should be on an ABCDE approach, assessment of the clinical picture and prompt transfer to general hospital.

Clues: angina, N&V, sweating, LVF, arrhythmias, Hx of IHD. Remember atypical pain and silent infarcts in DM, elderly or if ↓GCS.

ACS encompasses the following:

1 **STEMI:** ST elevation myocardial infarction.
2 **NSTEMI:** Non-ST elevation MI; troponin (T or I) +ve.
3 **UA(P):** Unstable angina (pectoris); troponin (T or I) –ve.

FOR ALL (SUSPECTED) ACS

- Arrange urgent transfer (999); patient may go to A&E or straight to catheter lab (particularly if STEMI).
- Perform a 12-lead ECG, but not if this delays transfer.
- Do not routinely administer O_2, but monitor O_2 sats using pulse oximetry as soon as possible to guide the use of supportive O_2 to maintain >94% (or 88%–92% if known T2RF).
- Aspirin: 300 mg po stat (chewable/dispersible form) unless CI.
- Offer iv or sc analgesia (morphine) if available.
- GTN: one to two sprays or SL tablets (300 micrograms to 1 mg). NB: can ⇒ ↓BP; do not give if systolic ≤100 mm Hg or inferior infarct (i.e. suspected RV involvement).

Further management will continue after transfer, which will include further medical Mx +/– primary PCI.

SECONDARY PREVENTION

Unless contraindicated, patients with ACS will require long-term dual antiplatelet medication, such as aspirin 75 mg + clopidogrel 75 mg or ticagrelor 90 mg BD[NICE] (both interact with carbamazepine, SSRIs, AChE inhibitors).

Patients will also usually be prescribed an ACE-i/ARB, beta-blocker and a high-dose statin (e.g. atorvastatin 80 mg).[NICE]

Lifestyle factors such as good diet, regular (daily) exercise and smoking cessation should always be encouraged.[NICE]

ACUTE ASTHMA

In the psychiatric setting, the onus should be on an ABCDE approach, assessment of the clinical picture, initiation of appropriate initial treatment and prompt transfer to general hospital if required.

Clues: SOB, wheeze, ↓PEF, RR ≥25/min, HR ≥110/min, cannot complete sentences in one breath, low O_2 saturation.

- Attach pulse oximeter.
- 40%–60% O_2 through high-flow mask, e.g. Hudson mask.
- Salbutamol 5 mg neb in O_2; repeat up to every 15 min.
- Corticosteroids (i.e. in adults, 5/7 of prednisolone 40–50 mg od).[NICE]

If the attack is severe or life threatening (PEF <50% of usual best), the patient will require urgent transfer to general hospital.

CHRONIC OBSTRUCTIVE PULMONARY DISEASE EXACERBATION

In the psychiatric setting, the onus should be on an ABCDE approach, assessment of the clinical picture, initiation of appropriate initial treatment and prompt transfer to general hospital if required.

Clues: SOB, wheeze, RR >25/min, HR >110.

- Attach pulse oximeter.
- Use controlled/targeted O_2 to achieve O_2 saturation >94% (eucapnic patients) or 88–92% (hypercapnic patients, i.e. patients with T2RF). Drowsiness may indicate worsening T2RF.
- Ipratropium 500 micrograms neb in O_2; repeat up to every 4 h if very ill (max 2 mg in 24 h).

- Salbutamol 5 mg neb in O_2; repeat up to every 15 min if very ill (seldom necessary >hourly).

Transfer to general hospital if unwell and/or not improving.

VENOUS THROMBOEMBOLISM

VTE encompasses DVT and PE which are on a spectrum ranging from clinically unimportant to mortality-causing.

↑*Risk:* ↑age, smoking, pregnancy, oestrogens, malignancy, surgery or immobility, travel, previous VTE, schizophrenia (pro-inflammatory), recent COVID-19, known coagulopathy.

The normal value of the D-dimer increases with age.

DEEP VEIN THROMBOSIS (DVT)

In the psychiatric setting, the onus should be on an ABCDE approach, assessment of the clinical picture, initiation of appropriate initial treatment and prompt transfer to general hospital if required.

Clues: swollen or painful leg, other causes ruled out by clinical examination.

If a DVT is suspected, Dx is aided by Wells' score:

Feature	Score
Malignancy w/ treatment within 6 months or palliative	+ 1
Paralysis, paresis or recent plaster immobilisation of the lower extremities	+ 1
Immobilisation ≥3 days OR surgery in the previous 12 weeks	+ 1
Localised tenderness over the deep veins	+ 1
Entire leg swollen	+ 1
Calf swelling ≥3 cm larger than asymptomatic side	+ 1
Pitting oedema only on the symptomatic leg	+ 1
Collateral superficial veins (non-varicose)	+ 1
Previously documented DVT	+ 1
An alternative diagnosis is at least as likely as DVT	− 2

If <2 (DVT unlikely):

- Check D-dimer. If result not available within 4 h, start interim therapeutic anticoagulation (see below).
- If D-dimer negative, DVT excluded.
- If D-dimer raised, organise a proximal leg vein Doppler. If result not available within 4 h, start/continue interim therapeutic anticoagulation (see below). If Doppler negative, DVT is ruled out. If positive, continue with anticoagulation.

If ≥2 (DVT likely):

- Organise a proximal leg vein Doppler. If result not available within 4 h, start interim therapeutic anticoagulation (see below).
- If Doppler negative, stop interim anticoagulation. Check D-dimer; if raised, patient will require one repeat proximal leg vein ultrasound scan 6 to 8 days later (no interim anticoagulation).
- If Doppler positive continue with anticoagulation.

Anticoagulation:

- *Interim:* start direct oral anticoagulant (DOAC) (e.g. apixaban or rivaroxaban) or, if not suitable, LMWH, e.g. dalteparin or enoxaparin.
- Once DVT confirmed, continue with DOAC (note dose changes after 1/52 apixaban and 3/52 rivaroxaban) or, if not suitable, continue with LMWH for at least 5/7, followed by dabigatran, edoxaban or LMWH concurrently for at least 5/7 whilst starting a vit K antagonist (VKA).[NICE]

Look for an alternative diagnosis if DVT ruled out and stop interim therapeutic anticoagulation. Do not stop anticoagulation commenced for other reasons.

Discuss with patients with an extensive iliofemoral DVT, VTE whilst already anticoagulated, unprovoked DVTs, VTE during pregnancy or in childbearing age, those who may be unsuitable for anticoagulation or patients with known thrombophilia with the relevant acute specialty.

PULMONARY EMBOLISM

In the psychiatric setting, the onus should be on an ABCDE approach, assessment of the clinical picture, initiation of appropriate initial treatment and prompt transfer to general hospital if required.

Clues: unexplained hypoxia, pleuritic chest pain, leg pain/swelling.

Usually RR >20 and $\downarrow O_2$ saturation.

- 60%–100% O_2 if hypoxic. Care if T2RF failure (e.g. COPD).
- *Analgesia:* if excess pain or distress, try paracetamol/ibuprofen first; consider opiates if severe or no response (☠ can ⇒ respiratory depression ☠).
- *Anticoagulation:* start DOAC (e.g. apixaban or rivaroxaban) or, if not suitable, LMWH, e.g. dalteparin or enoxaparin.
- Once PE confirmed, continue with DOAC (note dose changes after 1/52 apixaban and 3/52 rivaroxaban) or, if not suitable, continue with LMWH for at least 5/7, followed by dabigatran, edoxaban or LMWH concurrently for at least 5/7 whilst starting a VKA.[NICE]

In stable patients, Dx is aided by Wells' score:

Feature	Score
Clinical signs and symptoms of DVT	+ 3
PE is #1 diagnosis OR equally likely	+ 3
HR >100	+ 1.5
Immobilisation at least 3 days OR surgery in the previous 4 weeks	+ 1.5
Previous, objectively diagnosed PE or DVT	+ 1.5
Haemoptysis	+ 1
Malignancy w/ treatment within 6 months or palliative	+ 1

Only take D-dimer if PE unlikely (≤3).

Patient should have a lung scan (CT-PA or, if contrast allergy, severe renal impairment or risk from irradiation, a V/Q scan) if PE likely (Wells' >4) or if D-dimer elevated.

Urgent transfer to hospital if hypoxia or haemodynamically unstable.

SEPSIS (SEVERE OR SEPTIC SHOCK)

In the psychiatric setting, the onus should be on an ABCDE approach, assessment of the clinical picture, initiation of appropriate initial investigations and treatment and prompt transfer to general hospital.

Clues: evidence of infection + ↓BP (MAP <65 mm Hg), serum lactate >4 mmol/L, ↓urine output, ↑creatinine, ↑bilirubin and ↑INR.

Outcomes from sepsis are improved via prompt undertaking of the 'Sepsis 6' (O_2, iv antibiotics, blood cultures, iv fluids, measuring serum lactate, recording urine output). It will be hard to fully implement this in a psychiatric environment.

NB: end-organ dysfunction may manifest as, e.g. delirium.

Start treatment and resuscitation immediately.

- *Oxygen:* 100% via non-rebreathe mask aiming for O_2 saturation 94%–98%; caution – aim for 88%–92% in COPD/T2RF.
- Take bloods including cultures (if possible): FBC, U&Es, LFTs, clotting, venous glucose, CRP, lactate.
- *Fluid:* for sepsis-induced hypoperfusion, give 500 mL Hartmann's iv in 15 min (if not CI) and aim for ≥30 mL/kg of iv fluid within first 3 h; 1L over 30 min; if still ↓BP, consider further iv fluids (20 mL/kg) to achieve urine output >0.5 mL/kg/h (caution if LVF).

Response to fluids can also be monitored by resolution of ↑HR, altered consciousness, oliguria and hyperlactatemia.

(Significantly) Adapted from Surviving Sepsis Campaign: International guidelines for management of severe sepsis and septic shock: 2016. Intensive Care Medicine 2017;43:304–377.

↑ GLUCOSE

Hyperglycaemia covers a spectrum from asymptomatic and well to life-threatening, as in DKA, HHS or a stress response to other severe illness.

Clues: polydipsia, polyuria/incontinence, weight loss, recurrent UTI, recurrent fungal infections.

Diagnosis: fasting BG >7 mmol/L or random >11 mmol/L.

Causes (apart from new diagnosis of DM): acute illness, physical and emotional stress, rebound after ↓BG, dietary, ↓exercise, missing diabetic medications, corticosteroids, antipsychotics, hyperthyroidism.

If not a hyperglycaemic emergency, follow patient's 'sick day rules' and give necessary correction doses. Discuss with diabetes nurse/team if needed.

HYPEROSMOLAR HYPERGLYCAEMIC STATE (HHS)

In the psychiatric setting, the onus should be on an ABCDE approach, assessment of the clinical picture, initiation of appropriate initial treatment and prompt transfer to general hospital.

Clues: polyuria, polydipsia, nausea, confusion/↓GCS, dehydration, ↑↑↑ glucose.

Occurs mostly in older people but increasingly seen in younger patients. Can be the first presentation of T2DM. Mixed presentations of HHS and DKA do occur. HHS has a dire mortality of >20%.

Diagnostic criteria: hypovolaemia, ↑BG (≥30 mmol/L), no severe ketonaemia (i.e. <3 mmol/L) or metabolic acidosis (pH >7.3, bicarbonate >15 mmol/L), ↑serum osmolality (≥320 mOsm/kg).

If HHS is suspected, then urgently transfer to general hospital whilst initiating fluid resuscitation.

IV fluids: 0.9% saline according to patients needs (guided by HR, BP, urine output etc), but generally slower/more cautiously than in DKA (see below), i.e. initially 1 L over 1 h (consider more rapid if systolic BP <90 mm Hg or more slowly if elderly with heart failure). If BP remains <90 mmHg, repeat this but call for senior help.

- *Additional initial measures:* O_2 if hypoxic, iv cannula.
- *Initial Ix:* blood ketones, capillary +/– venous BG, U&Es, measured or calculated ($2 \times$ Na + urea + glucose) osmolality, FBC, CRP, blood cultures (if available), ECG and urinalysis + culture.

Medics will Rx with intravenous fluids and may start/increase hypoglycaemic agents but will also try to establish an underlying cause (infection, infarction, compliance) whilst watching out for complications (thrombosis, cerebral oedema/central pontine myelinolysis, foot ulcers).

DIABETIC KETOACIDOSIS (DKA)

In the psychiatric setting, the onus should be on an ABCDE approach, assessment of the clinical picture, initiation of appropriate initial treatment and prompt transfer to general hospital.

Clues: ketotic breath, Kussmaul's (deep/rapid) breathing, dehydration, confusion/↓GCS, gastric stasis/abdominal pain, polyuria, polydipsia, lethargy, dry mucous membranes, tachycardia, hypotension.

Occurs mostly in patients with T1DM, but also in those with T2DM or non-diabetic patients on SGLT2-I ('flozins').

Diagnostic criteria: serum BG >11.1 mmol/L, pH <7.3 and/or HCO_3 <15 mmol/L, +ve ketones (blood ≥3 mmol/L or urine dipstick ≥2+). In a psychiatric setting, however, guide diagnosis by clinical exam, CBG monitoring and urinalysis.

If DKA is suspected, then urgently transfer to general hospital whilst initiating fluid resuscitation.

IV fluids: initially 0.9% saline according to individual patient needs (guided by pulse, BP, urine output, etc). For example, if systolic BP <90 mm Hg: 500 mL over 15 min. If BP remains <90 mm Hg, repeat this but call for medical help.

- Additional initial measures: O_2 if hypoxic, iv cannula.

- Initial Ix: blood ketones, capillary +/– venous glucose, U&Es, FBC, CRP, blood cultures (if available), ECG and urinalysis + culture.

Medics will Rx with fluids and iv insulin once transferred.

↓GLUCOSE

In the psychiatric setting, the onus should be on an ABCDE approach, assessment of the clinical picture, initiation of appropriate initial treatment and prompt transfer to general hospital.

Treat if BG <3 mmol/L or if symptoms and BG <4 mmol/L: ↑sympathetic drive (↑HR, sweating, aggression/behavioural changes), seizures or confusion/↓GCS.

- Glucose orally: 15–20 g quick-acting carbohydrates, especially sugary drinks, mouth gel (e.g. **Hypostop/Glucogel/Dextrogel**) or dextrose tablets. Miss this step if severe, but useful if delays in iv access.
- Glucose 150–200 mL of 10% glucose iv or 75–100 mL of 20% glucose iv (over 10–15 min); beware of fluid overload if HF.
- Glucagon 1 mg im/iv stat if very low glucose or no iv access.

Give oral carbohydrate within 10–30 min to prevent recurrence. *NB: think of and correct any causes, especially excess antidiabetics, alcohol withdrawal, liver failure, aspirin OD (rarely Addison's disease, ↓T4).*

Reference information

GUIDELINES

British Association for Psychopharmacology (BAP)

The British Association for Psychopharmacology produces Consensus Guidelines for treatment of many psychiatric disorders, updated at regular intervals. They are extensively referenced in this book with[BAP]. They are freely available at https://www.bap.org.uk/guidelines.

Topic	BAP guideline	Publication date
Anxiety disorders	Evidence-based pharmacological treatment of anxiety disorders, post-traumatic stress disorder and obsessive-compulsive disorder	2014
Attention deficit hyperactivity disorder (ADHD)	Evidence-based guidelines for the pharmacological management of attention deficit hyperactivity disorder: update on recommendations	2014
Autism	Autism spectrum disorder: consensus guidelines on assessment, treatment and research	2018
Benzodiazepines	Benzodiazepines: risks and benefits. A reconsideration	2013
Bipolar affective disorder	Evidence-based guidelines for treating bipolar disorder: revised third edition recommendations	2016
Catatonia	Evidence-based consensus guidelines for the management of catatonia.	2023
Dementia	Clinical practice with anti-dementia drugs: a revised (third) consensus statement	2017
Depression	Evidence-based guidelines for treating depressive disorders with antidepressants: a revision of the 2008 guidelines	2015
Metabolic side effects	Guidelines on the management of weight gain, metabolic disturbances and cardiovascular risk associated with psychosis and antipsychotic drug treatment	2016

(continued)

Topic	BAP guideline	Publication date
Off-license prescribing	Use of licensed medicines for unlicensed applications in psychiatric practice, 2nd edition	2017
Off-license prescribing	Position Statement: off-label prescribing of psychotropic medication to children and adolescents	2016
Other	Withdrawal of, and alternatives to, valproate-containing medicines in people of childbearing potential who have a psychiatric illness	2018
Other	Use of monoamine oxidase inhibitors in psychiatric practice	2020
Perinatal psychiatry	Consensus guidance on the use of psychotropic medication preconception, in pregnancy and postpartum 2017	2017
Rapid tranquilisation	Joint BAP NAPICU evidence-based consensus guidelines for the clinical management of acute disturbance: de-escalation and rapid tranquillisation	2018
Schizophrenia	Evidence-based guidelines for the pharmacological treatment of schizophrenia: recommendations	2020
Sleep disorders	Consensus statement on evidence-based treatment of insomnia, parasomnias and circadian rhythm disorders	2019
Substance misuse	Evidence-based guidelines for the pharmacological management of substance abuse, harmful use, addiction and co-morbidity: recommendations	2012

National Institute for Health and Care Excellence (NICE)

Many NICE guidelines are also relevant to mental health and may be found at https://www.nice.org.uk/guidance/lifestyle-and-wellbeing/mental-health-and-wellbeing. In addition, several 'pathways' serving as interactive ways to navigate the guidelines may be found at this link. These and some NICE evidence articles are referenced with[NICE].

Other

Topic	NICE guideline	Code	Publication date
ADHD	Attention deficit hyperactivity disorder: diagnosis and management	NG87	2019
Alcohol	Alcohol-use disorders: diagnosis, assessment and management of harmful drinking and alcohol dependence	CG115	2011
Anxiety disorders	Generalised anxiety disorder and panic disorder in adults: management	CG113	2019
ASPD	Antisocial personality disorder: prevention and management	CG77	2013
Autism	Autism spectrum disorder in adults: diagnosis and management	CG142	2021
Autism (children)	Autism spectrum disorder in under 19s: recognition, referral and diagnosis	CG128	2021
Borderline PD	Borderline personality disorder: recognition and management	CG78	2009
BPAD	Bipolar disorder: assessment and management	CG185	2020
Care transition	Transition between inpatient mental health settings and community or care home settings	NG53	2016
Common mental health problems	Common mental health problems: identification and pathways to care	CG123	2011
Conduct disorder	Antisocial behaviour and conduct disorders in children and young people: recognition and management	CG158	2013
Delirium	Delirium: prevention, diagnosis and management	CG103	2019
Dementia	Dementia: assessment, management and support for people living with dementia and their carers	NG97	2018

(continued)

Topic	NICE guideline	Code	Publication date
Depression	Depression in adults: recognition and management	CG90	2009
Depression	Depression in adults with a chronic physical health problem: recognition and management	CG91	2009
Depression (children)	Depression in children and young people: identification and management	CG28	2019
Eating disorders	Eating disorders: recognition and treatment	NG69	2020
Forensic mental health	Mental health of adults in contact with the criminal justice system	NG66	2017
Learning disability	Mental health problems in people with learning disabilities: prevention, assessment and management	NG54	2016
Learning disability	Challenging behaviour and learning disabilities: prevention and interventions for people with learning disabilities whose behaviour challenges	NG11	2015
OCD	Deep brain stimulation for chronic, severe, treatment-resistant obsessive-compulsive disorder in adults		2021
OCD and BDD	Obsessive-compulsive disorder and body dysmorphic disorder: treatment	CG31	2005
Other	Rehabilitation for adults with complex psychosis		2020
Perinatal mental health	Antenatal and postnatal mental health: clinical management and service guidance	CG192	2020
Psychosis	Psychosis and schizophrenia in adults: prevention and management	CG178	2014

(*continued*)

Topic	NICE guideline	Code	Publication date
Psychosis (children)	Psychosis and schizophrenia in children and young people: recognition and management	CG155	2013
Psychosis and substance misuse	Coexisting severe mental illness (psychosis) and substance misuse: assessment and management in healthcare settings	CG120	2011
PTSD	NG116 Post-traumatic stress disorder	CG26	2018
Rapid tranquilisation	Violence and aggression: short-term management in mental health, health and community settings	NG10	2015
Self-harm	Self-harm in over 8s: short-term management and prevention of recurrence	CG16	2004
Social anxiety disorder	Social anxiety disorder: recognition, assessment and treatment	CG159	2013

Topic	Guideline	Publication date	Reference
Club drugs and novel psychoactive substances	Novel Psychoactive Treatment: UK Network (NEPTUNE) (http://neptune-clinical-guidance.co.uk)	2015	**NEPTUNE**
Prescribing in psychiatry	*The Maudsley Prescribing Guidelines in Psychiatry*, 14th edition	2021	**MPG**
Various	Scottish Intercollegiate Guidelines Network (SIGN) (https://www.sign.ac.uk)	Various	**SIGN**

USEFUL CONTACTS

CRISIS CONTACTS

Contact	Description	Website	Telephone number
CALM (Campaign Against Living Miserably)	For men in crisis	https://www.thecalmzone.net	0800 58 58 58 (5 p.m.–midnight)
ChildLine	Emergency counselling service	https://www.childline.org.uk	0800 1111 (24/7)
NHS 111	Helpline for urgent medical problems; can connect patients to onward care	https://111.nhs.uk	111 (24/7)
PAPYRUS	Suicide prevention line; accepts calls from concerned others	https://www.papyrus-uk.org	0800 068 4141 (24/7)
Samaritans	Crisis line for any issues	https://www.samaritans.org.uk	116 123 (24/7)

PATIENT INFORMATION/SUPPORT

Contact	Description	Website	Telephone number
NHS Patient Information	Reliable information on common mental health problems	https://www.nhs.uk/conditions	–
Mind	Mental health information and support	https://www.mind.org.uk	0300 123 3393 (Monday–Friday, 9 a.m.–6 p.m.)

(continued)

Contact	Description	Website	Telephone number
Alcoholics Anonymous	Peer support network for those wishing to stop drinking	https://www.alcoholics-anonymous.org.uk	0800 9177 650 (24/7)
Narcotics Anonymous	Peer support network for those wishing to stop using drugs	https://ukna.org	0300 999 1212 (10 a.m. until midnight)
Alzheimer's Society	Support for those with all types of dementia and their carers	https://www.alzheimers.org.uk	0300 222 1122 (Monday–Wednesday, 9 a.m.–8 p.m., Thursday and Friday, 9 a.m.–5 p.m. and weekends, 10 a.m.–4 p.m.)
BEAT Eating Disorders	Support for those with eating disorders	https://www.beateatingdisorders.org.uk	Adults: 0808 801 0677 (Monday–Friday, 12 p.m.–8 p.m., weekends, 4 p.m.–8 p.m.)
Mencap	Support for those with a learning disability and their families	https://www.mencap.org.uk	0207 454 0454 (Monday–Friday, 9 a.m.–5 p.m.)

PROFESSIONAL

Contact	Description	Website	Telephone number
National Poisons Information Service (NPIS)	Comprehensive information on management of drug overdoses	https://www.toxbase.org (requires institutional login)	0344 892 0111 (24/7)

(continued)

Contact	Description	Website	Telephone number
UK Teratology Information Service (UKTIS)	Drug monographs with detailed information on use in pregnancy	http://www.uktis.org	0344 892 0909 (24/7 for urgent requests)
UK Drugs in Lactation Advisory Service (UKDILAS)	Advice on prescribing in breastfeeding women	https://www.sps.nhs.uk/articles/advising-on-medicines-during-breastfeeding	0116 258 6491
Specialist Medicines Information Service for Psychiatry at the Maudsley Hospital	Advice from specialist mental health pharmacists for UK health professionals	–	020 3228 2317 (Monday–Friday, 9 a.m.–5 p.m.)
Medscape	Free professional medical information	https://reference.medscape.com	–
Mental Elf	Blog distilling mental health research	https://www.nationalelfservice.net/mental-health	–

REFERENCE VALUES

NB: normal ranges often vary between laboratories. The ranges given here are deliberately narrow to minimise missing abnormal results, but this means that your result may be normal for your laboratory's range, which should always be checked if possible.

Biochemistry

Na$^+$	135–145 mmol/L
K$^+$	3.5–5 mmol/L
Urea	2.5–6.5 mmol/L
Creatinine	70–110 micromole/L
Ca^{2+}	2.15–2.65 mmol/L
PO$_4$	0.8–1.4 mmol/L
Albumin	35–50 g/L
Protein	60–80 g/L
Mg^{2+}	0.75–1.0 mmol/L
Cl$^-$	95–105 mmol/L
Glucose (fasting)	3.5–5.5 mmol/L
LDH	70–250 iu/L
CK	25–195[a] units/L ($\neq$ in blacks)
Trop I	<0.4 ng/mL (= microgram/L)
Trop T	<0.1 ng/mL (= microgram/L)
D-dimers	<0.5[b] mg/L
Bilirubin	3–17 micromole/L
ALP	30–130 iu/L
AST	3–31 iu/L
ALT	3–35 iu/L
GGT	7–50[a] iu/L
Amylase	0–180 units/dL
Cholesterol	3.9–5.2 mmol/L
Triglycerides	0.5–1.9 mmol/L
LDL	<2 mmol/L
HDL	0.9–1.9 mmol/L
Urate	0.2–0.45 mmol/L
CRP	0–10 mg/L

[a] Sex differences exist: females occupy the lower end of the range.

[b] D-dimer normal range can vary with different test protocols: check with your lab.

Haematology

Hb male	13.5–17.5 g/dL
Hb female	11.5–15.5 g/dL
Pt	150–400 $\times 10^9$/L
WCC	4–11 $\times 10^9$/L
NØ	2–7.5 $\times 10^9$/L (40%–75%)
LØ	1.3–3.5 $\times 10^9$/L (20%–45%)
EØ	0.04–0.44 $\times 10^9$/L (1%–6%)
PCV (Hct)	0.37–0.54[a] L/L
MCV	76–96 fl
ESR	<age in years *(+10 in women)*/2
HbA$_{1C}$	<48 mmol/mol

[a] Sex differences exist: females occupy the lower end of the range.

Clotting

APTT	35–45 sec
APTT ratio	0.8–1.2
INR	0.8–1.2

Haematinics

Iron	11–30 micromole/L
Transferrin	2–4 g/L
TIBC	45–72 micromole/L
Serum folate	1.8–11 microgram/L
B$_{12}$	200–760 pg/mL (5 ng/L)

Arterial blood gases

PaO$_2$	>10.6 kPa
PaCO$_2$	4.7–6 kPa
pH	7.35–7.45

Arterial blood gases

HCO_3^-	24–30 mmol/L
Lactate	0.5–2.2 mmol/L
Base xs	±2 mmol/L

Thyroid function

Thyroxine (total T_4)	70–140 nmol/L
Thyroxine (free T_4)	9–22 pmol/L
TSH	0.5–5 mU/L

INDEX

NUMBERS